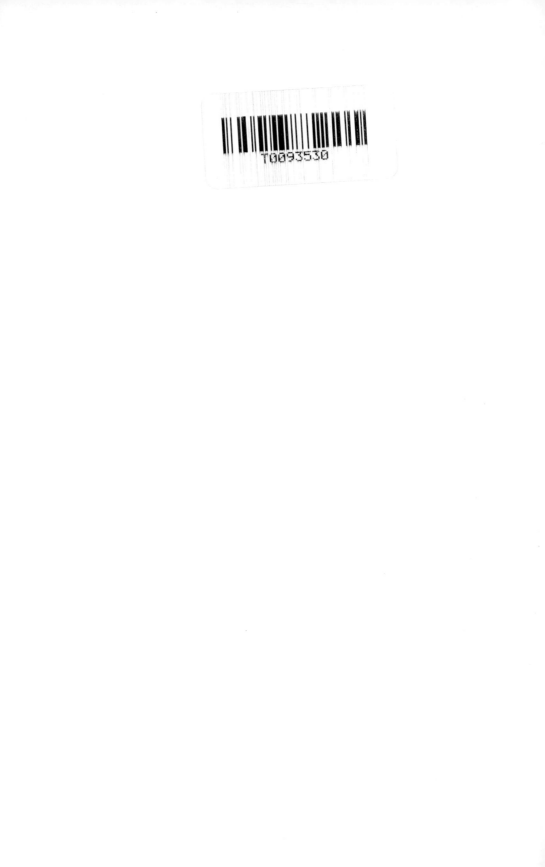

Laparoscopic Entry

Andrea Tinelli

Editor

Laparoscopic Entry

Traditional Methods,
New Insights and Novel Approaches

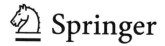 Springer

Editor
Andrea Tinelli, M.D.
Department of Obstetrics and Gynecology
Division of Experimental
Endoscopic Surgery, Imaging
Technology and Minimally Invasive Therapy
Vito Fazzi Hospital
Lecce, Italy

ISBN 978-0-85729-979-6   e-ISBN 978-0-85729-980-2
DOI 10.1007/978-0-85729-980-2
Springer London Dordrecht Heidelberg New York

British Library Cataloguing in Publication Data
A catalogue record for this book is available from the British Library

Library of Congress Control Number: 2011939576

Printed on acid-free paper

Springer is part of Springer Science+Business Media (www.springer.com)

This work is dedicated to my wife, Ughetta, who is my life, for her continuous support, for always believing in me and loving me.

And in love and gratitude to my parents, Francesco and Vivi, who have always been there through my growth and without whom I'd be nothing. They are simply the best parents of all time and I am blessed to be their son.

Every journey begins with a single step and this editorial journey is for all of you.

Foreword

In the last decades, surgery has been converted from tradition-based open surgery into evidence-based endoscopic surgery. Most surgical procedures today have endoscopic alternatives, and it seems that in the future only very few, elective laparotomies, like caesarean section, will remain.

It seems, however, that despite the considerable development of surgical instruments and methodologies surgery will continue to develop and to optimise.

One of the drawbacks of endoscopy, however, is that in most of the instruments the sensitivity of the fingertips has been abandoned in favour of the palms. Many surgeons insert the trocars into the abdomen while holding them with their fist.

Since the beginning of the twenty-first century, we have experienced another development, namely, tele-surgery. Tele-surgical equipment is getting more widely used with the advantages of precision, 3D vision, lack of tremor, and improved ergonomy but still lack of haptic sensation.

Our vision should therefore be targeted at the development of advanced telesurgical systems which will combine the usage of the sensitive fingertips with haptic sensation, which will bring about a renaissance of abdominal surgery. Such a system like, for example, the Telelap ALF-X, will enable evidence-based abdominal surgery with all the advantages of endoscopy. Every step in each operation should be subjected to analysis for its necessity and, if found essential, for its optimal way of performance. Therefore, we have to congratulate Andrea Tinelli on the courageous decision to edit this book, which is dedicated to one of the crucial steps in every endoscopic operation, namely, the entry to the body. Andrea Tinelli has managed to gather opinion-leading surgeons from Austria, Canada, Germany, Italy, the Netherlands, and the USA, who describe various aspects of this subject, starting with anatomical aspects and including several techniques and alternatives, risks, exciting observations far outranging technical issues concerning the endoscopic entry, new dimensions and ideas as well as future prospects. The reader will be confronted with a wide range of information which will help him or her to reconsider and optimise his/her own method.

Prof. Dr. Michael Stark, President
The New European Surgical Academy (NESA)
www.nesacademy.org

Prof. Dr. Antonio Malvasi
Department of Obstetric & Gynecology
Santa Maria Hospital
Bari, Italy

Contents

Contributors

Roberto Angioli, M.D. Division of Gynaecology, Department of Gynaecology, Campus Biomedico University, Rome, Italy

Tahar Benhidjeb, M.D. Department of General, Visceral and Thoracic Surgery, University Medical Center Hamburg-Eppendorf, Hamburg, Germany

The New European Surgical Academy (NESA), Berlin, Germany

Maurizio Brusati, M.D. Unit of Obstetrics and Gynecology, General Hospital of Chivasso, Turin, Italy

Maurizio Buscarini, M.D. Division of Urology, Department of Urology, Campus Biomedico University, Rome, Italy

Guilherme M. Campos, M.D., F.A.C.S. University of Wisconsin School of Medicine and Public Health, Madison, WI, USA

Shao-Chun R. Chang-Jackson, M.D. Minimally Invasive Gynecologic Surgery, St. Luke's-Roosevelt Medical Center, New York, NY, USA

Paul G. CurcilloII, M.D., F.A.C.S. Department of Surgical Oncology, Fox Chase Cancer Center, Philadelphia, PA, USA

Patrizio Damiani, M.D. Division of Gynaecology, Department of Gynaecology, Campus Biomedico University, Rome, Italy

Crisitina Falavolti, M.D. Division of Urology, Department of Urology, Campus Biomedico University, Rome, Italy

Nicola Gasbarro, M.D. Unit of Obstetrics and Gynecology, Santa Maria delle Grazie Hospital, Pozzuoli (Na), Italy

Sandro Gerli, M.D. Department of Obstetrics and Gynecology, University of Perugia, Perugia, Italy

Gernot Hudelist Department of Obstetrics and Gynecology, Endometriosis & Pelvic Pain Clinic, Wilhelminen Hospital, Vienna, Austria

Jakob R. Izbicki Department of General, Visceral and Thoracic Surgery, University Medical Center Hamburg-Eppendorf, Hamburg, Germany

Jörg Keckstein Abteilung Fur Gynakologie und Geburtshilfe, LandesKrankenHouse (LKH), Villach, Austria

Stephanie A. King, M.D. Department of Surgical Oncology, Fox Chase Cancer Center, Philadelphia, PA, USA

Pietro Lupo, M.D. Unit of Obstetrics and Gynecology, General Hospital of Chivasso, Turin, Italy

Antonio Malvasi, M.D. Department of Obstetrics and Gynecology, Santa Maria Hospital, Bari, Italy

Oliver Mann Department of General, Visceral and Thoracic Surgery, University Medical Center Hamburg-Eppendorf, Hamburg, Germany

Liselotte Mettler, M.D. Department of Obstetrics and Gynecology, Kiel School of Gynaecological Endoscopy, University Hospitals Schleswig-Holstein, Kiel, Germany

Farr R. Nezhat, M.D., F.A.C.O.G., F.A.C.S. Division of Gynecologic Oncology and Minimally Invasive Surgery, Department of Obstetrics and Gynecology, Columbia University, New York, NY, USA

Division of Gynecologic Oncology, Department of Obstetrics and Gynecology, St. Luke's-Roosevelt Medical Center, New York, NY, USA

Erica R. Podolsky, M.D. Department of Surgery, College of Medicine, Drexel University, Philadelphia, PA, USA

Charlotte Rabl, M.D. Paracelsus Private Medical University, Salzburg, Austria

Gian Carlo Di Renzo, M.D. Department of Obstetrics and Gynecology, University of Perugia, Perugia, Italy

Wael Sammur, M.D. Department of Obstetrics and Gynecology, German Medical Centre, DHCC, Dubai, UAE

Tom A.J. Schneider Department of Obstetrics and Prenatal Medicine, Erasmus MC University, Rotterdam, The Netherlands

Michael Stark, M.D. The New European Surgical Academy (NESA), Mallorca, Spain

The USP Hospital Palmaplanas of Mallorca, Mallorca, Spain

Artin Ternamian, M.D., F.R.C.S. Director of Gynecologic Endoscopy, Department of Obstetrics & Gynecology, Faculty of Medicine, University of Toronto, St. Joseph's Health Centre, Toronto, ON, Canada

Andrea Tinelli, M.D. Department of Obstetrics and Gynecology, Division of Experimental Endoscopic Surgery, Imaging, Technology and Minimally Invasive Therapy, Vito Fazzi Hospital, Lecce, Italy

Daniel A. Tsin, M.D. Division of Minimal Invasive Endoscopy, Department of Gynecology, The Mount Sinai Hospital of Queens, New York, USA

Chapter 1
Anatomy of the Abdominal Wall and Vaginal Entry in Relation to Complications of Access and Injury in Laparoscopy

Tom A.J. Schneider

Abdominal Wall Anatomy

In the early days of laparoscopic surgery in procedures such as diagnostic laparoscopy and tubal ligation, the Veress-needle and trocar were only placed in the relatively avascular midline (Fig. 1.1). Consequently, injuries of the abdominal wall vessels were rare. Vessel injuries of the abdominal wall have become more common

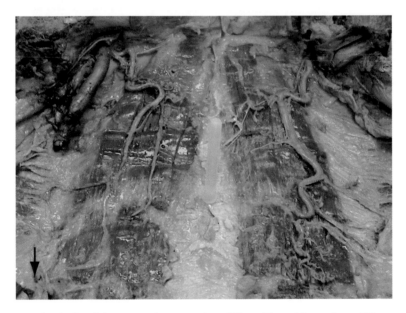

Fig. 1.1 Abdominal wall from posterior, avascular midline with marking at the umbilicus

T.A.J. Schneider
Department of Obstetrics and Prenatal Medicine, Erasmus MC University,
Rotterdam, The Netherlands

A. Tinelli (ed.), *Laparoscopic Entry*,
DOI 10.1007/978-0-85729-980-2_1, © Springer-Verlag London Limited 2012

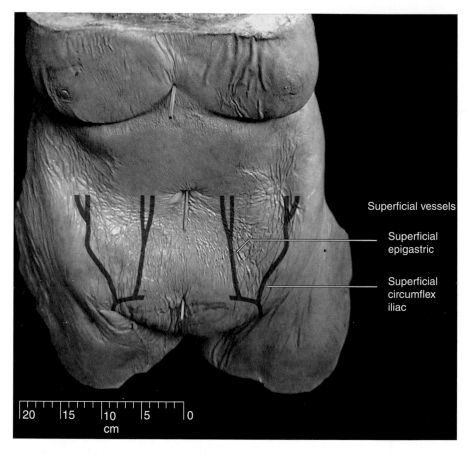

Superficial vessels

Superficial
epigastric

Superficial
circumflex
iliac

20   15   10   5   0
cm

Fig. 1.2 Superficial vessels of the abdominal wall

with the development of more complicated laparoscopic procedures with placement
of large-bore trocars laterally. The precise incidence of major and minor vascular
injury is unknown, but is reported to be 0.2–2% [1]. Abdominal vessels can be
divided into superficial (Fig. 1.2) and deep vessels. Veins with the same name
accompany the arteries and are not mentioned separately.

Superficial vessels in the abdominal wall can often be avoided by transillumination
of the abdominal wall with the laparoscope. This is especially true in light-skinned and
thin women. Blood vessels in the subcutaneous tissue that can be visualized in this
way are the superficial epigastric artery and the superficial circumflex iliac artery, both
of which are branches of the femoral artery that run to the level of the umbilicus. They
are both at risk of injury by lateral trocar placement.

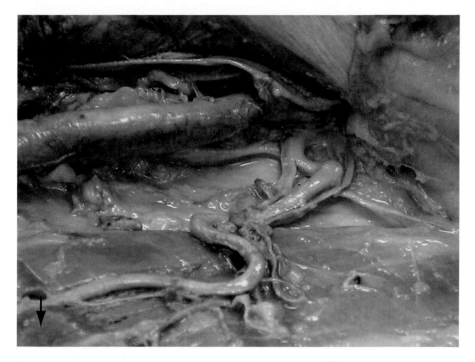

Fig. 1.3 Left inferior epigastric artery originating from the external iliac artery

The deep vessels of the inferior part of the anterior abdominal wall are the inferior epigastric artery (Fig. 1.3) placed medially, and the deep circumflex iliac artery placed laterally. Both originate from the external iliac artery. The inferior epigastric artery follows its course cranially on the posterior side of the m. rectus abdominis muscle, just covered by the peritoneum.

Because of the deep location of the inferior epigastric artery, it cannot be seen by transillumination, although occasionally it can be seen laparoscopically [2]. This peritoneal fold is known as the *lateral umbilical ligament*.

Damage to the Deep Abdominal Vessels

We used tattoo techniques for teaching purposes. To produce a model with the medial deep vessels visible on the skin, we copied the course of the inferior epigastric artery on paper. With the help of markers at xiphoid processus, umbilicus, and symphysis, we copied it on the skin again and made it permanent by tattooing the skin (Figs. 1.4–1.10).

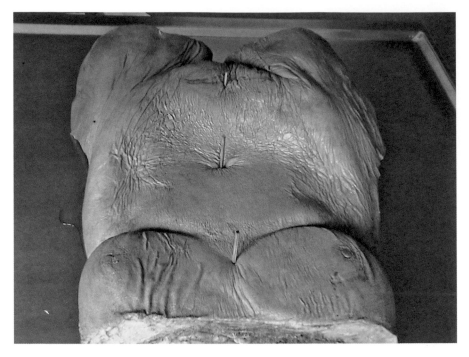

Fig. 1.4 Abdominal wall with markers at xiphoid processes, umbilicus, and symphysis

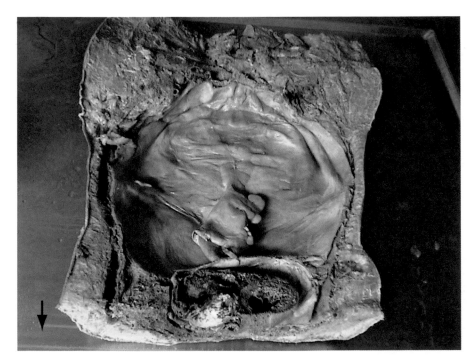

Fig. 1.5 Abdominal wall from posterior with peritoneum intact

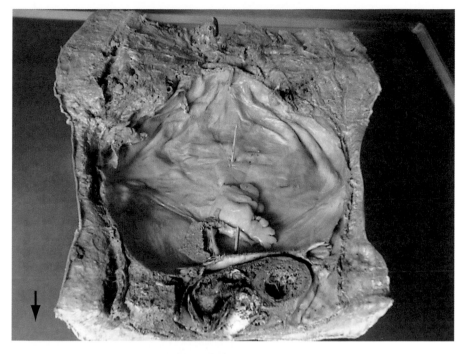

Fig. 1.6   Abdominal wall from posterior, markers at xiphoid, umbilicus, and symphysis

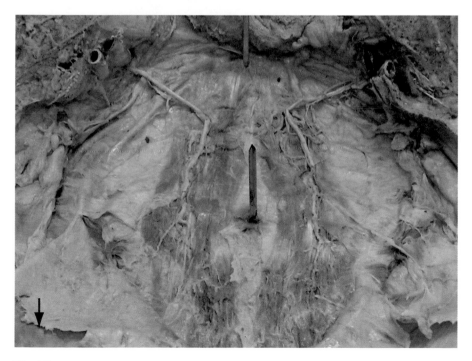

Fig. 1.7   Both inferior epigastric arteries on the posterior surface of the rectus muscles, markers at the umbilicus and symphysis

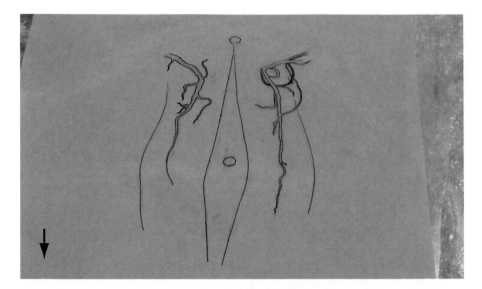

Fig. 1.8 Anatomy copied on paper

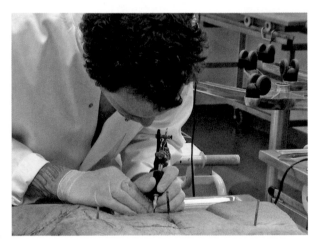

Fig. 1.9 Tattoo artist at work

Fig. 1.10 Course of both inferior epigastric arteries and borders of rectus abdominis muscle tattoo on the skin, markers at xiphoid, umbilicus, and symphysis

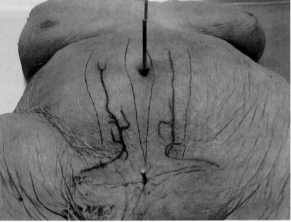

Trocar Placement Recommendations to Avoid Damage to Deep Abdominal Wall Vessels

In the past during procedures such as diagnostic laparoscopy and tubal ligation, trocars were placed almost exclusively in the midline, which did not place the anterior abdominal wall vessels at risk [3]. No branches of the inferior epigastric artery cross the midline. *Standard sites for midline trocar placement are subumbilical, 5 cm lower and above the symphysis* (Fig. 1.11).

Immediately above the symphysis, the superficial and inferior epigastric arteries are located approximately 5.5 cm from the midline. This location corresponds to the traditional location used for lateral trocar placement. Approximately at 7 cm from the midline at this level lies the superficial circumflex iliac artery. *To avoid both vessels, a safer location may be 8 cm above the symphysis and 8 cm from the midline* (Fig. 1.12).

The main stem of the inferior epigastric artery will be avoided if trocars are inserted [3] at >2/3 on the line [4] between the midline and the anterior superior iliac spine (ASIS) (Fig. 1.13). *Branches of the inferior epigastric artery are least frequently found in the lowest part af the abdomen, lateral to the artery.*

The ideal primary port lies in the ASIS plane in the midline. By inserting the lateral port at least 6 cm from the midline on either side in the same plane, the trocar is unlikely to damage the inferior epigastric artery. This measurement is a useful too for anyone required to place a drain safely through the abdominal wall (Fig. 1.14).

Another method to avoid injury is to stay out of the area 4-8 cm from the midline [5, 6]. This recommendation is independent of the BMI of the patient (Fig. 1.15).

Notwithstanding these recommendations, the anatomical variations and anastomoses among vessels make it impossible to know the location of every vessel in the abdominal wall.

Fig. 1.11 Standard sites for
midline trocar placement

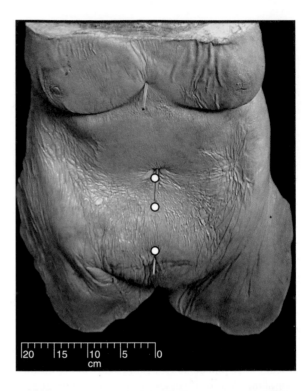

Fig. 1.12 Lateral trocar site
8 cm above symphysis, 8 cm
from midline

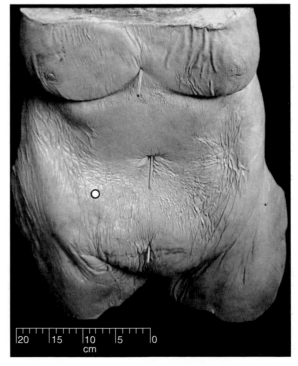

Fig. 1.13 Trocar site at >2/3 on the line between the midline and the anterior superior iliac spine (ASIS)

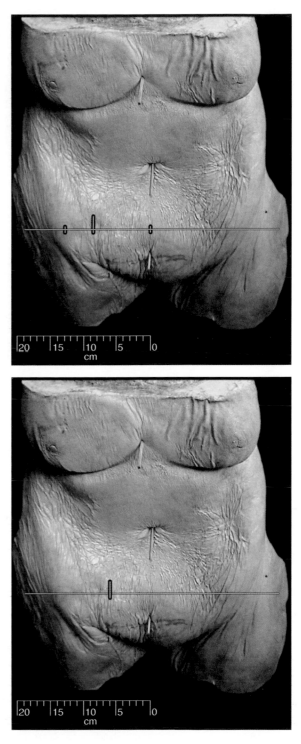

Fig. 1.14 Trocar site at the ASIS plane 6 cm from the midline

Fig. 1.15 Stay away area
4–8 cm from the midline

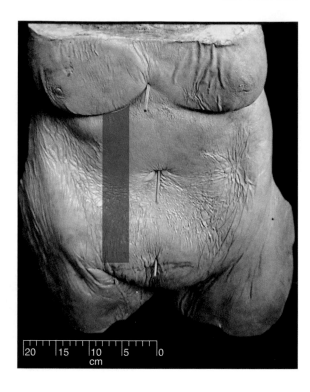

Injury to the Aorta, Iliac Arteries, and Viscera

Although uncommon, injury to major retroperitoneal vessels and viscera, mostly the bowel, is one of the most serious complications of the closed laparoscopic technique. It occurs in approximately 3 patients per 1,000 laparoscopies.

The open (Hasson) technique seems to lower the incidence, but not to zero [7].

In thin patients, the measurement of anterior–posterior distance from the umbilicus to the retroperitoneal vessels may be as little as 3–4 cm (Figs. 1.16 and 1.17). In the average patient, this distance can be increased to 8–14 cm by lifting the anterior abdominal wall with towel clips placed through the skin next to the incision. An angle of 45° in the sagittal plane should be used for the Veress needle in the umbilicus. It then misses the aorta and the iliac vessels no matter how deep it penetrates [5].

Piercing the Veress needle or cannula perpendicularly through the base of the umbilicus traverses the shortest distance (1.4±0.5 cm) to the abdominal cavity through the least vascular area of the abdominal wall. Sometimes the skin in this area is tough, and a sharp needle may be necessary. A small superficial stab incision with a No. 11 blade may facilitate entry [8].

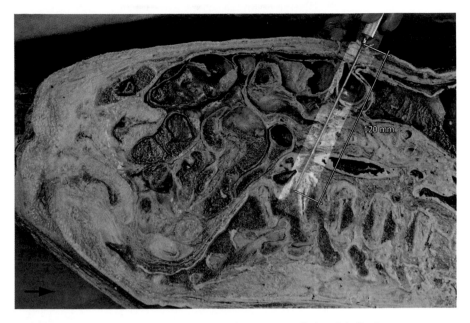

Fig. 1.16 Sagittal section of frozen specimen with Veress needle length indication

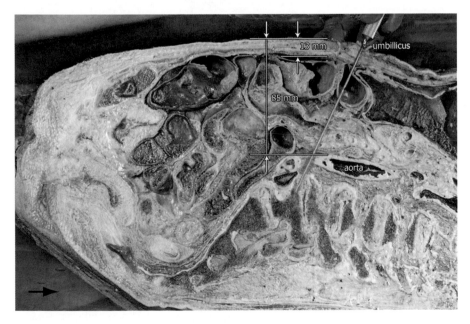

Fig. 1.17 Sagittal section: measurements with Veress needle in situ

Injuries to abdominal viscera can occur when the trocar penetrates too far into the abdominal cavity, or when the viscera (here the enlarged liver) are unusually close to the point of the insertion (Figs. 1.18 and 1.19).

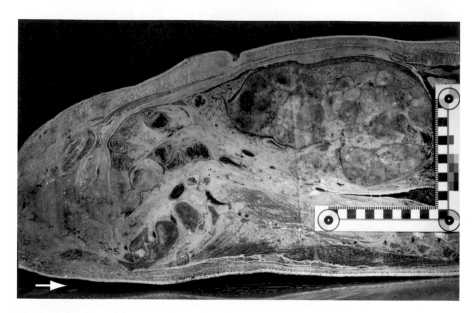

Fig. 1.18 Sagittal section with enlarged liver

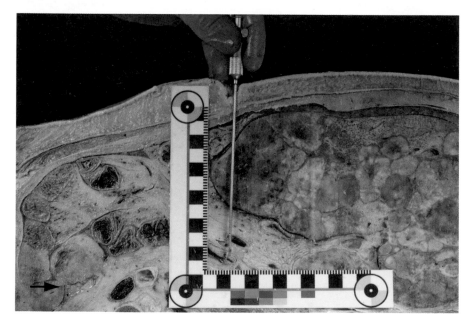

Fig. 1.19 Sagittal section with Veress needle at umbilicus

Preperitoneal Insufflation Has Occurred

Once insufflation is begun with the needle in the preperitoneal space, the peritoneum is pushed away from the abdominal wall, making subsequent entry more difficult. The peritoneum is firmly attached at the base of the umbilicus. This facilitates another entry into the peritoneal cavity (Figs. 1.20–1.22).

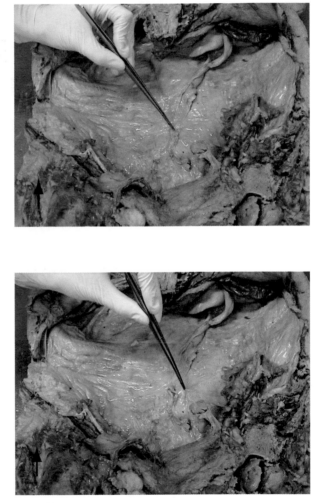

Fig. 1.20 Location of the umbilicus

Fig. 1.21 Peritoneum in the umbilical area: fixed

Fig. 1.22 Outside this area: more mobility

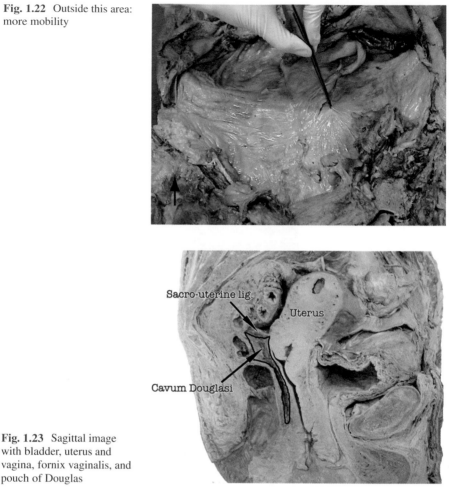

Fig. 1.23 Sagittal image with bladder, uterus and vagina, fornix vaginalis, and pouch of Douglas

Anatomy of the Posterior Vaginal Vault in Its Use as a Visual and Operative Vaginal Port

The fornix vaginalis is formed anatomically by the vagina around the cervix uteri. It is most spacious dorsally, where it is separated from the recto-uterine pouch of Douglas only by vaginal wall and peritoneum. The fornix to Douglas relation is not end-to-end.

Douglas continues for a smaller or longer distance along the posterior vaginal wall [9, 10]. In the embryological phase, the pouch of Douglas is deeper, reaching the perineum (Fig. 1.23).

It condensates later into the recto-vaginal septum as the cul-de-sac moves upward along the full length of the posterior vaginal wall. The recto-vaginal septum then extends from the caudal margin of the recto-uterine peritoneal pouch to the proximal

Fig. 1.24 Hegar dilators in the fornix vaginalis

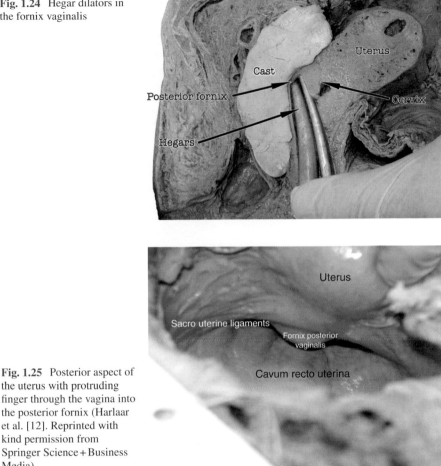

Fig. 1.25 Posterior aspect of the uterus with protruding finger through the vagina into the posterior fornix (Harlaar et al. [12]. Reprinted with kind permission from Springer Science + Business Media)

border of the perineal body (Figs. 1.24 and 1.25). It forms a fix point for the perineal body and stiffens the anterior rectal wall during defecation [9].

The Fornix Vaginalis as an Exit

The posterior fornix can serve as an exit for a laparoscopically removed specimen such as fibroids, the gallbladder, or a fallopian tube that cannot be removed through the abdominal wall without extension of the abdominal incision [11]. We measured the limits of capacity of this route [12]. The transversal and sagittal diameter of the fornix posterior was measured in 10 embalmed female human bodies that had not undergone any previous pelvic surgery (Fig. 1.26). The pouch of Douglas was filled to maximum capacity with moldable latex through the open abdomen.

Fig. 1.26 Impression of the fornix vaginalis in a Douglas pouch cast. Note that the connection is not with the deepest point (Harlaar et al. [12]. Reprinted with kind permission from Springer Science + Business Media)

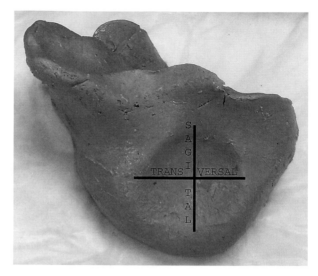

The imprint was measured in the transversal and sagittal direction. The mean fornix posterior diameter was 2.6 cm (±0.5 cm) with a range of 2.0–3.4 cm. Rigor mortis and the effect of embalming have an effect on this diameter. In living women the anatomical limits should be wider. When much bigger specimens are removed, the fixation point of the rectovaginal fascia nearby could be damaged. The rectovaginal fascia has a considerable clinical significance. If damaged, the anterior rectal wall may bulge during straining in defecation, resulting in functional disturbances of bowel movement with possible chronic retention of feces [9].

Histology of the Posterior Vaginal Vault

In order to study the histological structure, we took 3-mm full-depth biopsies of the posterior fornix vaginalis in embalmed female human bodies. The tissue was fixated and colored with hematoxylin-eosin, and paraffin sections were made (Fig. 1.27).

We found strong tissue, comprised of smooth muscle bundles in three directions that are united by connective tissue (Figs. 1.28 and 1.29). The muscle structure corresponded with that of the myometrium. The damage of bypassing the fornix with instruments is thus comparable with a perforation of the uterus, which we know is without consequences when there is no bleeding.

Acknowledgments The author would like to thank Rob Stoeckart, Edward Breedveld, Joris Harlaar, and Claire Pellikaan for their assistance.

Fig. 1.27 Overview: portio vaginalis, cervical glands, and fornices in a small ape

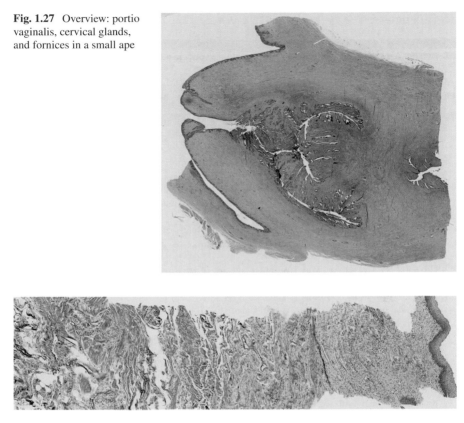

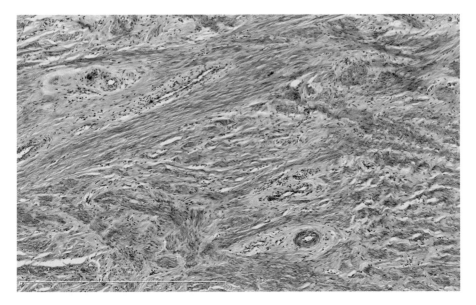

Fig. 1.28 Biopsy from the center of the fornix vaginalis posterior; bordered by epithelial lining (*right*) and peritoneal fat. In the center smooth muscle bundles united by connective tissue

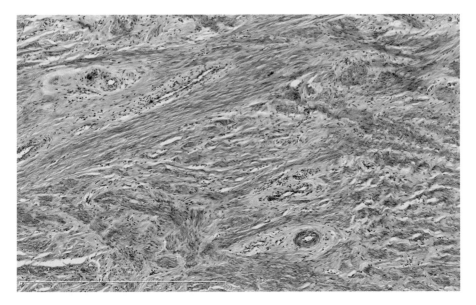

Fig. 1.29 Smooth muscle bundles in several directions

References

1. Schafer M, Lauper M, Krahenbuhl L. A nation's experience of bleeding complications during laparoscopy. Am J Surg. 2000;180:9–14.
2. Hurd WW, Amesse LS, Gruber JS, Horowitz GM, Cha GM, Hurteau JA. Visualization of the epigastric vessels and bladder before laparoscopic trocar placement. Fertil Steril. 2003;80:209–12.
3. Hurd WW, Bude RO, DeLancey JOL, Shewman J. The location of abdominal wall blood vessels in relationship to abdominal wall landmarks apparent at laparoscopy. Am J Obstet Gynecol. 1994;171:642–6.
4. Epstein J, Arora A, Ellis H. Surface anatomy of the inferior epigastric artery in relation to laparoscopic injury. Clin Anat. 2004;17(5):400–8.
5. Sriprasad S, Yu DF, Muir GH, Poulsen J, Sidhu PS. Positional anatomy of vessels that may be damaged at laparoscopy: new access criteria based on CT and ultrasonography to avoid vascular injury. J Endourol. 2006;20(7):498–503.
6. Saber AA, Meslemani AM, Davis R, Pimentel R. Safety zones for anterior abdominal wall entry during laparoscopy: a CT scan mapping of epigastric vessels. Ann Surg. 2004;239(2):182–5.
7. Chandler JG, Corson SL, Way LW. Three spectra of laparoscopic entry access injuries. J Am Coll Surg. 2001;192:478–90.
8. Roy GM, Bazzurini L, Solima E, Luciano AA. Safe technique for laparoscopic entry into the abdominal cavity. J Am Assoc Gynecol Laparosc. 2001;8(4):519–28.
9. Nichols D. Vaginal surgery. London: Williams & Wilkins; 1983.
10. Baessler K, Schuessler B. Anatomy of the sigmoid colon, rectum, and the rectovaginal pouch in women with enterocele and anterior rectal wall procidentia. Clin Anat. 2006;19(2):125–9.
11. Delvaux G, De Waele B, Willems G. Transvaginal removal of gallbladders with large stones after laparoscopic cholecystectomy. Surg Laparosc Endosc. 1993;3(4):307–9.
12. Harlaar JJ, Kleinrensink GJ, Hop WJC, Stark M, Schneider AJ. The anatomical limits of the posterior vaginal vault toward its use as route for intra-abdominal procedures. Surg Endosc. 2008;22:1910–2.

Chapter 2
Surgical Technique of Traditional Laparoscopic Access

Gernot Hudelist and Jörg Keckstein

Introduction

The primary aim of any surgical procedure in gynecology is either to repair or eradicate benign or malignant disorders of the female genital tract. Within this, the potential of minimal invasive surgery for operative treatment gynecological diseases has increased dramatically because intraoperative and postoperative complication rates of laparoscopic procedures appear to be equally or even less frequent compared with conventional abdominal techniques [1, 2]. Compared with open surgical procedures, laparoscopic surgery is less painful for the patient, postoperative cosmetic results from a reduction of scar length are more satisfying, and most important, recovery and return to everyday life are more rapid with the laparoscopic approach [1]. However, surgical procedures performed via laparoscopy require well-trained surgeons and standardized techniques in order to confer an advantage for the patient. Successful performance of laparoscopic access is an essential first step toward performance of efficient and safe laparoscopic surgery. Independent of the entry technique preferred by the surgeon, several basic principles of laparoscopic entry should be kept in mind and must be adhered to in order to minimize the risk of complications, such as bowel, bladder, or vessel injury during insertion of the insufflation needle and trocar [3].

G. Hudelist (✉)
Department of Obstetrics and Gynecology, Endometriosis & Pelvic Pain Clinic,
Wilhelminen Hospital, Vienna, Austria

J. Keckstein
Abteilung Fur Gynakologie und Geburtshilfe, LandesKrankenHouse (LKH), Villach, Austria

A. Tinelli (ed.), *Laparoscopic Entry*,
DOI 10.1007/978-0-85729-980-2_2, © Springer-Verlag London Limited 2012

Closed Technique for Laparoscopic Entry

In principle, the *closed technique* using nonoptical trocars is a blind approach in which the laparoscope is introduced via a trocar used to penetrate the abdominal wall layers after insufflation of the peritoneal cavity with CO_2 via a hollow needle (Veress needle) [1, 3]. In contrast, the *open technique* is associated with minilaparotomy to achieve entry to the peritoneal cavity with the trocar fixed to the abdominal wall with sutures [4].

When performing the *closed technique*, disinfection of the skin is followed by a midsagittal or transverse incision, which is performed at the lower end of the umbilical scar. The depth and length of the incision should depend on the size and diameter of the trocar to be further inserted. Although both sagittal and transverse incisions are appropriate for primary access, the sagittal incision often yields more satisfying postoperative cosmetic results compared with the transverse incision [5].

One exception is a flat umbilical scar, which is often associated with transverse folding of the skin. In these cases, we have observed a better cosmetic outcome following the performance of a transverse incision of the skin. Special care should be taken with the incision depth because perforation of the abdominal wall with the scalpel can cause injury to intraabdominal structures such as the bowel or the abdominal aorta, especially in low-weight patients with thin abdominal wall layers and reduced subcutaneous adipose tissue [1, 4, 5]. In order to avoid these complications, the scalpel should be held at a 30° angle to the patient's abdominal wall with the blade headed toward the surgeon (Fig. 2.1a, b).

Following this, the functionality of the Veress needle (Fig. 2.2a) should be checked before insufflation of the peritoneal cavity [6]. Usually, the spring-loaded blunt obturator is pushed back into the hollow needle, revealing its sharpened end when the needle passes through the tissue layers. The obturator springs back into its original position after entry into the peritoneal cavity and again protects the sharpened end, thereby avoiding injury of the intraabdominal contents [7]. Importantly, the patient should be positioned horizontally for needle and trocar insertion. The reason for this is the location of the pelvic vessels and a so-called "safety zone" that exists inferior to the sacral promontory and is bounded cephalad by the bifurcation of the abdominal aorta, laterally by the external iliac artery and vein, and posteriorly by the sacral bone. In a patient placed in the Trendelenburg position, the great vessels are positioned more cephalad and anterior [8].

As a consequence, these structures are more likely to be injured during the insertion process even if appropriate adjustments are made in the angle of needle and cannula insertion. In a patient positioned horizontally, insertion of the instruments usually happens within the "safety zone," because the great vessels are situated less cephalad and posterior [6–8].

For needle insertion, the surgeon should be positioned on the left side of the patient. The abdominal wall should be grasped and lifted with two hands at both sides of the umbilicus, which can be performed with the help of an assistant. The insufflation needle should be directed at a 45° angle to the patient's spine in a woman with average weight. In obese patients, insertion of the needle might be easier

Fig. 2.1 (**a**) Position of the scalpel for performance of periumbilical incision. (**b**) The incision should be performed at the level of the skin in order to avoid deep incision and perforation of the whole abdominal wall which can cause injury of intraabdominal structures such as the bowel or the abdominal aorta

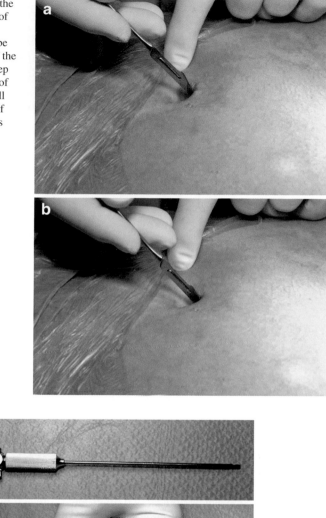

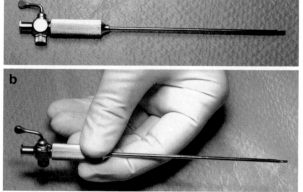

Fig. 2.2 (**a**) Insertion needle by Veress. A spring-loaded blunt obturator is pushed back into the hollow needle, revealing its sharpened end for perforation of the abdominal wall layers when the needle is pressed against tissue. The obturator again springs back into its basic position after entry of the peritoneal cavity which protects the sharpened end and therefore avoids injury of intraabdominal contents. The handle of the needle is connected to a tube for installing CO_2 insufflation gas. (**b**) Transumbilical insertion of the Veress needle: The needle can either be is hold by the tips of the fingers or at its free end

Fig. 2.3 (**a**) The needle should be guided steadily in the same 45° angle position. (**b**) Two "click"-like sounds can usually be noted and is created by perforating the abdominal wall fascia and the peritoneum

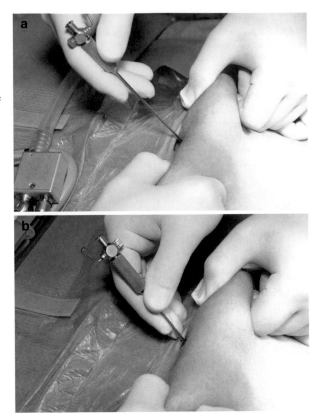

accomplished by positioning the needle more vertically for penetration of the subcutaneous fat. The needle is held by the tips of the fingers either at the needle's shaft or at its free end (Fig. 2.2b).

Importantly, the needle should be guided steadily in the same 45° angle position. When the needle passes through the abdominal wall fascia and the peritoneum, a "click"- like sound can be noticed two times and is created by perforating the mentioned structures and may help in addition to the tactile feedback given by perforation of the abdominal wall layers (Fig. 2.3a, b).

It should be mentioned that this "proprioceptive" feedback during needle insertion is less noted in single-use needles because of sharpness of the needle's blade. In these cases, passage of the abdominal wall with a single-use inflation needle must be performed with special caution to avoid puncture of the intestine or great abdominal vessels [9].

Safe insertion of the Veress needle is accomplished by guiding the needle via a movement out of the wrist. Prompt and aggressive insertion attempts performed by the whole forearm should be avoided. In addition, the needle must not be connected to the insufflation tube during the insertion process and the ventilator must be kept open until the needle has passed all anatomical layers. Puncture of the bowel or a large vessel may be noticed by blood or malodor passing back through the needle.

Fig. 2.4 After the insertion of the Veress' needle, the surgeon performs an "injection–aspiration test" before insufflation of the abdomen

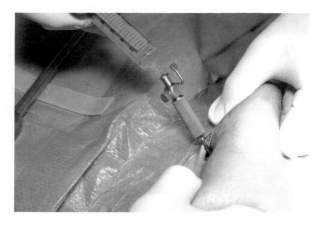

Following the insertion of the needle with the tip situated in the peritoneal cavity, the injection–aspiration test should be performed before insufflation of the abdomen (Fig. 2.4). Within this, a syringe is filled with 20 mL of NaCl and is connected to the needle. This is followed by aspiration to exclude puncture of a vessel or the bowel [8]. In this case, blood or stool may be aspirated. Next, NaCl is injected and reaspirated. If the tip is located in the peritoneal cavity, small gas bulbs may be visible. In case of re-aspiration of the fluid, the tip may either be situated between the abdominal wall layers or between peritoneal–intestinal adhesions where a small reservoir is created by the fluid injected primarily.

In patients with extensive or multiple previous abdominal surgery or those with large abdominal tumors reaching the level of the umbilicus, trocar insertion can also be carried out at the point described by Palmer [10].

Situated in the left hypochondrium just below the costal margin in the midclavicular line (Fig. 2.5a–c), this region is rarely involved in intraabdominal adhesions. In addition, insertion of the laparoscope at the Palmer's point often allows better visualization of the whole abdomen in case of a large intraabdominal mass [11].

If the technique described by Palmer fails, we have performed insufflation of the abdominal cavity via penetration of the posterior vaginal fornix and placement of the Veress needle in the pouch of Douglas [12]. However, this technique should only be performed by experienced laparoscopists because of the risk of bowel injury caused by the Veress needle.

To start insufflation, the Veress needle is connected to a tube with a flow of CO_2.

If the needle is appropriately positioned, lifting of the abdominal wall creates a negative pressure of 2–3 mmHg demonstrated by the digital pressure gauge on the insufflator. The intraabdominal pressure during insufflation should not be more than 5–10 mmHg and reflects the systemic resistance to the flow of CO_2. Higher pressure measurements are often associated with contact of the needle's tip with the omentum. A gentle movement backward may free the tip and allow proper insufflation. The needle never should be moved in a stirring manner because this could lead to extended injury of probably punctured anatomical structures such as the bowel.

Fig. 2.5 (**a**) Veress needle could be inserted at the Palmer's point, situated in the left hypochondrium just below the costal margin in the midclavicular line.
(**b**) Veress needle inserted at Palmer's point permits a correct pneumoperitoneum for laparoscope insertion.
(**c**) Trocar insertion at Palmer's point offers a better visualization of the intraabdominal contents, with a safe entry technique if extensive intraabdominal adhesions are expected or in patients with previous abdominal surgery

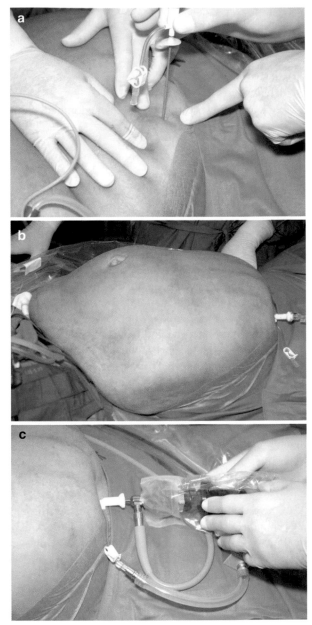

High insufflation pressures may also be explained by the extraperitoneal position of the insufflation needle. Again, proper position and functionality of the Veress needle should be checked. For insertion of the trocar, between 2 and 2.5 L of CO_2 should be allowed to flow into the abdominal cavity, depending on the stature of the patient. Signs of proper insufflation are regular percussion revealing a tympanic sound and symmetric distention of all four quadrants. Following this, the insertion needle is withdrawn carefully and the abdominal wall is gripped below the umbilicus at both sides with the help of an assistant and lifted for insertion of the trocar.

In principle, two classes of trocars can be used for penetration of the subumbilical wall layers—reusable trocars with a conic tip and disposable sharp-tipped trocars.

Whereas reusable trocars are inserted with screwlike movements and may be associated with a higher risk of injury of intraabdominal structures, disposable sharp-ending trocars should be inserted in a straightforward manner to reduce the size and diameter of the fascial incision [2].

However, it should be noted that the risk of large defects of the abdominal wall fascia and small vessel injury of the abdominal wall are higher with nonconic sharp-ending trocars. The maneuver should be performed with the surgeon's right hand formed to an index finger along the barrel of the trocar. Care must be taken to limit the depth of insertion because the abdominal aorta and vein are situated no more than 2 cm behind the umbilicus in slim patients. This can be achieved by situating the index finger on the trocar during the insertion process and avoiding sudden and deep insertion of the trocar in case of unexpected loss of resistance during insertion of the instrument. The trocar thereby will protrude no more than 2–3 cm into the abdominal wall (Fig. 2.6a–c).

After perforating all abdominal wall layers, CO_2 gas will be released from the insufflated abdomen via the trocar and hints at proper insertion and intraabdominal position. Following this, a warmed laparoscope is inserted and the middle and lower abdomen are visualized to exclude injury to anatomical structures such as the omentum, bowel, or large vessels. Examination of the abdomen and exclusion of complications is a precondition for situating the patient in the Trendelenburg position and continuation of the surgical procedure.

It should be noted that several Anglo-American authors prefer the technique described by Garry et al. [13], in which CO_2 flow is continued until intraabdominal pressure reaches 20–25 mmHg. Because of maximal distention of the abdominal wall, the distance is increased from the abdominal wall layers and intraperitoneal structures such as the bowel. The trocar is now inserted vertically without risking injury to the abdominal contents because the distance between the front and back of the abdomen is not reduced by the pressure applied on the trocar for abdominal wall perforation. Following the successful introduction of the instrument, intraabdominal pressure is reduced to 10–12 mmHg. This technique allows insertion of the trocar with both hands (because the abdominal wall is not lifted by the other hand), which is advantageous, especially for surgeons with small hands; however, possible disadvantages are anaesthetic and ventilation complications caused by high intraabdominal pressure and an excess of CO_2. However, a retrospective study conducted by Reich and colleagues [14] on the use of high-pressure trocar insertion in more than 3,000 patients reported only minor complication rates (two bowel perforations and no vascular injuries) using this technique.

Fig. 2.6 (**a**) Transumbilical insertion of the trocar. The instrument should be inserted with the index finger of the surgeon's hand along the barrel of the trocar. (**b**) By performing screwlike movements, the trocar protrudes through the abdominal wall layers. In order to limit insertion depth, the index finger rests on the trocar at all times during the insertion process. (**c**) As a consequence, the trocar will only protrude 2–3 cm into the abdominal wall, which will avoid injury of the big abdominal vessels

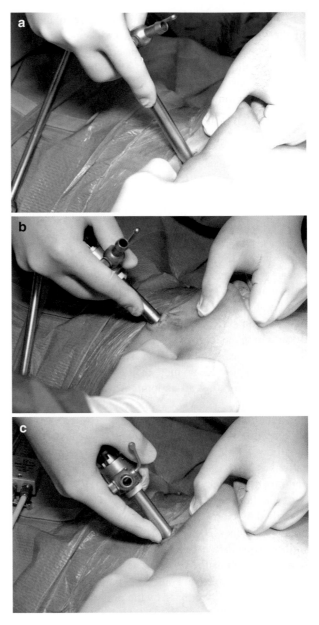

Open Technique for Laparoscopic Entry

In contrast to the closed technique for peritoneal entry, the open technique first described by Hasson [15] uses a small abdominal, predominantly subumbilical incision to protrude a blunt-tipped cannula into the abdominal cavity. After incising the skin, the subcutaneous fat tissue is dissected until the upper sheet of the rectal fascia can be visualized. Following this, the fascia is dissected in the midline and fixed at either side. Finally, the peritoneum is incised with a scalpel or divided with the two index fingers followed by insertion of the cannula under continuous visualization of the surrounding anatomical structures to avoid injury of the abdominal contents. The trocar is then fixed to the abdominal wall/ rectal fascia at both sides, after insufflation of the abdominal cavity via the trocar and insertion of the prewarmed laparoscope [16].

Although the open technique is less popular among gynecological surgeons and the majority of our colleagues prefer blind insertion of needle and trocars, there is a constant debate on the safety of either way of peritoneal entry. Several large retrospective studies on open versus closed establishment of pneumoperitoneum in general and gynecological surgery have given conflicting results regarding the safety of either technique [17, 18].

A retrospective review by Bonjer and colleagues [19] including a retrospective review of the literature and the author's experiences on closed laparoscopy in more than 489,000 cases and on open laparoscopy in more than 12,400 cases revealed significantly higher visceral and vascular complication rates of 0.083% and 0.075% after closed abdominal entry compared with 0.048% and 0% after open abdominal access. Similarly, a multicenter study of the Lap Group Roma [20], which included data on laparoscopic practice in 28 centers of laparoscopic surgery, revealed that the closed approach was the standard procedure for creation of a pneumoperitoneum (Veress needle and first trocar) in 82% of more than 12,900 laparoscopic procedures versus 9% of open technique cases and 9% of optical trocar use. However, complication rates differed significantly depending on the type of approach used. Among seven major vascular injuries (0.05%), nine minor vascular lesions (0.07%), and eight visceral injuries (0.06%), 0.27% were related to the use of optical trocars, 0.18% to the closed technique, and 0.09% to the open approach.

These results stand in contrast to the only systematic review of the safety and effectiveness of both methods, which was published by Merlin and colleagues [21]. They included data from standardized protocols of prospective, nonrandomized studies of open versus closed access from six bibliographic databases, the Internet, and reference lists. Although an open access slightly trended toward a reduced risk of major complications, these differences did not reach statistical significance. The authors finally concluded that data on major complications in studies directly comparing both techniques were inconclusive and the evidence on the comparative safety of both methods was not definitive. Based on these data and the experience of several other centers performing laparoscopic surgery, a consensus document published in 1999 [22] clearly expresses that to date a definitive conclusion regarding the safety of the use of open and/or closed abdominal access cannot be made based on the little evidence of an advantage in the Hasson technique.

In our experience, the open technique for laparoscopic access confers advantages in preoperated patients with a preexistent median laparotomy scar. In these patients, direct visualization of the abdominal wall layers and identification of possible adhesions might reduce complication rates. In addition, the longitudinal incision of the skin in a patient with previous abdominal surgery via a median laparotomy does not yield additional cosmetic disadvantages. However, the final decision to routinely use the open technique for abdominal entry should possibly be made by the surgeon and be based on personal experience [23–25].

Optical Trocars for Laparoscopic Entry

One alternative to the closed technique or abdominal access via the Hasson trocar is to use an optical Veress needle [26–28] and/or an optical trocar to enter the abdomen under direct view [29–31]. The use of insertion needles with an optical catheter system allows the surgeon to perform minimally invasive, predominantly diagnostic procedures via a 3-mm incision. The Visiport system (Autosuture Inc., Norwalk, CT) consists of an 11-mm trocar with a Plexiglas tip and an integrated scalpel that can pushed forward, revealing its sharpened end when the trocar passes through the tissue layers. The scalpel can be retracted into its original position after entry of the peritoneal cavity. To visualize protrusion of the trocar through the abdominal wall layers, a 10-mm laparoscope is inserted into the cannula [32].

Similar systems, such as Endopath Bladeless Trocars, have been designed (Ethicon Endosurgery, Johnson & Johnson, Somerville, NJ) that aim to reduce complication rates during entry in various laparoscopic procedures. To date we have conducted prospective, randomized trials to prove the possible advantages of this last technique [33–35].

Although some small retrospective studies have reported no major complications during abdominal access via the optical trocar [36–38], contrasting results have been published by Brown and colleagues [39], who described large bowel injuries in 2/96 consecutive cases in which the optical-access visual obturator trocar was used. Within this, it is questionable if the surgeon who protrudes the trocar under direct visual control can clearly differentiate between the anatomical structures of the abdominal wall and adhesive intraabdominal contents such as the bowel. In addition, the high costs of these single-use instruments confer an additional disadvantage and therefore another argument against the routine use of the optical trocar method.

Gasless Abdominal Access the Direct Trocar Technique

Direct insertion of the trocar without prior creation of a pneumoperitoneum is seen as an alternative approach to abdominal entry for laparoscopy especially in slim, nonobese patients [40–42].

Although the technique is only used by a expert surgeons and has not gained widespread popularity among gynecological laparoscopists, a small number of retrospective studies and a prospective, randomized trial by Agresta and co-workers [43] do report similar complication rates in the closed and the direct entry technique in patients with a body mass index (BMI) around 21. Based on the author's experiences, the direct trocar technique represents a safe approach to abdominal entry without creation of a pneumoperitoneum in nonobese patients.

However, since data on the use of this technique are limited, direct insertion of the trocar should only be performed by experienced and well-trained surgeons who are used to the method but cannot be recommended for general use [8, 44–46].

Insertion of Secondary and Additional Trocars

Even if performing solely diagnostic laparoscopic procedures, at least one additional port should be inserted to visualize both ovaries and the retroovarian region, as well as to move the bowel out of the pouch of Douglas. Usually, the second port is inserted via a midline incision 4–5 cm above the symphysis. Several surgeons vote against the use of a midline-inserted port and argue that the risk of bladder injury is too high to weigh out the benefits of a third instrument [47, 48].

In our experience, the risk of bladder injury caused by insertion of a midline trocar is very low in patients without previous abdominal surgery if the surgeon strictly adheres to the following basic principles. First, the bladder has to be catheterized preoperatively since an empty bladder lies behind the symphysis and can therefore not be punctured. Second, the trocar is inserted strictly 4–5 cm above the symphysis at the line described by Pfannenstiel incision. Third, the upper pole of the bladder should be visualized in patients with previous surgery, especially with prior Pfannenstiel incisions. Because the bladder might be situated more cephalad towing to the formation of postoperative adhesions, visualization of the filled bladder and its upper pole enables the surgeon to avoid injury of the organ by inserting the trocar under continuous visual control strictly above the vesical apex.

In operative laparoscopic procedures, two additional ports are inserted in the right and left lower abdomen, about 3–4 cm median and above the upper spine of the iliac bone. Insertion of additional trocars has to be performed under constant visualization of the trocar protruding into the abdominal wall, since injury to the external and common iliac arteries can happen if these trocars are inserted blindly and in an overly aggressive fashion. In addition, care must be taken to avoid puncture of vessels of the abdominal wall, especially the inferior epigastric artery [47]. This major vessel arises from the external iliac artery and anastomoses with the superior epigastric artery. The vessels are usually located 2–3 cm laterally from the midline and run in the rectus sheath. Sometimes small side branches of the inferior epigastric artery arise from the vessel just above the inguinal ligament and can also cause hematoma of the abdominal wall. Vessel puncture can be avoided by visualizing the arteries and concomitant veins via transilluminating the abdominal wall with the laparoscope [8]. However, this method only works well in nonobese patients with a relatively thin abdominal wall. In obese women, we suggest to insert the trocar strictly lateral to the rectus sheath in order to avoid puncture of the main vessel (inferior epigastric artery). In case of vessel injury, bleeding usually can be controlled by a laparoscopic mattress suture as described in the previous chapters.

In general, the surgeon should always be prepared to convert to laparotomy and should not hesitate to do so in case of intraoperative complications or if he is confronted with technical difficulties he might not be able to solve by laparoscopy.

References

1. Collinet P, Ballester M, Fauconnier A, Deffieux X, Pierre F. Risks associated with laparoscopic entry. J Gynecol Obstet Biol Reprod (Paris). 2010;39(8 Suppl 2):S123–35.
2. Garry R. The benefits and problems associated with minimal access surgery. Aust N Z J Obstet Gynaecol. 2002;42:239–44.
3. Chaudhuri T, Mandal K, Mandal D, Mondal J, Bose B, Basu A. Access in laparoscopy: an appraisal. J Indian Med Assoc. 2010;108(10):674–6.
4. Keren D, Rainis T, Stermer E, Lavy A. A nine-year audit of open-access upper gastrointestinal endoscopic procedures: results and experience of a single centre. Can J Gastroenterol. 2011;25(2):83–8.
5. Sasmal PK, Tantia O, Jain M, Khanna S, Sen B. Primary access-related complications in laparoscopic cholecystectomy via the closed technique: experience of a single surgical team over more than 15 years. Surg Endosc. 2009;23(11):2407–15.
6. Neudecker J, Sauerland S, Neugebauer E, Bergamaschi R, Bonier HJ, Cuschieri A, et al. The European Association for Endoscopic Surgery clinical practice guideline on the pneumoperitoneum for laparoscopic surgery. Surg Endosc. 2002;16(7):1121–43.
7. Vilos GA. The ABCs of a safer laparoscopic entry. J Minim Invasive Gynecol. 2006;13:249–51.
8. Vilos GA, Ternamian A, Dempster J, Laberge PY, The Society of Obstetricians and Gynaecologists of Canada. Laparoscopic entry: a review of techniques, technologies, and complications. J Obstet Gynaecol Can. 2007;29(5):433–65.
9. Shamiyeh A, Glaser K, Kratochwill H, Hormandinger K, Fellner F, Wayand WU, et al. Lifting of the umbilicus for the installation of pneumoperitoneum with the Veress needle increases the distance to the retroperitoneal and intraperitoneal structures. Surg Endosc. 2009;23: 313–7.
10. Palmer R. Safety in laparoscopy. J Reprod Med. 1974;13:1–5.
11. Agarwala N, Liu CY. Safe entry technique during laparoscopy: left upper quadrant entry using the ninth intercostal space: a review of 918 procedures. J Minim Invasive Gynecol. 2005;12:55–61.
12. Davila F, Tsin DA, Dominguez G, Davila U, Jesús R, Gomez de Arteche A. Transvaginal cholecystectomy without abdominal ports. JSLS. 2009;13(2):213–6.
13. Garry R. Various approaches to laparoscopic hysterectomy. Curr Opin Obstet Gynecol. 1994;6:215–22.
14. Reich H, Ribeiro SC, Rasmussen C, Rosenberg J, Vidali A. High-pressure trocar insertion technique. JSLS. 1999;3:45–8.
15. Hasson HM. Open laparoscopy. Biomed Bull. 1984;5:1–6.
16. Hasson HM, Rotman C, Rana N, Kumari NA. Open laparoscopy: 29-year experience. Obstet Gynecol. 2000;96(5 Pt 1):763–6.

17. Huang CC, Yang CY, Wu MH, Wang MY, Yeh CC, Lai IR, et al. Gasless laparoscopy-assisted versus open resection of small bowel lesions. J Laparoendosc Adv Surg Tech A. 2010;20(8): 699–703.
18. Wu JM, Yang CY, Wang MY, Wu MH, Lin MT. Gasless laparoscopy-assisted versus open resection for gastrointestinal stromal tumors of the upper stomach: preliminary results. J Laparoendosc Adv Surg Tech A. 2010;20(9):725–9.
19. Bonjer HJ, Hazebroek EJ, Kazemier G, Giuffrida MC, Meijer WS, Lange JF. Open versus closed establishment of pneumoperitoneum in laparoscopic surgery. Br J Surg. 1997;84: 599–602.
20. Catarci M, Carlini M, Gentileschi P, Santoro E. Major and minor injuries during the creation of pneumoperitoneum. A multicenter study on 12,919 cases. Surg Endosc. 2001;15:566–9.
21. Merlin TL, Hiller JE, Maddern GJ, Jamieson GG, Brown AR, Kolbe A. Systematic review of the safety and effectiveness of methods used to establish pneumoperitoneum in laparoscopic surgery. Br J Surg. 2003;90:668–79.
22. White JV. Consensus on laparoscopic surgery. J Laparoendosc Surg. 1992;2:195.
23. Agresta F, Mazzarolo G, Ciardo LF, Bedin N. The laparoscopic approach in abdominal emergencies: has the attitude changed? A single-center review of a 15-year experience. Surg Endosc. 2008;22(5):1255–62.
24. Kyung MS, Choi JS, Lee JH, Jung US, Lee KW. Laparoscopic management of complications in gynecologic laparoscopic surgery: a 5-year experience in a single center. J Minim Invasive Gynecol. 2008;15(6):689–94.
25. Wind J, Cremers JE, van Berge Henegouwen MI, Gouma DJ, Jansen FW, Bemelman WA. Medical liability insurance claims on entry-related complications in laparoscopy. Surg Endosc. 2007;21(11):2094–9.
26. Valtchev KL. Laparoscopic needle introducer. J Am Assoc Gynecol Laparosc. 2001;8(4):579–82.
27. Ghezzi F, Cromi A, Siesto G, Boni L, Uccella S, Bergamini V, et al. Needlescopic hysterectomy: incorporation of 3-mm instruments in total laparoscopic hysterectomy. Surg Endosc. 2008;22(10):2153–7.
28. Ikeda F, Vanni D, Vasconcelos A, Podgaec S, Abrão MS. Microlaparoscopy vs. conventional laparoscopy for the management of early-stage pelvic endometriosis: a comparison. J Reprod Med. 2005;50(10):771–8.
29. Tai HC, Lai MK, Chueh SC, Chen SC, Hsieh MH, Yu HJ. An alternative access technique under direct vision for preperitoneoscopic pelvic surgery: easier for the beginners. Ann Surg Oncol. 2008;15(9):2589–93.
30. Sabeti N, Tarnoff M, Kim J, Shikora S. Primary midline peritoneal access with optical trocar is safe and effective in morbidly obese patients. Surg Obes Relat Dis. 2009;5(5):610–4.
31. Hajdinjak T, Oakley NE. Use of optical dilating trocar for initial access during extraperitoneal laparoscopic radical prostatectomy. J Endourol. 2007;21(9):1089–92.
32. Pelosi MA, Pelosi 3rd MA. Laparoscopically assisted colpotomy with the Pelosi illuminator and Visiport trocar system. J Reprod Med. 1996;41(8):548–54.
33. Tinelli A, Malvasi A, Istre O, Keckstein J, Stark M, Mettler L. Abdominal access in gynaecological laparoscopy: a comparison between direct optical and blind closed access by Veress needle. Eur J Obstet Gynecol Reprod Biol. 2010;148(2):191–4.
34. Tinelli A, Malvasi A, Hudelist G, Istre O, Keckstein J. Abdominal access in gynaecologic laparoscopy: a comparison between direct optical and open access. J Laparoendosc Adv Surg Tech A. 2009;19(4):529–33.
35. Tinelli A, Malvasi A, Guido M, Istre O, Keckstein J, Mettler L. Initial laparoscopic access in postmenopausal women: a preliminary prospective study. Menopause. 2009;16(5):966–70.
36. Minervini A, Davenport K, Pefanis G, Keeley Jr FX, Timoney AG. Prospective study comparing the bladeless optical access trocar versus Hasson open trocar for the establishment of pneumoperitoneum in laparoscopic renal procedures. Arch Ital Urol Androl. 2008;80(3):95–8.

37. Rabl C, Palazzo F, Aoki H, Campos GM. Initial laparoscopic access using an optical trocar without pneumoperitoneum is safe and effective in the morbidly obese. Surg Innov. 2008;15(2):126–31.
38. Berch BR, Torquati A, Lutfi RE, Richards WO. Experience with the optical access trocar for safe and rapid entry in the performance of laparoscopic gastric bypass. Surg Endosc. 2006;20(8):1238–41.
39. Brown JA, Canal D, Sundaram CP. Optical-access visual obturator trocar entry into desufflated abdomen during laparoscopy: assessment after 96 cases. J Endourol. 2005;19:853–5.
40. Altun H, Banli O, Karakoyun R, Boyuk A, Okuducu M, Onur E, et al. Direct trocar insertion technique for initial access in morbid obesity surgery: technique and results. Surg Laparosc Endosc Percutan Tech. 2010;20(4):228–30.
41. Günenç MZ, Yesildaglar N, Bingöl B, Onalan G, Tabak S, Gökmen B. The safety and efficacy of direct trocar insertion with elevation of the rectus sheath instead of the skin for pneumoperitoneum. Surg Laparosc Endosc Percutan Tech. 2005;15(2):80–1.
42. Bernante P, Foletto M, Toniato A. Creation of pneumoperitoneum using a bladed optical trocar in morbidly obese patients: technique and results. Obes Surg. 2008;18(8):1043–6.
43. Agresta F, De Simone P, Ciardo LF, Bedin N. Direct trocar insertion vs Veress needle in non obese patients undergoing laparoscopic procedures: a randomized prospective single-center study. Surg Endosc. 2004;18:1778–81.
44. Ahmad G, Duffy JM, Phillips K, Watson A. Laparoscopic entry techniques. Cochrane Database Syst Rev. 2008;2:CD006583.
45. Perunovic RM, Scepanovic RP, Stevanovic PD, Ceranic MS. Complications during the establishment of laparoscopic pneumoperitoneum. J Laparoendosc Adv Surg Tech A. 2009;19(1): 1–6.
46. Kroft J, Aneja A, Tyrwhitt J, Ternamian A. Laparoscopic peritoneal entry preferences among Canadian gynaecologists. J Obstet Gynaecol Can. 2009;31(7):641–8.
47. Pickett SD, Rodewald KJ, Billow MR, Giannios NM, Hurd WW. Avoiding major vessel injury during laparoscopic instrument insertion. Obstet Gynecol Clin North Am. 2010;37(3):387–97.
48. Vilos GA, Vilos AG, Abu-Rafea B, Hollett-Caines J, Nikkhah-Abyaneh Z, Edris F. Three simple steps during closed laparoscopic entry may minimize major injuries. Surg Endosc. 2009;23(4):758–64.

Chapter 3
Laparoscopic Abdominal Entry by the Ternamian Threaded Visual System

Artin Ternamian

Introduction

The word endoscopy is of Greek derivation in which *endon* means internal, and *skopein* means to examine. Healers from Hippocrates' time have adapted primitive viewing instruments to peer into dark and yet-undiscovered body crevasses, in an attempt to understand and relieve human suffering [1]. Despite considerable technologic advancements, endoscopy retains three principal elements to accomplish its objective. The first comprises a flexible or rigid viewing tube endoscope to transmit light into the body cavity and convey back images for the surgeon to observe. The second consists of an array of ancillary surgical instruments to enable the operator to perform minimally invasive diagnostic and therapeutic tasks. The third is an anchored access system that leads instruments in and out of body compartments without loss of distention or orientation. These conduits (ports) are either surgically created temporary invariant entry points (thoracoscopy, laparoscopy, culdoscopy), through natural orifices, without requiring entry wounds (bronchoscopy, colonoscopy, hysteroscopy) or through contemporary hybrid conduits (Natural Orifice Transluminal Endoscopic Surgery [NOTES]). Endoscopy is now practiced in most specialties and is the preferred method of managing several gynecological conditions. It is a technology driven, dynamic discipline that challenges conventional surgical practice and teaching. It offers inventive solutions to render robotic surgery, remote tele-presence surgery, frameless stereotactic surgery, and other innovative advances possible. Reduced patient disability, diminished costs, and early recovery are among important advantages of minimally invasive surgery compared with open laparotomy (estimated overall complications risk 8% versus 15%) [2, 3]. Endoscopy has become a popular operative approach around the world, and in North America, more than 2 million laparoscopies are performed annually [4].

A. Ternamian
Director of Gynecologic Endoscopy, Department of Obstetrics & Gynecology,
Faculty of Medicine, University of Toronto, St. Joseph's Health Centre, Toronto, ON, Canada

A. Tinelli (ed.), *Laparoscopic Entry*,
DOI 10.1007/978-0-85729-980-2_3, © Springer-Verlag London Limited 2012

33

It is anticipated that with the advent of robotic surgery and NOTES, these numbers will increase further in the foreseeable future. As a result, more than 6 million ports are created annually in the Unites States alone, and according to Medical Data International, global volume is estimated to rise at a compounded annual growth rate of 4.8% (Medical Data International, Inc., 1999, U.S. Markets for Endo-Laparoscopic Surgery Products). Given this increasing popularity of laparoscopic procedures and number of access devices used, the total public health burden of "uncommon," yet potentially disastrous entry related misadventures is considerable. Despite significant advances in endoscopy and patient safety, major operative complications with serious consequences continue to occur at about 1/1,000 procedures [5, 6]. Several large multicenter studies and metaanalyses demonstrated that more than 50% of bowel (0.4/1,000) and major vessels (0.2/1,000) injuries occur during initial peritoneal entry, in which 80% are attributed directly to primary port (trocar and cannula) application [4, 7, 8]. Actually, push-through trocars and cannulas are the most common type of laparoscopic device causing injuries. Regrettably. more than two-thirds of these mishaps are not recognized until some time after the conclusion of the operation (http://www.piaa.us/ LaparoscopicInjuryStudy/pdf/PIAA_2000). Accordingly, the U.S Food and Drug Administration (FDA), in a Laparoscopic Trocar Injuries report, recommends surgeons performing endoscopic operations to be well versed in alternate laparoscopic access methods and instruments to address evolving patient expectations and societal safety requirements [9]. The Institute of Medicine Committee report on Patient Safety in the USA publication suggests that more than 90% of unintended medical mishaps are human error–related [10]. Accordingly, surgeons and industry now recognize the need for less hazardous laparoscopic port options with imbedded safety redundancies to avert mishaps, especially in high-risk situations. It appears that the real prevalence of entry-related vascular and visceral injury remains imprecise and possibly is much higher than suspected, as the majority of accidents are unpublished or omitted from retrospective analysis. Besides, often entry-related injuries are misunderstood and erroneously attributed to incorrect etiologies [11, 12]. In effect, vessel-related accidents are the second most common cause of death during laparoscopy, second to anesthetic mortality. Consequently, medical instruments and methods that can anticipate avoid or at the very least recognize inadvertent injury are preferred, in which error recovery is possible, before permanent patient harm occurs [13]. Misperceptions and unrealistic expectations about accident causation and incidence of human error during endoscopic surgery complications in general and port creation in particular, often results in assumption of incompetence, guilt, and litigation. Generally, body cavity entry and exit has three distinct and different aspects to consider, peritoneal port creation Method, port creation Instrument, and port creation Site, MIS (Table 3.1). In addition, port instruments can be single use, multiple use, or hybrid. They can be blind or visual, sharp-tipped, or blunt-ended. In turn, each of these instrument models can be deployed by several methods and at different port sites. Often, investigators fail to appreciate these important yet fundamental distinctions when describing their observations or discussing ways to improve laparoscopic access safety, and end up confusing both their results as well as their readers. Most peritoneal entry-related publications are limited to small studies in which high-risk patients are usually excluded. In addition, these papers are

Table 3.1 Different aspects of port creation: Methods, Instruments, and port Sites

Port creation	
Method	Closed conventional insufflated, open noninsufflated, direct noninsufflated, visual, etc.
Instrument	Sharp/blunt conventional trocar and cannula, radially expanding trocar & cannula, open trocar & cannula, optical trocar and cannula, threaded visual cannula, single/multiple use, SILS, LESS.
Site	Sub, intraumbilical, supraumbilical, lower quadrant, left upper quadrant, intercostal, suprapubic, etc.

clearly underpowered and do not include experience with the Ternamian Threaded Visual Cannula (TVC) system. A metaanalysis of 17 randomized controlled trials, evaluating 3,040 laparoscopic operations, failed to validate superiority of one port system over the other [14]. Given the infrequency of these adverse events, it is highly unlikely that a randomized trial will reliably and scientifically determine which method, instrument, or site is the least accident prone. To demonstrate a 50% difference in entry bowel injury (from 0.04% to 0.02%) would require a study population of more than 800,000 patients. Consequently, surgeons must practice what they are schooled in and become versed in more than one entry method, instrument, and site [15, 16]. This chapter introduces the Ternamian Threaded Visual Cannula: EndoTIP method, instrument, and application sites, emphasizing its characteristics and safe deployment to render primary and ancillary port creation less perilous. This port system allows error archiving, recall, and examination, to understand better body cavity entry accident causation. As with all visual entry systems, knowledge of anatomy, appreciation of navigational cues (perceptual blindness), and correct recognition of displayed monitor images (situational awareness), are essential competencies for safe deployment [17]. Irrespective, patients with previous abdominal surgery and known or suspected abdominal adhesions present a higher risk for peritoneal entry complications [18]. Consenting high-risk patients must be informed of the possibility of an alternate entry method (visual or open entry), the probability of a different access site (left upper quadrant, LUQ), or the likelihood of conversion to laparotomy [4].

Dynamics of Peritoneal Entry

Conventional push-through body cavity entry systems have relied on a simple concept since time immemorial (Fig. 3.1). This primitive and simple push-through mechanical model comprises a central pointed or sharp obturator, *trocar*, sheathed into a hollow conduit, *cannula*. (Origin: 1700–1710. French *trocart: trois*, three [Old French, from Latin *trēs;* Indo-European roots] + *carre*, side of an object [Old French, from *carrer*, meaning square, from the Latin *quadrāre;* Indo-European roots], *quadrum*, square; The American Heritage Dictionary of the English Language, 4th ed 2010, Houghton Mifflin Harcourt.)

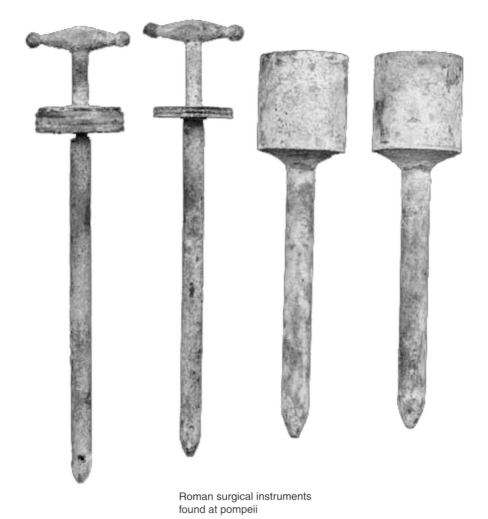

Roman surgical instruments
found at pompeii

Fig. 3.1 Roman surgical instruments, *trocar and cannula*, found in Pompeii

Operators require knowledge of anatomy, location of pathology, and proprioception to navigate instruments safely toward a target body area. Healers used this archetype to access the vascular system, the cerebrospinal space, the pericardial compartment, and the thoracic cavity, among others. Endoscopists seconded this very same concept and instrument to develop primary and ancillary peritoneal ports with little modification or thought about potential and real hazards associated with their use (Fig. 3.2). There are three fundamental variables to consider when creating a laparoscopic port. First is the different body tissue layers that have to be traversed en route to the target compartment in which surgery is performed (anterior abdominal or intercostals wall), second is the instrument trajectory design that is applied to

Fig. 3.2 Conventional push-through sharp trocar and vented cannula

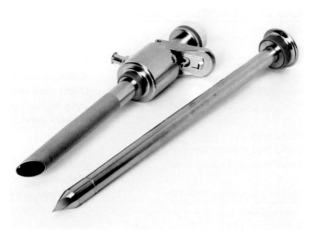

create the port (sharp, blunt, visual), and third is the penetration force (direction, amount, rate, control, recruitment) required to safely deploy the port. The anterior abdominal wall is a dynamic body organ that comprises interposed tissue layers, to offer essential trunk containment. It is generally the platform in which primary, ancillary, and hybrid temporary ports are anchored to perform extra-, intra-, or retroperitoneal operations. Knowledge of this important anatomical environment and understanding of the functional anatomy of every component from skin, subcutaneous fat, fascia, muscle, peritoneal membrane, vessel, nerve, and osseous scaffolding will guarantee effective and safe port application irrespective of method, instrument, and port site. Some of the important difference between open and laparoscopic surgery include size of surgical wound, visual fidelity (magnification, illumination, depth perception), and haptic (force + tactile feedback). It is important to appreciate that a fixed port entry point in relation to a dynamic surgical field creates a significant ergonomic challenge for surgeon and assistant alike [19]. Unlike open conventional surgery, the fulcrum effect during laparoscopic port-centered operations, necessitates paradoxical field and instrument movement, limited excursion, suboptimal work ergonomics, and altered haptic, and alters the operator's body posture relative to the surgical target [20, 21]. Although open surgery allows the surgeon's hand two degrees of freedom (DOF) of movement, for each of the nine interphalangeal joints, conventional laparoscopic operative instruments, with the exception of contemporary robotic arms, offer only four DOFs [19]. In addition, the surgeon's body allows six trunk DOF movements, three rotations at the shoulders, one at the elbow and one in the forearm, with two at the wrist. Long straight or curved operative instruments pivot at port sites to create force transmission variances according to the extra- or intracorporeal instrument length ratio. Additionally, short extracorporeal length diminishes mechanical advantage, whereas long extracorporeal length induces the operator to assume awkward nonergonomic forearm and shoulder positions [22]. Instrument tip excursion differs from that of instrument handle unless the instrument pivots exactly at its midpoint [23]. In addition, because

Table 3.2 Methods of primary laparoscopic peritoneal entry

Blind entry	
Insufflated	Closed trocar and cannula entry
	High-pressure trocar and cannula entry
	Radially expanding trocar and cannula entry
Noninsufflated	Direct trocar and cannula entry
	Open Hasson's trocar and cannula entry
	Hybrid laparoscope ports LESS, SILS, NOTES
Visual entry	
Visual Veress minilaparoscopic entry	
Visual trocar and cannula entry	EndoPath OptiView trocar and cannula entry
	Visiport trocar and cannula entry
Visual cannula entry EndoTIP	Endoscopic threaded imaging port

laparoscopic operating instruments have reduced grasping surfaces and diminished mechanical advantage, the force required to effectively grasp tissue is estimated to be six times greater than the force necessary to operate with open conventional surgical instruments. Given the current suboptimal ergonomic physical environment (operating room setup and endoscopic instruments), surgeons often wrestle with unnecessary technical difficulty, unwarranted overuse fatigue, and needless operative morbidity during laparoscopic more than open surgery [24]. Consequently, minimally invasive procedures are generally significantly more stressful and require additional operator concentration compared with open laparotomy [25]. It is recognized that a suboptimal surgical environment and other stressors (such as sleep deprivation) can impede surgical dexterity and increase the likelihood of inadvertent operative error [26, 27]. Interestingly, despite multiple stresses, surgeons are less likely to acknowledge the effects of stress on their operative performance than individuals in other equally demanding and safety critical disciplines [28]. Primary peritoneal port insertion methods can be either blind or visual (Table 3.2). Visual entry requires a zero-degree laparoscope mounted into the access instrument during port creation, whereas blind entry requires no laparoscope during placement. Entry is also described as closed entry (applied after CO_2 insufflation) or open/direct entry (deployed without preinsufflation) [29]. When applying visual ports, recognition of the cascade of different anterior abdominal wall layers is particularly important as they create a real-time navigational guide to safe port placement and offer the unique advantage of recognizing inadvertent access injury if and when they occur. The peritoneal cavity is a sealed compartment, often described as a "virtual cavity" in which viscera occupy the entire area save for a few milliliters of peritoneal fluid. Generally, operators palm the conventional push-through trocar and cannula with the dominant hand and apply significant linear force, generated by the shoulder and trunk muscles, toward the body part to access. This linear propulsion requirement dictates instrument design to have a pointed or sharp end, to decrease entry force necessary to transect different tissue layers during port placement [30]. Evidence indicates that more than 30 commercially available port systems have a specific reproducible, characteristic and predictable penetration force profile, and that

Fig. 3.3 Performance
shaping factors: penetration
force, access instrument, and
port site

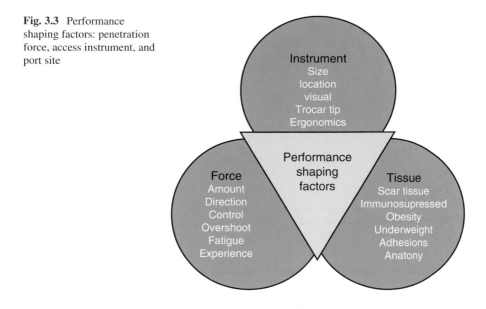

required to penetrate the thin loosely bound peritoneal membrane is significant when compared with that of the taught thicker anterior rectus fascia, causing considerable tenting or tissue deformation. In addition, once the peritoneal layer is transfixed, an immediate sudden loss of resistance is registered [12]. The more sudden (200–300 ms) and uncontrolled is this loss of resistance, the higher is the extent of trocar overshoot and the likelihood of loss of control and inadvertent injury. Often conventional trocars are blind, with no ability to avert instrument overshoot; no mechanism to anticipate, avoid, or recognize injury; and no mechanism to control penetration [17]. In effect, successful primary port insertion represents one of the fundamental core competencies required for safe endoscopic surgery. This single task remains the most important and potentially dangerous first step in laparoscopy [31, 32]. Failure of satisfactory peritoneal access or strategic port placement can undermine the laparoscopic approach or render the procedure unsafe for patient and surgeon alike [33]. Conventional push-through trocar and cannula application at primary and ancillary ports offers limited safety redundancy when applying uncontrolled linear entry force to a sharp blind trajectory toward the viscera, with no mechanism to temper penetration force, gage insertion depth, and avoid sudden uncontrolled overshoot. Accident causation and error analysis studies identified specific performance shaping factors (PSF), which are shown to influence inadvertent entry mishaps, irrespective of a surgeon's skill, instruments, and method of application (Fig. 3.3). The compilation of potentially dangerous PSFs during primary port insertion renders accessing less forgiving and sets the stage for inadvertent injury. Deconstructing and reengineering port creation without the identified access PSFs introduces increments of access safety, to individually or collectively render peritoneal entry less hazardous [34].

Fig. 3.4 The Ternamian threaded visual cannula EndoTIP with telescope stopper

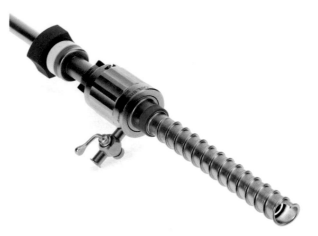

Ternamian Threaded Visual Cannula EndoTIP Method

Application of the Ternamian Threaded Visual Cannula EndoTIP system (Karl STORZ GmbH Tuttlingen, Germany) entails a complete departure from the conventional push-through trocar and cannula peritoneal entry method (Fig. 3.4). Significant differences define this new body cavity access method. The first is elimination of the sharp or pointed trocar and use of a blunt cannula only as access tool. The second is trading blind for visual entry to archive and retrieve entry information. The third is conversion of uncontrolled excessive linear to moderate radial penetration force. The fourth is introduction of incremental measured entry instead of sudden and uncontrolled entry to avoid overshoot. The fifth is conversion of the push-through to pull-up entry [35]. By redirecting penetration entry force from linear to radial, the need of a sharp or pointed trocar is obviated. When a cannula without a sheathed trocar (sharp, cutting, blunt, others) is used, inadvertent "trocar" injury is eliminated and tissue integrity is better preserved along the port tract. Instead of transecting fascia and muscle fibers, the blunt TVC cannula parts different tissue layers, ensuring safe port placement and securing tissue competence and recoil at port retrieval. Application of the TVC requires a clear understanding that this method is different from the conventional push-through entry systems in which the advancing trocar and cannula dents (funneling) the anterior abdominal wall forwards toward the peritoneum. Instead, during TVC application the reverse occurs, in which the cannula tip, with the sheathed zero-degree laparoscope, engages the fascial tissues and tents successive abdominal wall layers up the cannula's outer thread with little downward pressure. Penetration force is redirected radial rather that axial or linear until the peritoneal cavity is entered incrementally under visual oversight, avoiding cannula overshoot. The ability to observe instrument, tissue, and force dynamics in real time during insertion and retrieval of ports tempers the amount of entry force recruited and allows immediate error recognition and repair, if inadvertent injury occurs [36, 37]. The first to advocate visual primary port insertion was Professor K. Semm of Kiel University. His teaching discouraged blind abdominal entry with sharp trocars and used bevelled vented cannulas to insert primary ports under visual control [38].

Closed Laparoscopic Access with the Ternamian Threaded Visual Cannula EndoTIP

Safe umbilical application of the TVC as primary port with closed preinsufflation involves the following steps. Careful inspection of the supine nondraped abdomen for previous surgical scars, palpation of the abdominal wall, and identification of the five invariant abdominal bony landmarks (suprapubic bone, anterior superior iliac spine, iliac crest, sacral promontory, and subcostal angle) must precede each laparoscopic port placement, irrespective of entry method, instrument, or access site. This important measure develops a 3D spatial conceptualization of the anatomical relationships between the abdominopelvic organs and peripheral osseous scaffolding for safe port placement irrespective of the patient's BMI and anatomy. As recommended at the Middlesbrough Consensus Document on Laparoscopic Entry, patients are to remain in the horizontal supine position until successful insufflation and primary TVC port insertion [5]. To date, most visual entry systems require use of a zero-degree laparoscope sheathed into the port system, unless if a contemporary variable vision laparoscope is used. This new, rigid endoscope, the Endocameleon (ECAM, Karl STORZ GmbH, Tuttlingen, Germany) is developed to combine beneficial features of rigid and flexible endoscopes, where the viewing direction can be adjusted as required between 0° and 120°. Generally, manufacturers recommend their visual entry systems to be deployed with preinsufflation until surgeons appreciate the fundamental differences between conventional push-through methods and visual entry system and are versed in their safe application. Using a No. 15 surgical blade, a generous (sub-, intra-, or infraumbilical) skin incision is preferred to accommodate the TVC's outer diameter and avoid skin dystocia. This minimizes unnecessary friction between the outer surface of the rotating cannula and tissue along the port tract during insertion and removal. Use of ribbon retractors facilitates paring of the periumbilical subcutaneous fatty tissue off the anterior rectus fascia using "peanut sponges." Exposure of the white anterior rectus fascia is very important before cannula application because this will avoid drawing loose subcutaneous fatty tissues into the TVC's inner space during rotation and obscuring tissue visualization. Understandably, CO_2 leakage around a cannula has very little to do with skin incision size and everything to do with anterior rectus fascial application and tissue recoil relative to the cannula's outer diameter. Gynecologists prefer a sub- or intraumbilical primary port incisions because of training and cosmesis rather than evidence. An initial Veress needle entry pressure of <10 mmHg with a CO_2 insufflation pressure of up to 25–30 mmHg is described as being less hazardous [6, 39]. A recent Canadian gynecologist's survey demonstrated that 45% of practitioners use 25 mmHg of CO_2 insufflation pressure at primary port insertion, 28.8% of respondents use 20–25 mmHg, and 16.2% use 16–19 mmHg [40]. Determining correct Veress placement before insufflation remains a very important step, because failure to achieve and maintain adequate pneumoperitoneum is a common cause of procedural failure. To date, the most reliable indicator of correct peritoneal placement remains an initial intraperitoneal pressure reading of <10 mmHg (range 4–10 mmHg). Only when intraperitoneal needle placement is secure is the CO_2 insufflation flow rate safely cranked to high flow [41, 42]. High CO_2 insufflation pressure ($\geq$25–30 mmHg) is an alternate closed entry method in which the elevated intraperitoneal pressure is purported to brace the abdominal wall to counter axial penetration force and the inevitable overshoot that accompanies all push-through trocar and cannula entry methods by interposing a larger gas envelope between the advancing trajectory and great vessels, viscera, or retroperitoneum [43, 44]. What is certain is that anterior abdominal tissue layer deformation is significantly reduced at 10 mmHg compared with 0 mmHg of intraperitoneal CO_2 pressure [12]. Once the TVC primary cannula is placed and correct insertion verified, intraperitoneal pressure must be lowered and maintained at about 10–15 mmHg. Abdominal palpation to gage sufficient insufflation is sometimes preferred to determine adequacy of distention, because instilled gas volume measurement can be unreliable. Obesity does not generally adversely affect insufflation volume for a given intraabdominal pressure because the actual intraabdominal volume is a finite value, and 94% of this capacity is attained at an abdominal pressure of 55 mmHg [43, 45].When adequately insufflated, retrieve the Veress, and apply the TVC instrument. It is important to maintain the median plane during Veress and primary port insertion and not rely on umbilical positioning relative to termination of the aorta as your only topographic landmark. A zero-degree laparoscope is defogged (UltraStop sterile antifog solution, Sigmapharm, Vienna), and sheathed into the hollow TVC cannula, locked with the Telescope Stopper 1 cm short of the cannula's distal end and camera focused to beam real-time port images during insertion and removal of the cannula (Fig. 3.5). The surgeon holds the sheathed zero-degree laparoscope with the non dominant hand perpendicular to the supine abdomen and the TVC cannula with the dominant hand, resting on the anterior rectus fascia at the primary port site. The surgeon faces the monitor with shoulders at rest and forearms held at right angle to the arms (Fig. 3.6). It is important to minimize unintentional downward force: The idea is to allow the wrist muscles (weaker muscle = less penetration force applied) to do the rotation with minimal downward arm movement (stronger muscle = more penetration force applied) [44]. As the TCV is rotated using the dominant hand, the cannula tip engages the white anterior rectus fascia and parts the fascial fibers to transpose them onto the cannula's outer threads. The next layer to part and move up is the red rectus muscle, followed by the white posterior fascia and translucent peritoneal membrane as the cannula enters the insufflated peritoneal cavity (Fig. 3.7). Once in the cavity, an inspection survey of the entire cavity is conducted before the Trendelenburg position is assumed. When applying the TVC at a primary port in closed peritoneal entry, the CO_2 insufflated peritoneal cavity will transilluminate and look grayish in color unless parietal, bowel, or omental adhesions are present, at which time the intense laparoscopic light will reflect back and appear white in

Fig. 3.5 The Ternamian threaded visual cannula with sheathed zero-degree laparoscope and magnified distal end

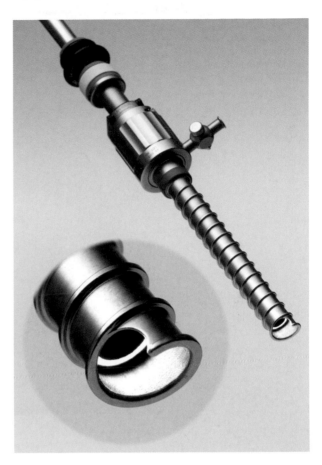

color. Although bowel adherent to the parietal port-site remains susceptible to injury irrespective of access method, the TVC entry methods offer varying degrees of prediction, prevention, and real-time injury recognition capabilities (Fig. 3.8) [37]. In high-risk patients, a preliminary umbilical inspection is possible when the TVC EndoTIP, the visual Veress micro-laparoscope, or other visually guided system is applied through the left upper quadrant to safely map periumbilical or other visceral–parietal peritoneal adhesions and place additional ancillary ports accordingly [47]. One has to remember that successful peritoneal access on first passage of a Veress needle through a conventional sites does not necessarily exclude the possibility of umbilical adhesions or subsequent bowel injury upon insertion of conventional trocars. The SCAR study demonstrated that the clinical burden is considerable, because 60–90% of women who have previously undergone major gynecologic surgery have some postoperative peritoneal adhesions [48]. The incidence of periumbilical adhesion is <0.03%; however, it may be as high as 68% in patients with previous laparotomy, especially those in whom a midline surgical scar extends to

Fig. 3.6 Hold laparoscope with nondominant hand ND and rotate the threaded visual cannula with dominant hand DH. *TS* Telescope Stopper

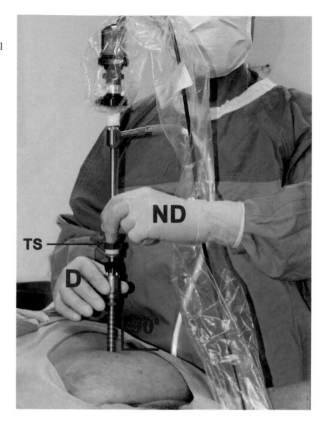

the umbilical region [49]. Patients with known peritoneal adhesions, those with a history of more than one previous laparotomy, morbidly obese patients, those with history of previous failed laparoscopy or insufflation, and others in special high-risk situation, may be candidates for combined application alternatives such as peritoneal entry with the TVC, applied without preinsufflation through the left upper quadrant [50]. It is recommended to keep the CO_2 stopcock shut during closed TVC application to avoid unnecessary gas loss upon peritoneal entry until the CO_2 stopcock is connected and insufflation is initiated. When insufflation is complete and telescope stopper released, the laparoscope is advanced into the peritoneal cavity to perform surgery. Appreciation of tissue sequencing off the monitor is an important competency of safe visual port placement. Surgeons intuitively look at the abdominal port site during cannula deployment instead of observing peritoneal entry images off the monitor. Successful visual entry gaze-transference from port site to monitor is an integral learning curve with TVC and other visual entry methods for safe application. The average time required to insert a primary TVC port is about 1–4 min, depending on the patient's specifics and the surgeon's dexterity. Increased BMI does not appear to add significantly to insertion ease or time [51].

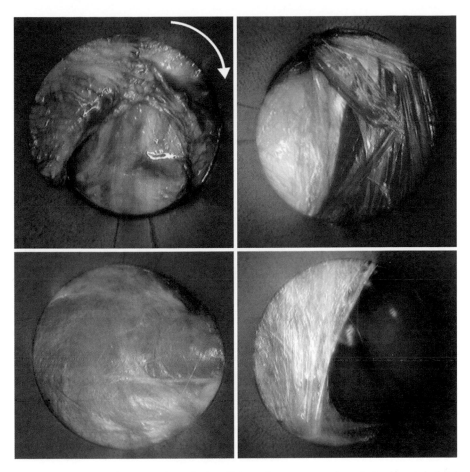

Fig. 3.7 A cascade of anterior abdominal wall tissue layers as seen through the threaded visual cannula during primary umbilical entry. White anterior fascia, red rectus muscle, white posterior fascia, yellow pre-peritoneal layer, gray-white peritoneal membrane

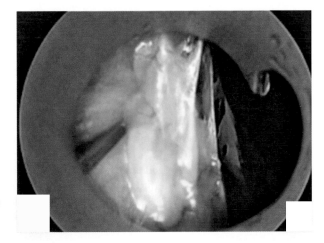

Fig. 3.8 The Ternamian threaded visual cannula can predict, prevent or recognize when parietal adhesions are encountered

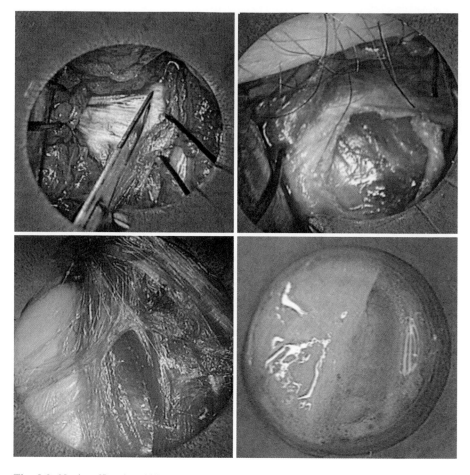

Fig. 3.9 Noninsufflated umbilical application of the threaded visual cannula at umbilicus with anterior abdominal wall tissue sequencing

Open or Direct Laparoscopic Access with the Ternamian Threaded Visual Cannula EndoTIP

When applying the TVC at the primary port in open or direct peritoneal entry, without CO_2 preinsufflation, a similar subumbilical skin incision is performed using a No. 15 surgical blade. The skin incision must allow adequate visualization of the white anterior rectus fascia, especially in obese patients, in whom use of 1-cm ribbon retractors and "peanut sponges" can facilitate exposure. A small 3-mm vertical anterior rectus fascial incision will facilitate cannula application (Fig. 3.9). A zero-degree laparoscope is defogged and sheathed into the hollow TVC cannula, locked with the telescope stopper 1 cm short of the cannula's distal end and camera focused to beam real-time port images during insertion and removal of the cannula. The surgeon holds the sheathed zero-degree laparoscope with the nondominant hand

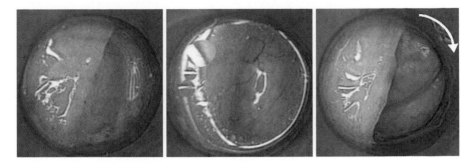

Fig. 3.10 Upon noninsufflated peritoneal entry, the threaded visual cannula tip rests on the bowel. CO_2 insufflation lifts the anterior abdominal wall to safely advance the cannula

perpendicular to the supine abdomen and the TVC cannula with the dominant hand resting on the anterior abdominal wall rectus fascia at the primary port site. The surgeon faces the monitor with shoulders at rest and forearms held at right angles to the arms. It is important to avoid downward force, especially during noninsufflated application of the TVC because the distance between the instrument's tip and viscera or retroperitoneal large vessels is minimal. To avoid inadvertent injury, a pair of Khockers or fascial holding stitches is applied at 3 and 9 o'clock, to steady and lift the fascia during cannula insertion [46]. Upon TCV rotation using the dominant hand, the cannula tip engages the white anterior rectus fascial incision and parts the fascia to transpose it onto the TVC outer threads. Next to part and move up is the red rectus muscle, followed by the white posterior fascia. Once the pre-peritoneal fatty layer is cleared, before peritoneal entry, bowel peristalsis or omentum can be observed through the intact thin transparent peritoneal membrane, moving in synch with the respiratory movements of the patient. Further rotation will part the peritoneum and allow room air to stream into the peritoneal cavity through the open TVC CO_2 stopcock. At this very moment, rotation is stopped and CO_2 insufflation initiated under visual control. As the CO_2 fills the peritoneal compartment, the cannula's tip that was resting on bowel or omentum lifts up with the rising anterior abdominal wall (Fig. 3.10). When insufflation is complete and the telescope stopper is released, the laparoscope is advanced into the peritoneal cavity to insert ancillary ports and perform surgery. Although bowel adherent to the parietal port-site remains susceptible to injury irrespective of access method, TVC entry methods offer prediction, prevention, and real-time injury recognition capabilities. Appreciation of tissue sequencing off the monitor is an important competency of safe visual port placement. Of particular importance in visual port entry (in closed, open or direct TVC application) is the ability to distinguish between extraperitoneal and intraperitoneal transition off the monitor. Sometimes the images can be deceptive and the only reliable way to tell is insufflation of CO_2 gas in low pressure, to identify the peritoneal window (Fig. 3.11). In high-risk patients, a preliminary umbilical inspection is possible when the TVC EndoTIP, the visual Veress micro-laparoscope, or other visually guided systems are applied through the left upper quadrant with or without insufflation, to safely map periumbilical or other visceral/parietal peritoneal adhesions and place additional ancillary ports accordingly.

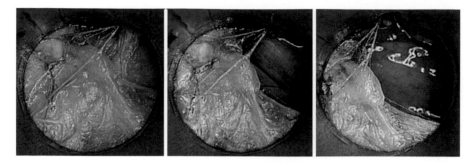

Fig. 3.11 Upon noninsufflated peritoneal entry, the threaded visual cannula tip rests on bowel. Distinguishing extra to intra peritoneal transition

Ancillary Peritoneal Entry with the Ternamian Threaded Visual Cannula EndoTIP

Ancillary port insertion is also a critical step in its own right. It plays a very important role during laparoscopic operations. It is through these strategically placed ports that endoscopists introduce sophisticated and specialized instruments to perform various complex operations. Their insertion method, instrument design, site, and number depend on several strategic factors, including the patient's anatomy, surgical history, and type of procedure performed, as well as the surgeon's preference and training. Intuitively surgeons advocate insertion of all ancillary ports under visual observation through the already inserted primary port, to minimize inadvertent injury [52]. Some endoscopists consider doing otherwise irresponsible, although there are no randomized trials demonstrating patient safety benefits. Curiously, these very same surgeons feel perfectly comfortable inserting sharp blind trocars directly into noninsufflated abdomens without hesitation during direct trocar and cannula use. Knowledge and careful attention to intraperitoneal visceral and vascular anatomy is very important, because injury to the deep epigastric vessels in particular, is the single most common vascular injury sustained during laparoscopic operations. In effect, a comprehensive Canadian study demonstrated that 22% if unintended bowel and vessel injuries happened during ancillary port insertion [53]. Location of the epigastric vessels in the lower abdominal wall is quite predictable and easily identifiable. The inferior epigastric artery and veins (last branch of the external iliac vessels) curl around the origin of the round ligament and the superficial epigastric artery and vein transilluminates (first branch of the femoral vessels) as it reverts north over the inguinal ligament. Downward abdominal pressure with the advancing push-through trajectory tip or the TVC blunt cannula tip indents access site and delineates possible risk along port tract. Redirection of entry axis or moving of port location will avert unintended injury. Sometimes the inferior epigastric vessel is difficult to identify by abdominal transillumination, especially in morbidly obese patients, those having several previous surgical scars, patients with cosmetic anterior abdominal operations, and those with abdominal adhesions. These vessels invariably course lateral to the umbilical

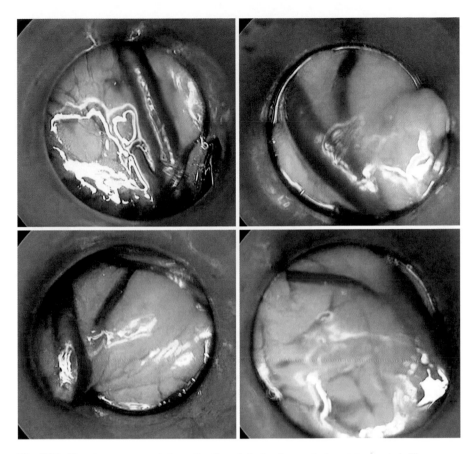

Fig. 3.12 Vessels encountered along the threaded visual cannula is not transected. They move laterally out of harm's way

ligaments, on either side of the bladder, just medial to the internal inguinal ring. This is important to know because they can bleed quite profusely if unexpectedly injured. To avoid vascular injury, ancillary ports must be inserted lateral to the internal inguinal ring or medial to the umbilical ligaments. Avoiding this triangular region between the two lines if possible is important. In the case of vascular injury, an easy temporary method for hemostasis, until assistance and equipment is recruited, is firm compression by a grasping laparoscopic instrument at the lateral base of the ipsilateral round ligament to arrest the torrent. Interestingly, when the TVC encounters vessels along the primary and ancillary port tract, they tend to move radially out of harm's way during cannula rotation and recoil back to position upon visual port removal, instead of being transected by a pointed or sharp trocar (Fig. 3.12). Applying the TVC EndoTIP requires an adequate skin incision along Langer's lines after palpation of the anterior superior iliac spines, iliac crests, and suprapubic spine for orientation and safe port application, especially when the patient is draped and repositioned in a

Fig. 3.13 Ancillary
Ternamian Threaded Visual
Cannula EndoTIP must
remain perpendicular to
distended abdomen until it
passes through peritoneal
membrane

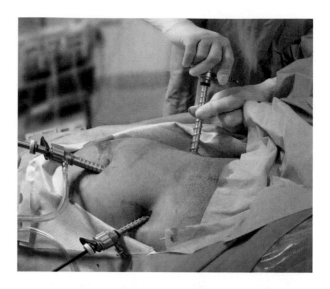

darkened operating room. Considering that apposition of the peritoneal membrane in
the lower half of the abdominal wall is less so than the upper abdomen or periumbilical region, application of the blunt-tipped TVC suprapubically can be difficult sometimes. The ancillary port must remain strictly perpendicular to the distended abdomen
until it passes through the peritoneal membrane to avoid peritoneal tenting (Fig. 3.13).
Sometimes, a pointed laparoscopic instrument can be used to perforate the loosely
apposed parietal peritoneum before the blunt cannula tip and tread take up the loosely
applied peeled peritoneum. Needless to say, suprapubic port application is always
preceded by urinary bladder emptying [37].

Peritoneal Exit with the Ternamian Threaded
Visual Cannula EndoTIP

As important as peritoneal entry is, safe port removal is recognized as an equally
critical step at the end of all laparoscopic surgery, which requires special mention
when describing port methods. Compared with the incidence of ventral hernia after
laparotomy, the incidence of laparoscopic port hernia is rare, ranging between 11%
and 20%, versus an estimated 0.02% incidence for port site herniation [54]. The
published incidence of port herniation following all laparoscopic operations varies
from 0.3% to 3%. However, most publications refer to their occurrence following
conventional push through trocar and cannula use and none include TVC applications. The incidence following laparoscopic cholecystectomy is quoted to be 0.14–
0.77% [55–57]. Several important steps are practiced to minimize the likelihood of
inadvertent port removal complication. By far the most important maneuver is retrieval
of all primary and ancillary ports under visual control while maintaining the CO_2

valve in the closed position. This allows surgeons to observe port sites for bleeding and avoid visceral entrapment along the port tract. Evidently, access-device tip design is a very important PSF when assessing port-related injury causation and port competence. Unlike sharp beveled push-through trocar and cannula tips, conical trocars have pointed nonbladed but sharp ends with no cutting lateral edges; these require infinitely higher penetration force, because abdominal wall layers must part radially to house the cannula's diameter [58]. A conical trocar with a sharp pointed tip has to exact a direct vascular hit to cause bleeding, whereas a similar diameter pyramidal or bladed trocar can cause significant bleeding even when a vessel is only partly sliced along its path [59]. More importantly, Leibl and co-workers established that port-site incisional hernia risk is ten times greater when single-use cutting pyramidal trocar and cannulas are used in lieu of multiple-use conical trocars (1.83% versus 0.17%) [60]. It is believed that outward pressure during cannula removal can entrap small bowel or suck up omentum into the cannula's tract that may result in hernia formation. This is particularly likely when the conventional push-through trocar and cannula are swiftly withdrawn at the same time as the peritoneal cavity is deinsufflating with the CO_2 valve open, at the end of a laparoscopic procedure. Primary fascial port closure of all sites larger than 5 mm is clearly intended to decrease these complications. However, suture securing of laparoscopic ports may minimize but not necessarily eradicate hernia occurrences. Port events can still occur, especially in high-risk patients (immunosuppressed patient, those with port site infections, oncologic post-radiation patients, those with multiple port reinsertions and excessive port site manipulation, and others) [61]. In a recent prospective multicenter analysis of more than 10 years of TVC use in gynecological cases, using different diameter cannulas at different sites, no port-related hernias were reported and no port competence events were observed [50]. This may not be unexpected because the TVC design allows tissue along the port's tract to part during insertion and recoil shut upon removal. In a randomized, observer-blinded comparative study, six conventional push through sharp trocar and cannula systems demonstrated significantly larger fascial and muscle defects at the port site when compared with the TVC EndoTIP system, as the formers' bladed, pyramidal, or cutting tips transacted tissue layers along the trajectory's path, disrupting tissue shutter recoil mechanism at the port site. They confirmed that TVC created a smaller fascial wound area and inflicted less muscle damage, and more importantly, required less penetration force compared with the Ethicon Endopath TriStar pyramidal cutting trocar of the same diameter. In addition, as the TVC is rotated to access and exit, fascial, muscle, and peritoneal wounds are not aligned, the likelihood of incisional hernia is thereby potentially minimized [36, 58]. Although oblique push-through trocar and cannula insertion at the lateral abdominal wall is thought to prohibit herniation in adults, there is no evidence to suggest that that same is true for TCVs, because here applications remain perpendicular to the abdominal tissues and oblique application is not recommended unless an extraperitoneal procedure is performed. In pediatric surgery, ancillary port diameters are comparatively miniscule (2–3 mm), and only the larger 5-mm primary port needs to be secured with a fascial suture. The abdominal muscles in preschool children are weak and thin, and Z or oblique push-through trocar and cannula insertion

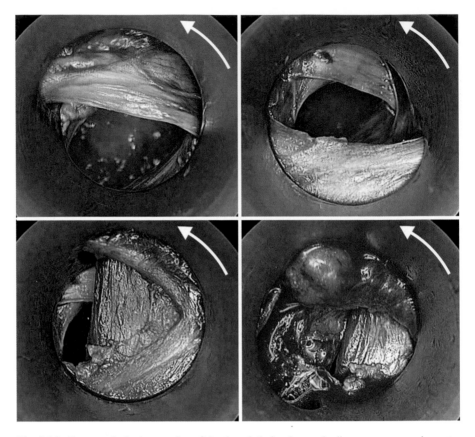

Fig. 3.14 Counter clockwise rotation of the threaded visual cannula disengages successive anterior abdominal wall tissue layers

passes straight through the anterior abdominal wall. Therefore, the abdominal wall wounds in the different layers are not essentially misaligned to discourage port herniation, as would with true oblique or Z insertion channels [62]. Removal of TVC involves the following; the defogged zero-degree laparoscope is drawn 1 cm into the primary TVC port, the telescope stopper locked, and the camera is held perpendicular to the supine abdomen with the operator's nondominant hand. The CO_2 insufflation tubing is disconnected and the cannula is rotated counterclockwise with the surgeon's dominant hand till the peritoneal membrane is seen at the cannula's edge. The peritoneal cavity is now deinsufflated while observing the abdominal wall recede until the cavity is deemed empty. The CO_2 valve is closed and the cannula is unwound further counterclockwise to disengage the TVC incrementally off the port tract, under visual control. The operator observes the cascade of successive recoiling tissue layers in reverse order until the cannula is released (Fig. 3.14). One must remember that when anterior rectus fascia is extended to retrieve surgical specimens, fascial sutures must be applied to that TVC entry site to further secure port competence.

Fig. 3.15 EndoCone,
for single port access surgery

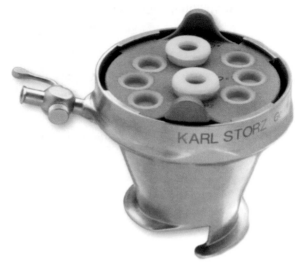

Table 3.3 Different approaches to minimally invasive surgery

1. Conventional laparoscopy
2. Robotically assisted laparoscopy
3. Laparoendoscopic single site surgery (LESS)
    a. Single skin incision with single laparoscopic inline operating channel
    b. Single skin incision with several fascial ports
    c. Single skin incision with single fascial incision but several ancillary inline portals
4. Natural orifice trans luminal endoscopic surgery (NOTES)

Peritoneal Entry with the Ternamian Threaded Visual Cannula EndoTIP as the Single Port

More recently, the TVC method has been adapted to offer ergonomic single port access surgery opportunities where a shorter and wider version EndoCone (Karl STORZ GmbH, Tuttlingen, Germany), is applied at the umbilicus with several ancillary instrument conduits at its proximal end (Fig. 3.15). At a recent consensus meeting on single port access surgery at The Cleveland Clinic, there was general agreement to use the acronym LESS (Laparo-endoscopic Single-Site Surgery) to describe this contemporary form of laparoscopic operations [63]. In effect, the evolutionary progress of minimally invasive surgery now offers four different and distinct approaches to achieve safe and less disabling endoscopic operations: conventional laparoscopic surgery, robotically assisted surgery, LESS and NOTES (Natural Orifice Transluminal Endoscopic Surgery) (Table 3.3). Single-site surgery in turn has three applications where through a single skin incision, different laparoscopic port methods are used to access the peritoneal cavity. The first method is application of a single conventional port and use of a laparoscope with an inline operative channel, the second method is

Fig. 3.16 Distal end of the Ternamian Threaded Visual Cannula EndoTIP with sheathed zero-degree laparoscope

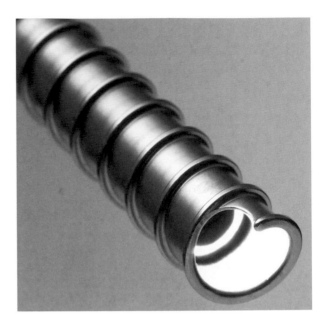

applications of several smaller ports through a single skin incision with several fascial incisions, and the third method is application of a single port designed to accommodate several ancillary portals applied through a single skin and fascial incision [64]. To date the TVC method has been successfully used with all three above applications; however, insertion of several smaller cannulas through the anterior fascia in such close proximity through a single skin incision must be regarded with caution because the collective effect of several fascial wounds in the same vicinity may undermine tissue recoil and the ability to restore port competence. Once the port shutter mechanism is compromised, the likelihood of incisional hernia becomes real. It is important to remember that present scientific evidence regarding emerging port technologies, including some of these more contemporary LESS applications in general, is lacking and too limited to draw any firm conclusions regarding their long-term outcomes and benefits [65].

The Ternamian Threaded Visual Cannula EndoTIP Instrument

The Ternamian TVC EndoTIP is a peritoneal port instrument that comprises a hollow threaded cannula with no central trocar. It is presently available in multiple use or single use hybrid form, in different diameters and lengths for human and animal use. It is used during conventional, robotic, or LESS laparoscopic surgery, in closed or open entry, as primary or ancillary ports, and to perform intraperitoneal or retroperitoneal operations [66]. It consists of a proximal valve and distal stainless steel hollow-threaded cannula section. The single thread, winding diagonally on its outer surface, ends distally in a blunt notched tip (Fig. 3.16). A reusable retaining ring,

Fig. 3.17 The Ternamian
Threaded Visual Cannula
EndoTIP with sheathed
zero-degree laparoscope and
telescope stopper

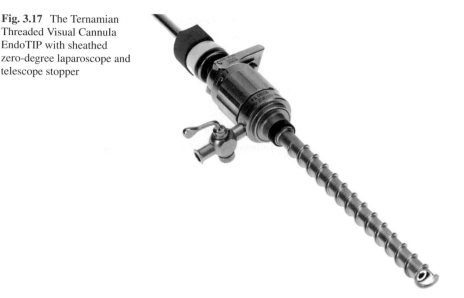

telescope stopper keeps the sheathed zero-degree laparoscope from sliding out of focus during insertion and cannula removal (Fig. 3.17). They are available with a CO_2 stopcock, mounted on a rotating cuff to allow the cannula to revolve while still connected to the CO_2 insufflators tubing. Alternatively, they come without a CO_2 stopcock for ancillary and other applications. In addition, they can have a flapper, silicon, or hybrid valve form, with a single use adaptation to facilitate effective tissue retrieval and suturing. By far, the most important body cavity access innovation of the TVC EndoTIP instrument is the lack of a trocar component and the proprietary cannula tip design that is essentially blunt and an extension of the cannula thread. These aspects of the instrument make it amenable to varied human and animal surgical applications with a potential use in remote expert guided robotic access in unsupported environments. The LESS modification of the TVC EndoCone, entails a shorter cone shaped wider reusable cannula with a single thread winding to a blunt distal tip. Proximally, a CO_2 stopcock is mounted and several ancillary access openings are present on the detachable valve section. This single port TVC is applied preferably through a larger umbilical skin incision in which the subcutaneous fat is first dissected off the anterior rectus fascia and then fascia and peritoneal membrane are incised and cannula applied under visual control before insufflation.

Threaded Visual Cannula Application Sites

When umbilical placement of a Veress needle or primary port is unsafe, such as in high-risk patients known to have umbilical adhesions, alternate peritoneal entry locations are preferred. Theoretically, any part of the abdominal cavity can act as a primary port site, if the anatomy allows and the entry method and instrument is unobtrusive. A French gynecologist, Raoul Palmer, first introduced the concept of an alternate primary port location when he popularized left upper quadrant peritoneal entry. "Palmer's point," is located 3 cm below the left costal margin at mid clavicular line, and is a safe alternative for insufflation and primary TVC port application in high risk situations [50, 67]. Once the patient is anesthetized, a nasogastric tube is first inserted to prevent inadvertent gastric injury, as sometimes the stomach may be distended with aesthetic gases during bagging, prior to intubation. Surgeons must be particularly careful in patients with splenomegaly or hepatomegaly in portal hypertension, gastropancreatic masses, or when left upper abdominal pathology exists [68]. Some high-risk patients may require preliminary intraperitoneal inspection, with the TVC EndoTIP, Veress microlaparoscope, or other visually guided system, introduced through the left upper quadrant, with or without insufflation, to map intra peritoneal visceral adhesions before additional ancillary ports are inserted. Patient abdominal anatomy and surgical characteristics dictates position and number of ancillary TVC ports required, determined by the surgeon's training and pathology involved.

Conclusion

Latent peritoneal port PSFs lies in wait with all surgical systems, instrument, or operative sites to extract injury at human instrument and force interface. Clearly, all humans err, and surgeons are no exception, and those who claim to perform error-free are destined to fail. Surgeons need to be particularly attentive to avoid unintended mishaps as patient safety is an important tenet of contemporary practice. Unfortunately in health care, when a nonsurgical medical error occurs, colleagues instinctively ask, "what happened;" however, when a surgical error occurs, we spontaneously ask, "who did it." High reliability organizations (HRO) appreciate and accept the reality that conditions inherent in tasks will predictably lead to recurrent failure with similar untoward outcomes unless events and conditions are isolated and altered. When faced with serious but very infrequent devastating industrial accidents such as a nuclear accident or chemical spills, HROs do not have the luxury of conducting randomized controlled trials. Instead, they manage rare adverse events by applying tested and proved accident causation strategies, and error analysis knowhow to deconstruct events and re-engineer tasks to render them less hazardous. Modeling and simulation plays a dramatic function in this regard. Surgical root-cause analysis is possible during body cavity entry, including peritoneal port placement, only when visual ports such as the TVC is used to capture, recall, and review events at port, tissue and force interface. The TVC EndoTIP systems is redesigned to eliminate the need of a central trocar, render entry and exit visual, and relocate the entry point from the trocar's central pointed or sharp tip to the cannula's peripherally placed blunt end. This converts the penetration force from linear to radial and entry becomes incremental and controlled as opposed to sudden and forceful, eliminating port overshoot. Consequently, the trajectory's entry path through the anterior rectus fascia, muscle, posterior fascia, and peritoneal membrane is not aligned or stacked, along a straight linear axis. Instead, they are scattered along a wider perimeter, thereby theoretically enhancing port competence and discourage incisional hernias. Additionally, when using TVC during port insertion and removal, surgeons electronically capture, recall, and review archived adverse port events to improve their understanding and performance. This develops a robust laparoscopic port placement database that encourages investigators to conduct real-time data mining and interpretation. A better understanding by surgeons of port dynamics will result in continuous quality improvement initiatives. In addition, it can improve our ability to construct good fidelity port simulation for robotic applications, teaching, error analysis, and research to enhance patient safety. Understanding body cavity port dynamics and port creation competencies can be particularly useful in the future when contemplating remote access robotic surgery. It is our observation that primary peritoneal access using the TVC, creates a zero fault tolerance environment by introducing three important patient safety redundancies that render laparoscopy less perilous. It allows real-time recognition of port injury (heightened situational awareness), offers mishap archiving opportunities for objective accident causation analysis (eliminates hind sight bias) and develops error aversion techniques (warning annunciation) that other trocar and cannula entry methods fail to offer.

References

1. Robinson V. Preface. In: Leonardo R, editor. History of gynecology. New York: Forben Press; 1944.
2. Nieboer TE, Johnson N, Lethaby A, et al. Surgical approach to hysterectomy for benign gynaecological disease. Cochrane Database Syst Rev. 2009;25(1):CD003677.
3. Chapron C, Fauconnier A, Coffinet F, et al. Laparoscopic surgery is not inherently dangerous for patients presenting with benign gynecologic pathology: results of a meta-analysis. Hum Reprod. 2002;17:1334–42.
4. Fuller J, Ashar BS, Carey-Corrado J. Trocar-associated injuries and fatalities: an analysis of 1399 reports to the FDA. J Minim Invasive Gynecol. 2005;12:302–7.
5. Garry R. A consensus document concerning laparoscopic entry techniques: Middlesbrough. Gynecol Endosc. 1999;8:403–6.
6. Vilos GA, Ternamian A, Dempster J, et al. Laparoscopic entry: a review of techniques, technologies, and complications. J Obstet Gynaecol Can. 2007;29:433–65.
7. Garry R. Toward evidence based laparoscopic entry techniques: clinical problems and dilemmas. Gynecol Endosc. 1999;8:315–26.
8. Vilos GA, Hancock G, Penava DA, Kozak I, Davies W. Nine cases of bowel injury during 3472 laparoscopies. J Obstet Gynecol Can. 1999;21:144–50.
9. Laparoscopic trocar injuries: a report from a U.S. Food and Drug Administration (FDA). Center for Devices and Radiological Health (CDRH) Systematic Technology Assessment of Medical Products (STAMP) Committee. (Cited 2003 Nov 7). Available from: URL: http://www.fda.gov/cdrh/medicaldevicesafety/stamp/trocar.html.
10. Institute of Medicine. To err is human. Building a safer health system. Washington, DC: National Academy Press; 1999.
11. Philip PA, Amaral JF. Abdominal access complications in laparoscopic surgery. J Am Coll Surg. 2001;192(4):525–36.

12. Passerotti CC, Begg N, Penna FJ, et al. Safety profile of trocar and insufflation needle access systems in laparoscopic surgery. J Am Coll Surg. 2009;209(2):222–32.
13. Bogner MS. Medical devices and human error. In: Mouloua M, Parasuraman R, editors. Human performance in automated systems: current research and trends. Hillsdale: Lawrence Erlbaum; 1994. p. 64–7.
14. Ahmad G, Duffy J, Phillips K, et al. Laparoscopic entry techniques. Cochrane Database Syst Rev. 2008;2:CD006583.
15. Garry R. Surgeons may continue to use their chosen entry technique. Gynecol Surg. 2009;6: 87–92; discussion 91–2.
16. Vilos GA, Vilos AG, Abu-Rafea B, et al. Three simple steps during closed laparoscopic entry may minimize major injuries. Surg Endosc. 2009;23:758–64.
17. Ternamian A. Laparoscopic access. In: Jain N, editor. State of the art atlas of endoscopic surgery in infertility and gynecology: Laparoscopic access, vol. 2. New Delhi: Jaypee Bros; 2010. p. 20–33.
18. String A, Berber E, Foroutani A, et al. Use of the optical access trocar for safe and rapid entry in various laparoscopic procedures. Surg Endosc. 2001;15:570–3.
19. Patkin M, Isabel L. Ergonomics, engineering and surgery of endosurgical dissection. J R Coll Surg Edinb. 1995;40:120–32.
20. Cuschieri A. Whither minimal access surgery: tribulations and expectations. Am J Surg. 1995;1:9–19.
21. Hanna GB, Shimi SM, Cuschieri A. Optimal port locations for endoscopic intracorporeal knotting. Surg Endosc. 1997;11:397–401.
22. Quick NE, Gilette JC, Shapiro R, et al. The effect of using laparoscopic instruments on muscle activation patterns during minimally invasive training procedures. Surg Endosc. 2003;17: 462–5.
23. Emam TA, Hanna GB, Kimber C, et al. Effect of intracorporeal-extracorporeal instrument length ratio on endoscopic task performance and surgeon movements. Arch Surg. 2000;135: 62–5.
24. Beurger R, Forkey D, Smith WD. Ergonomic problems associated with laparoscopic surgery. Surg Endosc. 1999;13:466–8.
25. Beurger R, Smith WD, Chung YH. Performing laparoscopic surgery is significantly more stressful for the surgeon than open surgery. Surg Endosc. 2001;15:1204–7.
26. Moorthy K, Munz Y, Dosis A, et al. The effect of stress-induced conditions on the performance of a laparoscopic task. Surg Endosc. 2003;17:1481–4.
27. Taffinder N, McManus IC, Gul Y, et al. Objective assessment of the effect of sleep deprivation on surgical psychomotor skill. Lancet. 1999;353:1191.
28. Sexton JB, Thomas EJ, Helmreich RL. Error, stress, and teamwork in medicine and aviation: cross-sectional survey. BMJ. 2000;320:745–9.
29. Ternamian A. Endoskopische abdominalchirurgie in der Gynäkologie. In: Mettler L, editor. Stuttgart: Schattauer; 2002. p. 175–80.
30. Corson SL, Batzer FR, Gocial B, et al. Measurement of the force necessary for laparoscopic trocar entry. J Reprod Med. 1989;34(4):282–4.
31. Singh S, Marcoux V, Ternamian A, et al. Core competencies for gynecologic endoscopy in residency training: a national consensus project. J Minim Invasive Gynecol. 2009;16(1):1–7.
32. Raymond E, Ternamian A, Tolomiczenko G. Endoscopy teaching in Canada: a survey of obstetrics and gynecology program directors and graduating residents. J Minim Invasive Gynecol. 2006;13:10–6.
33. Munro MG. Laparoscopic access: complications, technologies and techniques. Curr Opin Obstet Gynecol. 2002;14(4):365–74.
34. Ternamian A. Port creation during laparoscopic hysterectomy. In: Mettler L, editor. Manual for laparoscopic and hysteroscopic gynecological surgery. New Delhi: Jaypee Brothers Medical Publishers (P) Ltd; 2007. p. 175–80.
35. Ternamian AM. Laparoscopy without trocars. Surg Endosc. 1997;11:815–8.

36. Glass KB, Tarnay CM, Munro MG. Intra-abdominal pressure and incision parameters associ-
    ated with a pyramidal laparoscopic trocar-cannula system and the EndoTIP cannula. J Am
    Assoc Gynecol Laparosc. 2002;9(4):508–13.
37. Ternamian AM. A trocarless, reusable, visual-access cannula for safer laparoscopy: an update.
    J Am Assoc Gynecol Laparosc. 1998;5(2):197–201.
38. Mettler L, Schmidt E, Frank V, Semm K. Optical trocar systems: laparoscopic entry and its
    complications (a study of cases in Germany). Gynaecol Endosc. 1999;8:383–9.
39. Vilos GA. The ABCs of a safer laparoscopic entry. J Minim Invasive Gynecol. 2006;13:249–51.
40. Kroft J, Aneja A, Ternamian A, et al. Laparoscopic peritoneal entry preferences among
    Canadian gynaecologists. J Obstet Gynecol Can. 2009;31:641–8.
41. Teoh B, Sen R, Abbott J. An evaluation of four tests used to ascertain Veress needle placement
    at closed laparoscopy. J Minim Invasive Gynecol. 2005;12:153–8.
42. Abu-Rafea B, Vilos GA, Vilos AG. High-pressure laparoscopic entry does not adversely affect
    cardiopulmonary function in health women. J Minim Invasive Gynecol. 2005;12:475–9.
43. Phillips G, Garry R, Kumar C, et al. How much gas is required for initial insufflation at lap-
    aroscopy? Gynaecol Endosc. 1999;8:369–74.
44. Reich H, Robeiro SC, Rasmussen C, et al. High-pressure trocar insertion technique. J Soc
    Laparoendosc Surg. 1999;3:45–8.
45. McDougall E, Figenshau RS, Clayman RV. J Laparosc Surg. 1994;4:6.
46. Ternamian A. How to improve laparoscopic access safety: ENDOTIP. Min Invas Ther Allied
    Technol. 2001;10(1):31–9.
47. Audebert AJ. The role of micro-laparoscopy in the diagnosis of peritoneal and visceral adhe-
    sions and in the prevention of bowel injury associated with blind trocar insertion. Fertil Steril.
    2000;73:631–5.
48. Lower AM, Hawthorn RJS, Ellis H, et al. The impact of adhesions on hospital readmissions
    over ten years after 8849 open gynaecological procedures: an assessment from the Surgical
    and Clinical Adhesions Research Study. Br J Obstet Gynecol. 2000;107:855–62.
49. Childers JM, Brzechffa PR, Surwit EA. Laparoscopy using the left upper quadrant as the pri-
    mary trocar site. Gynaecol Oncol. 1993;50:221–5.
50. Ternamian AM, Vilos GA, MacLeod NT, et al. Laparoscopic peritoneal entry with the reusable
    threaded visual cannula. J Minim Invasive Gynecol. 2010;17:461–7.
51. Ternamian A, Deitel M. Endoscopic threaded imaging port (EndoTIP) for laparoscopy: experi-
    ence with different body weights. Obes Surg. 1999;2:44–7.
52. Sutton C. A practical approach to diagnostic laparoscopy. In: Sutton C, Diamond M, editors.
    Endoscopic surgery for gynaecologists. London: WB Saunders; 1993. p. 21–7.
53. Yuzpe A. Pneumoperitoneum needle and trocar injuries in laparoscopy. A survey on possible
    contributing factors and prevention. J Reprod Med. 1990;35:485–90.
54. Luijendijk RW, Hop WCJ, van den Tol MP. A comparison of suture repair with mesh repair for
    incisional hernia. N Engl J Med. 2000;343:392–8.
55. Montz FJ, Holschneider CH, Munro MG. Incisional hernias following laparoscopy: a survey of
    the American Association of Gynecologic Laparoscopists. Obstet Gynecol. 1994;84:881–4.
56. Mayol J, Garcia-Aguilar J, Ortiz-Oshiro E, De-Diego Carmona J, Fernandez Represa JA.
    Risks of the minimal access approach for laparoscopic surgery: multivariate analysis of mor-
    bidity related to umbilical trocar insertion. World J Surg. 1997;21:529–33.
57. Azurin DJ, Go LS, Arroyo LR, et al. Trocar site herniation following laparoscopic cholecystec-
    tomy and the significance of incidental preexisting umbilical hernia. Am Surg.
    1995;5:419–21.
58. Tarnay CM, Glass KB, Munro MG. Entry force and intra-abdominal pressure associated with
    six laparoscopic trocar-cannula systems: a randomized comparison. Obstet Gynecol. 1999;94:
    83–8.
59. Hurd WW, Wang L, Schemmel MT. A comparison of the relative risk of vessel injury with
    conical versus pyramidal laparoscopic trocars in a rabbit model. Am J Obstet Gynecol.
    1995;173:1731–3.

60. Leibl BJ, Schmedt CG, Schwarz J, et al. Laparoscopic surgery complications associated with trocar tip design: review of literature and own results. J Laparoendosc Adv Surg Tech A. 1999;9:135–40.
61. Leonard F, Lecuru F, Rizk E, et al. Perioperative morbidity of gynecological laparoscopy: a prospective monocenter observational study. Acta Obstet Gynecol Scand. 2000;79:129–34.
62. Paya K, Wurm J, Fakhari M, et al. Trocar-site hernia as a typical postoperative complication of minimally invasive surgery among preschool children. Surg Endosc. 2008;22:2724–7.
63. Gill IS, Advincula AP, Aron M, et al. Consensus statement of the consortium for laparoscopic single-site surgery. Surg Endosc. 2010;24:762–8.
64. Uppal S, Frumovitz M, Escobar P, et al. Laparoscopic single-site surgery in gynecology: review of literature and available technology. J Minim Invasive Gynecol. 2011;18(1):12–23.
65. Romanelli JR, Earle DB. Single-port laparoscopic surgery: an overview. Surg Endosc. 2009;23: 1419–27.
66. Andou M, Yoshioka K, Ternamian A. A new approach for accessing retroperitoneal space using a 5 mm visual access cannula. Surg Endosc. 2003;17:1158–61.
67. Palmer R. Safety in laparoscopy. J Reprod Med. 1974;13:1–5.
68. Chapron C, Pierre F, Harchaoui Y, et al. Gastrointestinal injuries during gynaecological laparoscopy. Hum Reprod. 1999;14:337.

Chapter 4
Initial Access to the Peritoneal Cavity for Laparoscopic Surgery in Obese Patients

Charlotte Rabl and Guilherme M. Campos

Introduction

With the increasing incidence of obesity [1–3], a growing number of obese patients (body mass index, BMI, greater than 30 kg/m^2) are treated for common intra-abdominal diseases and also undergo weight loss or bariatric surgery [4, 5]. The use of laparoscopic techniques for general and bariatric surgery is preferred because it is associated with less postoperative pain, lower rates of wound infection and incisional hernias, faster recovery, shorter hospital stay, and earlier return to work [1, 6–10]. Obtaining safe access to the peritoneal cavity to create a pneumoperitoneum is a crucial step to start a laparoscopic operation, and it is, however, technically challenging and associated with more complications in obese and morbidly obese people [11]. To date, there is no clear consensus about the optimal method of entry into the peritoneal cavity, and therefore different techniques are available.

This chapter describes technical aspects and the risks and benefits of the different options for initial access to the peritoneal cavity for laparoscopic surgery in obese and morbidly obese patients.

C. Rabl
Paracelsus Private Medical University,
Salzburg, Austria

G.M. Campos (✉)
University of Wisconsin School of Medicine and Public Health,
Madison, WI 53792-7375, USA

A. Tinelli (ed.), *Laparoscopic Entry*,
DOI 10.1007/978-0-85729-980-2_4, © Springer-Verlag London Limited 2012

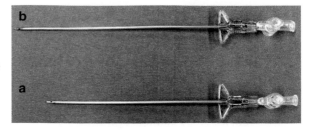

Fig. 4.1 The Veress needle is a sharp, hollow needle with a spring-loaded blunt obturator: (**a**) standard length of the Veress needle (120 mm), (**b**) extra-long Veress needle (150 mm); both for single use (Surgineedle™, Covidien, Norwalk, CT, USA)

The Veress Needle Technique

Veress Needle

The Veress needle is a sharp, hollow needle with a spring-loaded blunt obturator. It was developed by Janos Veres in 1938 as a safer access to create a therapeutic pneumothorax in the treatment of tuberculosis and to puncture the abdomen for ascites [12, 13]. It was later adopted for initial access to the peritoneal space and creation of a pneumoperitoneum for most laparoscopic surgical procedures [12].

In morbidly obese patients, the standard length of the Veress needle (120 mm) may be too short to reach the peritoneal cavity because of the thicker subcutaneous adipose tissue, especially at the level of the umbilicus. Extra-long Veress needles (150 mm) are available (Fig. 4.1).

Veress Needle Insertion Technique

The most used location for insertion of the Veress needle is the umbilical area in the midsaggital plane. In the morbidly obese, insertion of the needle in the left upper quadrant below the costal arch (Palmer's point) is preferred by many, because the subcutaneous adipose tissue of the abdominal wall is thicker at the umbilical area than higher in the abdomen [14, 15]. After a skin incision, the Veress needle is introduced with or without stabilizing or lifting the abdominal wall. In the morbidly obese, lifting the abdominal wall can be difficult. The angle recommended for Veress needle insertion differs according to the patient's body habitus: it should be inserted at 45° in nonobese patients and at 90° in obese patients to avoid both preperitoneal insufflation and major vessel injury [16]. This is because of different anterior abdominal wall thickness and distance from the base of the umbilicus to the retroperitoneal vessels and different position of the umbilicus with respect to the aortic bifurcation with increasing weight. A study [17] using computerized axial tomography in 38 women showed that the umbilicus is located caudally to the aortic bifurcation and that the average distance of the umbilicus to the aortic bifurcation increases with increasing BMI: 0.4 cm in patients with normal weight (BMI < 25 kg/m^2), 2.4 cm in overweight patients (BMI 25–30 kg/m^2), and 2.9 cm in the obese. In all patients the umbilicus was located cephalad to where the common iliac vein crossed the midline [15, 17].

After the subcutaneous tissue has been entered, the needle is pushed through the layers of the abdominal wall, during which the blunt tip is retracted into the needle while offering the sharp cutting edge. When the peritoneal cavity is being penetrated, the needle no longer encounters resistance and the blunt tip should emerge, thus protecting the bowel and other intra-abdominal or retroperitoneal organs from injuries from the sharp cutting edge.

Veress Needle Safety Tests

Safety tests are used to examine the correct intraperitoneal placement of the Veress needle. These safety tests include the double click sound of the Veress needle, the aspiration test, and the hanging drop of saline test.

In the double-click test, the passage of the Veress needle through the different layers of the abdominal wall twice causes an audible "click," the first while the needle is passing through the anterior rectus sheath and the second as the needle passes through the peritoneum. While passing these two structures, the blunt tip is retracted into the needle to offer the sharp cutting edge because of the increased resistance. When the resistance is overcome, the spring-loaded blunt tip emerges with a "click."

In the aspiration test, a small syringe (empty or partially filled with normal saline) is attached to the Veress needle. To determine if the needle is in the peritoneal space, the plunger is pulled back. If the needle is in the correct location, nothing should be aspirated, but blood or bowel contents are signs of organ perforation. If nothing is aspirated, a couple of milliliters of the saline solution is injected; and should flow through the needle into the peritoneal cavity with only minimal resistance. Finally, the plunger is pulled back again. Returning saline can be a sign of fluid trapped by adhesions or location of the needle in the preperitoneal tissue.

In the hanging drop of saline test, a drop of saline solution is placed on the top of the Veress needle. When the needle is correctly positioned in the peritoneal cavity, the saline solution should move into the Veress needle because of the negative intraperitoneal pressure and the force of gravity [15, 18, 19].

Although used routinely, these safety tests do not completely prevent intra-abdominal organ injury [19]. In a prospective study [19], laparoscopy was performed in 345 female patients and safety tests were used in 99% of the patients. Complications occurred in 19% of patients as a result of suboptimal placement of the Veress needle. The complications were minor and did not need further treatment and included omental emphysema (13%), preperitoneal insufflation (5.5%), and superficial gastric injury (0.3%). This study has shown that the sensitivity of the three safety tests is low (double-click test 39%, aspiration test 0%, hanging drop of saline test 16%), and is likely worse in the morbidly obese.

Another indicator of the correct placement of the Veress needle is the pressure measured by the carbon dioxide (CO_2) insufflation device just after starting insufflation [15, 19]. If the Veress needle is placed correctly, the intra-abdominal pressure measured should be low (less than 5 mmHg) [18]. This may not be an accurate test in the morbidly obese though, as many morbidly obese people have an increased intra-abdominal pressure (7–14 mmHg) caused by the larger abdominal wall [14]. Waggling the needle from side to side to check the free intraperitoneal mobility and to shake off possible attached tissue should be avoided because it can enlarge a perforation caused by the Veress needle if one is present [15].

Pneumoperitoneum

After the insertion of the Veress needle, the pneumoperitoneum is established by connecting the Veress needle to the CO_2 insufflation device. The definition of an adequate pneumoperitoneum pressure prior to insertion of the first trocar is controversial. We recommend insufflation of 1–4 L of CO_2 or an intraperitoneal pressure of 10–15 mmHg before inserting the first trocar [15].

First Trocar Insertion

After creation of a pneumoperitoneum by insufflation, a 5–12-mm trocar with or without a safety shield may be introduced blindly or using the direct visualization technique into the peritoneal cavity.

Different types of trocars are in use, and can be reusable or for single-use only (Fig. 4.2). Trocar systems include a central perforator and a trocar tube. Different perforator tips are available and therefore blunt trocars and cutting trocars can be differentiated. Sharp cutting trocars are usually for single use and equipped with a spring-loaded perforation shield, which protects the cutting device after it has entered the peritoneal cavity. For the direct visualization technique, special optical viewing trocars are available to allow visual passage through the layers of the abdominal wall into the peritoneal cavity (Fig. 4.3). No trocar has been proven to be superior to any other, and visceral and vascular injuries are not completely avoided by use of any trocar [15].

Complications

The blind insertion of the Veress needle and the insertion of the first trocar are associated with risk of injury of the bowel and abdominal vessels [18, 20–25]. These injuries seem to be rare, but the true incidence of vascular and intestinal injuries caused by the

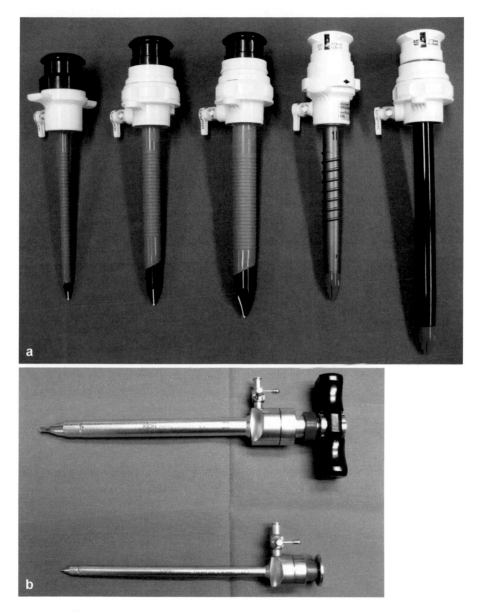

Fig. 4.2 Different types and sizes of trocars are available: (**a**) single-use trocars with bladeless and bladed obturators (Versaport™, Covidien, Norwalk, CT, USA); (**b**) reusable trocars (Xion, Germany)

Veress needle or the first trocar is unknown and may be higher than reported in the literature, because most injuries are not published [18]. The estimated incidence is 0.04–0.18% for bowel injuries and 0.03–0.3% for major abdominal vessel injuries. These injuries are often associated with conversion to open procedures, other complications, and mortality [18]. Existing adhesions from previous abdominal surgery are also

Fig. 4.3 Optical trocars allow visual passage through the layers of the abdominal wall into the peritoneal cavity: (**a**) bladeless optical trocars (Endopath® Xcel™, 5 mm and 11 mm, Ethicon Endo-Surgery, Cincinnati, OH, USA, also available with a handle), (**b**) bladed optical trocar (Visiport™, 5–11 mm, Covidien, Norwalk, CT, USA)

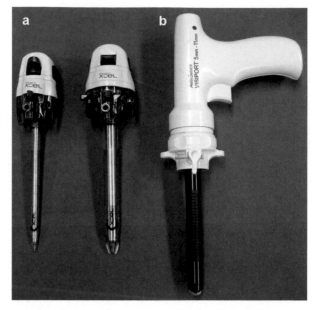

thought to increase the risk of intra-abdominal damage when the peritoneal cavity is entered to create the pneumoperitoneum [26]. Major vascular injuries are associated with a mortality rate of 15% [18], and can be caused by the Veress needle or by the trocar insertion. The risk of these injuries is higher for thin people than for obese people because the distance between the anterior abdominal wall and the retroperitoneal vessels is shorter in thin people. The distal aorta and the right common iliac artery are especially endangered because of their anatomic closeness to the umbilicus. Indications of a major vessel injury can be visualization of free blood or a retroperitoneal hematoma or hypotension. In cases of a major vascular injury, the anesthesiologist has to be immediately informed about the complication to be prepared for an adequate fluid or blood resuscitation. Most injuries of the major vessels cannot be repaired laparoscopically; thus, a laparotomy has to follow without hesitation.

Minor vascular injuries are reported in the literature with an incidence of 0.1–1.2% [23]. Minor vascular injuries involve vessels other than the aorta, inferior vena cava, or iliac vessels. Injuries of the minor vessels such as mesenteric and omental vessels are often the reason for reoperation, blood product transfusion, or conversion to the open technique [18].

The Hasson Technique or Open Access Technique

In 1971, Hasson [27] first described the open entry technique. The aim of this technique was to reduce intra-abdominal organ injuries and to prevent gas embolism and preperitoneal insufflation.

Hasson Trocar

The Hasson trocar is a blunt trocar which is inserted into the peritoneal cavity after making a small laparotomy under direct view and which is used for insufflation and introduction of a laparoscope.

Open Technique

A longitudinal or transverse minilaparotomy is performed. The incision has to be long enough to be able to dissect down to the fascia, which is incised and then the peritoneal cavity is entered under direct vision. This allows open control of the surrounding intraperitoneal space and a controlled insertion of the first trocar. The trocar with the inserted blunt obturator is passed into the peritoneal cavity. To seal the abdominal wall incision and thereby to avoid escape of gas, sutures on either side of the trocar are placed in the abdominal fascia and attached to the trocar or are purse-stringed around the cannula [15, 18]. Then the laparoscope is introduced into the trocar and the insufflation devise is connected to establish a pneumoperitoneum. At the end of the operation, the minilaparotomy has to be closed.

Complications

Although the Hasson technique has the potential advantage of visualization of the peritoneal entry and the surrounding intraperitoneal space, this method does not completely eliminate complications. There seems to be a lower incidence of major vascular injuries than for the Veress needle technique [15, 22, 24]. On the other hand, the incidence of bowel injuries is reported to be higher for the open technique than for the Veress needle technique [15]. This higher incidence of bowel injuries is likely influenced by selection bias, because the open technique is more commonly used in patients with previous abdominal surgery and thus there will be more adhesions to the abdominal wall.

Open Technique and Obesity

In obese and morbidly obese patients the open technique is difficult or sometimes impossible. The creation of a very large incision to traverse the tissue planes under direct view may be necessary and the fascial closure at the end of the procedure is difficult and time-consuming [28]. In addition, this larger incision may lead to a cumbersome leakage of CO_2 during the laparoscopic procedure, which results in an inadequate pneumoperitoneum with a reduced visualization of the operative field and an increased risk of the surgical procedure itself [18].

The Direct Trocar Insertion Technique Without Prior Creation of a Pneumoperitoneum

Another technique for entering peritoneal cavity in laparoscopic surgery is the direct insertion of the first trocar without prior creation of a pneumoperitoneum. This technique was first described by Dingfelder in 1978 [15]. Possible advantages were thought to be the avoidance of complications caused by the use of the Veress needle, such as preperitoneal insufflation, intestinal insufflation, and CO_2 embolism [15], and the reduction of the number of blindly inserted instruments from two (Veress needle and trocar) to only one (trocar) [15, 29].

Trocars

The trocars recommended for this technique are disposable and have a tip shielded by a plastic sheath [18], which is spring-loaded and retracts during the passage through the abdominal wall and protrudes automatically when the peritoneal cavity is entered.

Direct Trocar Insertion Technique

After complete muscular relaxation of the patient, decompression of the stomach and bladder, and a skin incision, the anterior abdominal wall should be elevated for the trocar insertion. Constant downward pressure is applied to the shielded cutting trocar until the peritoneal cavity is entered, indicated by the click sound of the shield. Then the obturator is removed and the CO_2 insufflation is started [29].

Complications

Although this technique has been reported in non-obese patients [22, 30–36], there are few reports for obese and morbidly obese patients [29]. Altun et al. [29] described the direct trocar insertion technique with a shielded cutting trocar in 155 morbidly obese patients prior to laparoscopic adjustable gastric banding. In this study, no major vascular or visceral injury occurred. Minor complications included extraperitoneal insufflation (3.2%), gastric serosal laceration (0.6%), and left liver lobe laceration (0.6%).

The Direct Trocar Insertion Technique Using an Optical Viewing Trocar Without Prior Creation of a Pneumoperitoneum

This technique evolved from the direct trocar insertion technique without prior creation of a pneumoperitoneum by adding real-time visualization of the abdominal wall layers while inserting the trocars. It is our preferred method in the obese and morbidly obese.

Trocars

With this technique, optical viewing trocars are inserted into the peritoneal cavity without prior abdominal insufflation. Different types of optical trocars are available; two of the most commonly used are the bladeless optical trocar and the bladed optical trocar.

Bladeless optical trocars (Endopath® Xcel™, 5 mm, 11 mm, and 12 mm, Ethicon Endo-Surgery, Cincinnati, OH, USA) are disposable blunt-tip trocars that accommodate a 5- or a 10-mm laparoscope inside. The trocars are guided in a stepwise fashion through the abdominal wall, providing controlled and direct visualization of the planes of the abdominal wall that is being dissected.

Bladed optical trocars (Visiport™, 5–11 mm and 5–12 mm, Covidien, Norwalk, CT, USA) are disposable instruments with a spring-loaded blade that is activated by a trigger controlled by the surgeon. Bladed optical trocars accommodate a 10-mm laparoscope.

The use of bladeless optical trocars without prior creation of a pneumoperitoneum in morbidly obese patients has been reported to be safe by many authors [11, 28, 37, 38]. Although the insertion of bladed optical trocars without creation of a pneumoperitoneum has been reported, their use is recommended by the manufacturers only after insufflation of the pneumoperitoneum [39, 40].

The Direct Trocar Insertion Technique Using a Bladeless Optical Trocar in the Morbidly Obese Patient [37]

One important aspect before starting the insertion of the bladeless optical trocar is to ascertain that the patient has complete muscular relaxation and that the patient's stomach and bladder have been decompressed. The initial entry site is either a 5-mm

Fig. 4.4 Proper assembly and handling of the Endopath® Xcel™ bladeless trocar, 11 mm (Ethicon Endo-Surgery, Cincinnati, OH, USA) and a zero-degree 10-mm laparoscope

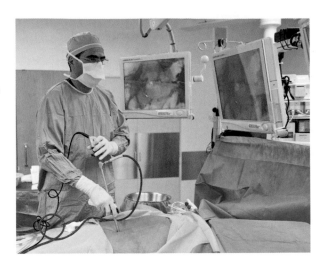

Fig. 4.5 View through the optical access trocar just before entry in the subcutaneous tissue

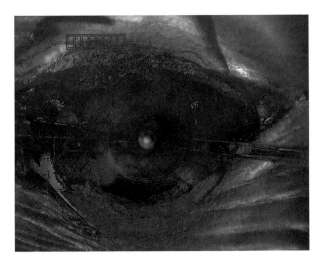

or a 10–11-mm skin incision to accommodate the preferred trocar. We prefer the 11-mm trocar. The incision is made just above and to the left side of the umbilicus, aimed to the medial side of the anterior rectus sheath. It is not necessary to dissect to and open the fascia. The bladeless optical trocar is inserted into the abdomen under constant direct visualization by using a zero-degree 5- or 10-mm laparoscope, which is assembled within the trocar (Fig. 4.4). The trocar is moved through the subcutaneous fat with a twisting motion and a steady and gentle pressure is applied downward (Figs. 4.5 and 4.6). This is done until the anterior rectus sheath is reached and identified, after which the pressure applied to the trocar is released. Then the trocar is moved with the same motion to traverse the next layer, the rectus abdominis muscle (Fig. 4.7), and the pressure is applied and released again. This procedure is repeated for all the other layers—the posterior rectus sheath, the preperitoneal fat, and the

Fig. 4.6 View through the optical access trocar while passing through the subcutaneous tissue

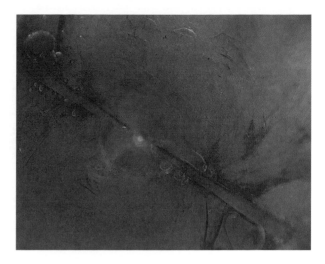

Fig. 4.7 View through the optical access trocar after passing through the anterior sheath of the rectus abdominis muscle and thereby reaching the muscle fibers

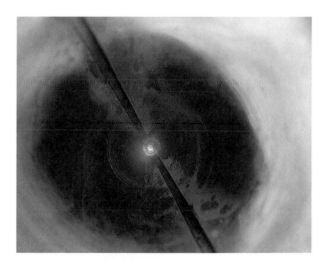

peritoneum (Figs. 4.8 and 4.9)—until the peritoneal cavity (Fig. 4.10) is reached. At this point, the 0° laparoscope and the blunt dissecting obturator of the trocar are removed and low-flow CO_2 insufflation is started. The 0° laparoscope without the obturator is reinserted to check for proper position of the trocar cannula. If the tip of the trocar cannula is found to be partially in the preperitoneal space, the insufflation is stopped; the 0° laparoscope is removed, reinserted in the obturator, and carefully advanced further using the same principles as described above. Then a CO_2 pneumoperitoneum is created and a 30° or 45° laparoscope is introduced through the cannula immediately, and the entry site and adjacent viscera are inspected promptly. At the end of the laparoscopic procedure, the trocar is removed. The fascial defect does not need to be routinely closed.

Fig. 4.8 View through the optical access trocar after passing the rectus abdominis muscle (displaced on the *right side*) and reaching the posterior rectus sheath

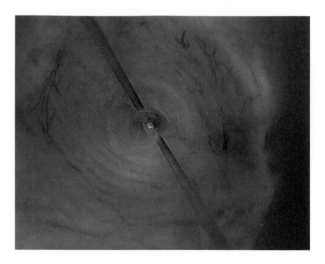

Fig. 4.9 View through the optical access trocar after passing the posterior rectus sheath and entering the preperitoneal fat

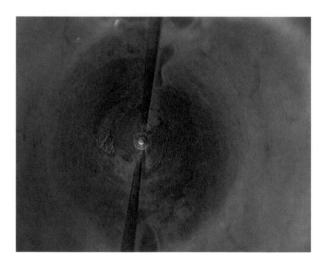

Variations of the Direct Trocar Insertion Technique Using an Optical Trocar

Variations of the direct insertion using an optical trocar are reported in the literature, such as using the optical trocar after creation of a pneumoperitoneum with the Veress needle [41, 42], after blunt dissection into the fascia and positioning two stay sutures in the anterior rectus sheath [43], and using the optical trocar in combination with a subcutaneous lifter [44].

Fig. 4.10 View through the optical access trocar after starting low-flow CO_2 insufflation while entering the peritoneal cavity

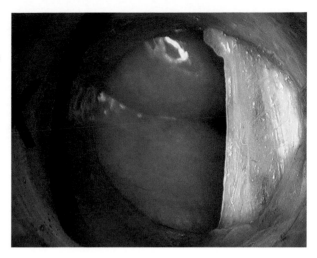

Complications

The direct trocar insertion technique using an optical trocar without prior creation of a pneumoperitoneum seems to be a safe and effective way to access the peritoneal cavity in morbidly obese patients. Many case series reported no hollow viscus or major vascular injury when a bladeless optical trocar was used and no conversion to other techniques was necessary [11, 28, 37, 38]. However, publication bias should be taken into account as the possibility of injury is always present when a rigid instrument is introduced into the abdominal cavity. Minor complications, such as superficial injuries of the small bowel mesentery or greater omentum with or without bleeding, are reported in 0–1.5% of cases [11, 37]. Because of the direct visualization of the peritoneal entry, these minor injuries were recognized and, if necessary, repaired immediately. No trocar injury was associated with further complications. Table 4.1 summarizes published articles reporting use of a bladeless optical trocar or a bladed optical trocar without prior creation of a pneumoperitoneum in the morbidly obese, the complication rates, and the trocar insertion time.

Severe complications from using the direct trocar insertion technique with an optical trocar during laparoscopy for general surgical and gynecologic procedures have been described in one review of three large databases: Medline, the Medical Device Reporting (MDR) database, and the Manufacturer and User Facility Device Experience (MAUDE) [45]. Eighty-two serious complications were found, and were major vascular injuries in 46.8% of cases and bowel injuries in 30.4% of cases, and four of these injuries resulted in patient deaths. A bladeless optical trocar was used in 32.9% of the cases and a bladed optical trocar was used in 67.1% of the cases. An important limitation of that study was the lack of specific information about the total number of patients and other patient characteristics, the risk factors (including whether the patients were obese), the exact technique that was used with the optical access trocar, and whether the technique was used appropriately [37].

Table 4.1 Summary of published articles reporting use of the direct trocar insertion technique in the morbidly obese using an optical viewing trocar without prior creation of a pneumoperitoneum

Authors	Type of optical trocar	Number of patients	Trocar insertion time (s)	Major[a] complication	Minor[a] complication	Type of complication
Sabeti et al. [40]	Bladed (Visiport[b], 5–12 mm)	2,207	NA	4 (0.18%)	0 (0%)	Three cases of vascular injury of the small bowel mesentery needing conversion (0.14%) One case of retroperitoneal bleeding (0.04%)
Bernante et al. [39]	Bladed (Visiport Plus[b], 5–12 mm)	200	20 (10–50)[c]	0 (0%)	0 (0%)	
Rabl et al. [37]	Bladeless (Endopath Xcel[d], 11 mm)	196	NA	0 (0%)	3 (1.5%)	Two cases of superficial laceration of the small mesentery (1.0%) One case of laceration of a vessel in the greater omentum (0.5%)
Madan and Menachery [11]	Bladeless (Endopath[d], 12 mm)	228	25 (10–60)[e]	0 (0%)	0 (0%)	
Rosenthal et al. [28]	Bladeless (Endopath[d], 12 mm)	849	NA	0 (0%)	0 (0%)	
Berch et al. [38]	Bladeless (Optiview[d], 12 mm)	327	28 ± 1.2[f]	0 (0%)	0 (0%)	

NA not available

[a]Major and minor complications related to the optical trocar insertion technique

[b]Covidien, Norwalk, CT, USA

[c]The trocar insertion time was defined as the time to place the trocar into the peritoneal cavity after skin incision; recorded in the last 70 cases

[d]Ethicon Endo-Surgery, Cincinnati, OH, USA

[e]The trocar insertion time was defined as the time to place the trocar into the peritoneal cavity, including infiltration of local anesthesia and incision; recorded in the last 50 cases

[f]The trocar insertion time was defined as the time from incision to CO_2 insufflation; recorded in ten cases

To minimize the possibility of complications, it is of utmost importance to closely follow all the technical steps described above, including patient preparation, determination of the location for trocar insertion, motions and pressure applied, and identification and visualization of all abdominal wall planes.

Advantages of the Direct Insertion Technique Using an Optical Trocar

In contrast to the Hasson technique, which is associated with problems such as losing CO_2, and the potential of being a time-consuming procedure in obese people, the direct trocar insertion technique is fast and no leakage of CO_2 occurs. The advantages of the direct insertion technique using an optical trocar in the morbidly obese are as follows:

- Short trocar placement time.
- No leakage of CO_2.
- Direct visualization of each layer of the abdominal wall.
- Direct visualization of the peritoneal entry.
- Immediate identification and repair of a possible injury of an intra-abdominal organ and avoidance of adverse consequences.
- Avoidance of the need for routine fascial closure with the bladeless, blunt-tip optical trocar.
- Abdominal wall vascular injury may be prevented with the bladeless, blunt-tip optical trocar.
- Previous lower abdominal or laparoscopic surgery is not a formal contraindications for the technique.

Madan and Menachery [11] reported an average trocar placement time (defined as the time to place the trocar into the peritoneal cavity, including the time for infiltration of local anesthesia and incision) of 25 s (range, 10–60 s) in morbidly obese patients. In addition, if damage of an intra-abdominal organ occurs, this injury can be recognized and repaired immediately and adverse consequences can possibly be avoided [41, 46].

Another advantage of blunt-tip trocars is the avoidance of the need for routine fascial closure [28, 37, 38], which can be a difficult and time-consuming procedure in obese patients. The use of the bladeless blunt-tip trocar allows muscle and fascia to be separated rather than cut, which may help prevent trocar site hernia and abdominal wall vascular injury [47–49]. The reported risk of port site hernias when using an 11-mm bladeless optical trocar after a median follow-up period of 18 months in morbidly obese patients is low (0–0.2%) [28, 37, 38]. Development of bleeding at a bladeless optical trocar insertion port site has not been reported [37].

Two studies reported the use of the direct insertion of a bladeless optical trocar without prior creation of a pneumoperitoneum in morbidly obese patients who had undergone previous abdominal operations [37, 38], which were most commonly a gynecologic lower abdominal procedure [37], and concluded that previous lower abdominal or laparoscopic surgery is not a formal contraindication for the technique.

Conclusion

Laparoscopic technique for general and bariatric surgery in the obese and morbidly obese patient is preferred because of several advantages. Obtaining safe access to the peritoneal cavity to create a pneumoperitoneum is technically challenging in obese and morbidly obese people. Two techniques for initial entry are preferred; the Veress needle in the Palmer's point and the direct trocar insertion technique using a bladeless optical trocar. Adherence to standardized technical principles is essential to reproduce the optimal results from published series.

References

1. Eisenberg D, Duffy AJ, Bell RL. Update on obesity surgery. World J Gastroenterol. 2006; 12:3196–203.
2. Buchwald H, Oien DM. Metabolic/bariatric surgery worldwide 2008. Obes Surg. 2009; 19:1605–11.
3. Fried M, Hainer V, Basdevant A, et al. Interdisciplinary European guidelines for surgery for severe (morbid) obesity. Obes Surg. 2007;17:260–70.
4. Santry HP, Gillen DL, Lauderdale DS. Trends in bariatric surgical procedures. JAMA. 2005;294:1909–17.
5. Steinbrook R. Surgery for severe obesity. N Engl J Med. 2004;350:1075–9.
6. Cottam DR, Nguyen NT, Eid GM, Schauer PR. The impact of laparoscopy on bariatric surgery. Surg Endosc. 2005;19:621–7.
7. Campos GM, Ciovica R, Rogers SJ, et al. Spectrum and risk factors of complications after gastric bypass. Arch Surg. 2007;142:969–75; discussion 976.
8. Sekhar N, Torquati A, Youssef Y, et al. A comparison of 399 open and 568 laparoscopic gastric bypasses performed during a 4-year period. Surg Endosc. 2007;21:665–8.
9. Nguyen NT, Hinojosa M, Fayad C, et al. Use and outcomes of laparoscopic versus open gastric bypass at academic medical centers. J Am Coll Surg. 2007;205:248–55.
10. Nguyen NT, Goldman C, Rosenquist CJ, et al. Laparoscopic versus open gastric bypass: a randomized study of outcomes, quality of life, and costs. Ann Surg. 2001;234:279–89; discussion 289–91.
11. Madan AK, Menachery S. Safety and efficacy of initial trocar placement in morbidly obese patients. Arch Surg. 2006;141:300–3.
12. Radojcic B, Jokic R, Grebeldinger S, Meljnikov I, Radojic N. et al. History of minimally invasive surgery. Med Pregl. 2009;62:597–602.
13. Bridgewater FH, Mouton WG. Rationale and intended use for the Veress needle: a translation of the original descriptive article. Surg Laparosc Endosc Percutan Tech. 1999;9:241–3.
14. Schwartz ML, Drew RL, Andersen JN. Induction of pneumoperitoneum in morbidly obese patients. Obes Surg. 2003;13:601–4; discussion 604.

15. Vilos GA, Ternamian A, Dempster J, et al. Laparoscopic entry: a review of techniques, technologies, and complications. J Obstet Gynaecol Can. 2007;29:433–65.
16. Hurd WH, Bude RO, DeLancey JO, et al. Abdominal wall characterization with magnetic resonance imaging and computed tomography. The effect of obesity on the laparoscopic approach. J Reprod Med. 1991;36:473–6.
17. Hurd WW, Bude RO, DeLancey JO, Pearl ML. The relationship of the umbilicus to the aortic bifurcation: implications for laparoscopic technique. Obstet Gynecol. 1992;80:48–51.
18. Philips PA, Amaral JF. Abdominal access complications in laparoscopic surgery. J Am Coll Surg. 2001;192:525–36.
19. Teoh B, Sen R, Abbott J. An evaluation of four tests used to ascertain Veres needle placement at closed laparoscopy. J Minim Invasive Gynecol. 2005;12:153–8.
20. Champault G, Cazacu F, Taffinder N. Serious trocar accidents in laparoscopic surgery: a French survey of 103,852 operations. Surg Laparosc Endosc. 1996;6:367–70.
21. Dunne N, Booth MI, Dehn T. Establishing pneumoperitoneum: Verres or Hasson? The debate continues. Ann R Coll Surg Engl. 2011;93:22–4.
22. Merlin TL, Hiller JE, Maddern GJ, et al. Systematic review of the safety and effectiveness of methods used to establish pneumoperitoneum in laparoscopic surgery. Br J Surg. 2003;90:668–79.
23. Catarci M, Carlini M, Gentileschi P, Santoro E. Major and minor injuries during the creation of pneumoperitoneum. A multicenter study on 12,919 cases. Surg Endosc. 2001;15:566–9.
24. Bonjer HJ, Hazebroek EJ, Kazemier G, et al. Open versus closed establishment of pneumoperitoneum in laparoscopic surgery. Br J Surg. 1997;84:599–602.
25. Azevedo JL, Azevedo OC, Miyahira SA, et al. Injuries caused by Veress needle insertion for creation of pneumoperitoneum: a systematic literature review. Surg Endosc. 2009;23:1428–32.
26. van Goor H. Consequences and complications of peritoneal adhesions. Colorectal Dis. 2007;9 Suppl 2:25–34.
27. Hasson HM. A modified instrument and method for laparoscopy. Am J Obstet Gynecol. 1971;110:886–7.
28. Rosenthal RJ, Szomstein S, Kennedy CI, Zundel N. Direct visual insertion of primary trocar and avoidance of fascial closure with laparoscopic Roux-en-Y gastric bypass. Surg Endosc. 2007;21:124–8.
29. Altun H, Banli O, Karakoyun R, et al. Direct trocar insertion technique for initial access in morbid obesity surgery: technique and results. Surg Laparosc Endosc Percutan Tech. 2010;20:228–30.
30. Yerdel MA, Karayalcin K, Koyuncu A, et al. Direct trocar insertion versus Veres needle insertion in laparoscopic cholecystectomy. Am J Surg. 1999;177:247–9.
31. Byron JW, Markenson G, Miyazawa K. A randomized comparison of Verres needle and direct trocar insertion for laparoscopy. Surg Gynecol Obstet. 1993;177:259–62.
32. Nezhat FR, Silfen SL, Evans D, Nezhat C. Comparison of direct insertion of disposable and standard reusable laparoscopic trocars and previous pneumoperitoneum with Veres needle. Obstet Gynecol. 1991;78:148–50.
33. Borgatta L, Gruss L, Barad D, Kaali SG. Direct trocar insertion vs. Verres needle use for laparoscopic sterilization. J Reprod Med. 1990;35:891–4.
34. Olvera D, Gomez JR. Pneumoperitoneum: its alternatives. Surg Laparosc Endosc. 1997;7:332–4.
35. Jarrett 2nd JC. Laparoscopy: direct trocar insertion without pneumoperitoneum. Obstet Gynecol. 1990;75:725–7.
36. Altun H, Banli O, Kavlakoglu B, et al. Comparison between direct trocar and Veress needle insertion in laparoscopic cholecystectomy. J Laparoendosc Adv Surg Tech A. 2007;17:709–12.
37. Rabl C, Palazzo F, Aoki H, Campos GM. Initial laparoscopic access using an optical trocar without pneumoperitoneum is safe and effective in the morbidly obese. Surg Innov. 2008;15:126–31.

38. Berch BR, Torquati A, Lutfi RE, Richards WO. Experience with the optical access trocar for safe and rapid entry in the performance of laparoscopic gastric bypass. Surg Endosc. 2006; 20:1238–41.
39. Bernante P, Foletto M, Toniato A. Creation of pneumoperitoneum using a bladed optical trocar in morbidly obese patients: technique and results. Obes Surg. 2008;18:1043–6.
40. Sabeti N, Tarnoff M, Kim J, Shikora S. Primary midline peritoneal access with optical trocar is safe and effective in morbidly obese patients. Surg Obes Relat Dis. 2009;5:610–4.
41. Swank DJ, Bonjer HJ, Jeekel J. Safe laparoscopic adhesiolysis with optical access trocar and ultrasonic dissection. A prospective study. Surg Endosc. 2002;16:1796–801.
42. Jirecek S, Drager M, Leitich H, et al. Direct visual or blind insertion of the primary trocar. Surg Endosc. 2002;16:626–9.
43. Hallfeldt KK, Trupka A, Kalteis T, Stuetzle H. Safe creation of pneumoperitoneum using an optical trocar. Surg Endosc. 1999;13:306–7.
44. Angelini L, Lirici MM, Papaspyropoulos V, Sossi FL. Combination of subcutaneous abdominal wall retraction and optical trocar to minimize pneumoperitoneum-related effects and needle and trocar injuries in laparoscopic surgery. Surg Endosc. 1997;11:1006–9.
45. Sharp HT, Dodson MK, Draper ML, et al. Complications associated with optical-access laparoscopic trocars. Obstet Gynecol. 2002;99:553–5.
46. String A, Berber E, Foroutani A, et al. Use of the optical access trocar for safe and rapid entry in various laparoscopic procedures. Surg Endosc. 2001;15:570–3.
47. Liu CD, McFadden DW. Laparoscopic port sites do not require fascial closure when nonbladed trocars are used. Am Surg. 2000;66:853–4.
48. Shalhav AL, Barret E, Lifshitz DA, et al. Transperitoneal laparoscopic renal surgery using blunt 12-mm trocar without fascial closure. J Endourol. 2002;16:43–6.
49. Hamade AM, Issa ME, Haylett KR, Ammori BJ. Fixity of ports to the abdominal wall during laparoscopic surgery: a randomized comparison of cutting versus blunt trocars. Surg Endosc. 2007;21:965–9.
50. Dingfelder JR. Direct laparoscope trocar insertion without prior pneumoperitoneum. J Reprod Med 1978, 21(1):45–47.

Chapter 5
The Direct Optical Access: A Feasible, Reliable, and Safe Laparoscopic Entry

Andrea Tinelli

Introduction

Access to the peritoneal cavity is the most crucial phase of laparoscopy, and fatal complications of laparoscopic surgery are related to first entry. The primary access- or trocar-related complications generally are underreported, and the true incidence may be higher than studies show. There is no clear consensus as to the optimal method of entry into the peritoneal cavity.

Although usually safe, a small minority of patients experiences life-threatening complications, including injuries to the blood vessels (0.9/1,000 procedures) and the bowel (1.8/1,000 procedures). Laparoscopic injuries frequently occur during the blind insertion of needles, trocars, and cannulae through the abdominal wall, hence, the period of greatest risk is from the start of the procedure until visualization within the peritoneal cavity has been established.

Over the past 50 years, developments in electronic and optical technologies have meant that it has become possible to perform many gynaecological operations laparoscopically. The unique feature distinguishing laparoscopic from open abdominal or vaginal surgery is the need to insert needles, trocars, and cannulae for initial entry into the abdomen. This may result in bowel, bladder, or vascular injury, suchas major abdominal vessels and anterior abdominal-wall vessels. Other less serious complications can also occur, such as postoperative infection, subcutaneous emphysema, and extraperitoneal insufflation [1].

The history of entry related complications is interesting and began with a letter in 1996 sent by the Food and Drug Administration (FDA) to the manufacturers of trocars, with the subject being shielded trocars and needles used for abdominal access during laparoscopy. The FDA requested manufacturers and distributors, in

A. Tinelli
Department of Obstetrics and Gynecology, Division of Experimental Endoscopic Surgery, Imaging, Technology and Minimally Invasive Therapy, Vito Fazzi Hospital, Lecce, Italy
e-mail: andreatinelli@gmail.com

A. Tinelli (ed.), *Laparoscopic Entry*,
DOI 10.1007/978-0-85729-980-2_5, © Springer-Verlag London Limited 2012

the absence of clinical data showing reduced incidence of injury, to eliminate safety claims from labeling of shielded trocars and needles, although the FDA did not object to labeling these devises as shielded trocars [1].

Nevertheless, the injuries to retroperitoneal structures appear to be associated with the angle of insertion rather than the type of trocar used [2]. Moreover, the subjectivity of technique used was another factor to include in this entry-related complication analysis, because different doctors use different specialized instruments and techniques [3]. The last review of Cochrane found no evidence that any single technique or specialized instrument used to enter the abdomen helped to prevent life threatening complications [4].

Laparoscopic entry could be blind by Veress needle or by direct access entry, viewable by open laparoscopy technique or by visual entry systems.

But all these methods have the same problems: the surgeon does not know the distance of the anterior peritoneum from the most adjacent bowel before lifting and after lifting, and the eventual presence of adhesions under entry point.

Two studies, one with ultrasonography (US) and the other with computed tomography (CT), determined the distance of the peritoneum from the bowel before lifting and after lifting. In the US investigation the fascia was elevated with towel clips in ten patients and the distance from the nearest bowel was 1.2 cm [5]. In the CT study, the fascia was elevated with sutures in ten laparoscopic cholecystectomy patients and the distance from the nearest bowel was 1.9 cm [6].

In both studies the space in between was taken up by omentum and, looking at the superficial omental vessels, they are large, unprotected, and fragile and you can see where they might be easily damaged. Another study used a suprapubic port to compare the efficacy of manual lifting below the umbilicus and of towel clips placed within and 2 cm from the umbilicus. The author concluded that lifting the abdominal wall with towel clips placed at the edges of the intraumbilical incision achieves the greatest distance between the parietal peritoneum of the abdominal wall and underlying viscera, thus maximizing the margin of safety in protecting peritoneal organs and retroperitoneal vessels from injury of the primary trocar insertion [7].

Umbilical Incision and Entry

The umbilicus is the ideal site of introduction of the lens, due to its thin, nonvascularized skin, also because it provides access to all the areas of the pelvis and abdomen. The inner face of the umbilicus, in fact, is adjacent to the middle line; upwards it is adjacent to the falciform ligament, downwards to the urachus cord, downwards and obliquely at 45° to the two fibrous cords of the left and right umbilical arteries [8].

About the umbilical skin incision, the Royal College Guidelines of 2008, according to the principle of Langer, stated, "In most circumstances the primary incision for laparoscopy should be vertical from the base of the umbilicus (not in the skin below the umbilicus). Care should be taken not to incise so deeply as to enter the peritoneal cavity" [9].

Langer published an anatomic textbook at the turn of the century. The lines of Langer are associated with skin and are still the principle by which plastic surgeons do their work. If a surgeon does not follow the Langer Principle, theoretically, he or she would get more scarring.

There are physicians who make a semicircular or half-moon incision below the umbilicus, but going at the innermost base of the umbilicus could be best both for cosmesis and because of the thin nature of the abdominal wall at that point. On the contrary, starting from the most inner base of the umbilicus and incising caudally, a surgeon will be able to better control the total length of the incision and minimize how close it goes to the more visible inferior edge of the umbilicus.

Starting from the inferior aspect of the outer edge of the umbilicus and then incising cranially, there is a greater risk of entering the abdomen with the scalpel in an uncontrolled manner if the surgeon slips, and the incision may be longer and less cosmetic because the surgeon doesn't know how far out he has to start from the base of the umbilicus to achieve the necessary length for the trocar. Moreover, during the insertion of the needle in the abdomen, excessive lateral movement of the needle should be avoided, as this may convert a small needlepoint injury in the wall of the bowel or vessel into a more complex tear [9]. There has been a great deal of debate about this issue in Europe.

Surgeons who support the use of the "waggle test" say that an inability to move the Veress needle back and forth laterally indicates retroperitoneal placement and that it should be partially withdrawn before insufflation to avoid the rare but deadly complication of intravascular insufflation.

Surgeons who oppose the use of the waggle test are concerned that it will enlarge any injury that has been made to vessel or bowel. Anyway, moving the needle laterally could increase the size of an injury.

Moreover, the angle of entry of the needle differs on the basis of the patient's body mass index (BMI). For heavier patients, the surgeon needs to use a near-vertical insertion angle to get through the abdominal wall. However, for thin patients the distance from the umbilicus to the vessels can be much smaller, and most vessel injuries happen in thin patients. For this reason it is recommend that the angle of insertion should be 45° from horizontal in patients with a BMI of <30 kg/M [10].

Some surgeons use the Z technique for thin patients, and it works particularly well. The Z technique should only be used with the Veress needle and not the trocar; otherwise the tip of the trocar and, as such, the laparoscope is in the cul-de-sac. The Consensus Document from Middleborough from 1999 recommends a perpendicular insertion of the Veress needle in all patients [11]. However, this document affirms, at the same time, the site of insertion should be stabilized by either lifting the umbilicus by hand or with a towel clip, even if that recommendation was made before anyone looked at the anatomy of the abdominal wall. Unfortunately, in patients who have a BMI of <25 kg/m^2, the average distance from the umbilicus to the vessels is 2–4 cm [12]. For patients who are at the highest risk for vessel injury, it is advised to use a 45° angle on thin patients to avoid vessel injury [1].

Some surgeons pull the lower abdominal wall below the umbilical caudally, essentially shifting the umbilicus away from the aortic bifurcation and sacral promontory, tethering the abdominal wall and inserting the Veress needle more perpendicularly in all patients. But if the surgeon is afraid of entry on an obese patient, use the left upper quadrant technique, as reported in the literature [13]. The left upper quadrant (LUQ) could be suggested as the technique of choice if you fail to obtain access via the umbilicus. Alternative sites include transfundal, cul-du-sac, and suprapubic.

The use of the LUQ is recommended in case of obesity and in difficulty, because this location works especially well with obese patients. In the literature not a single case is noted wherein they could not insufflate with the left upper quadrant using Dr. Raoul Palmer's technique. The patient is first placed in the supine position, the surgeon places a hand on the LUQ and pulls down to make the skin taut; then about 3 cm from the midline and 2 cm below the costal margin, the surgeon inserts the needle in cephalad.

Even if the original description was with use of two fingerbreadths from the midclavicular line and 15° cephalad, currently there are several recommendations for insertion angle at Palmer's point but there is no consensus. The only suggestions using Palmer's point are to place a nasogastric tube, but this is contraindicated if the patient has had surgery in the upper left quadrant. The LUQ is a logical choice, especially after three failed attempts at the umbilicus [13].

Another problem is if the attempts to entry by Veress were made by doctors in training. The height of the table in relation to the force and the ability to control the introduction of the Veress needle or trocar into the abdomen is one of the problems. Generally a senior laparoscopist teaches the residents to adjust the height of the table to the comfort of the operator because if the table is too high, young surgeon may deviate laterally and increase the risk of vascular injury. If the assistant surgeon is inserting the trocar or Veress needle, the table or step stool should be adjusted for the assistant. To decrease the risk of vascular injury, the patient should be flat during placement of the umbilical needle or trocar. Insert the laparoscope and inspect the omentum and bowel for possible injury before putting the patient into the Trendelenburg position.

Proper position is one of the most important factors for decreasing the risk of major vessel injury during trocar insertion. When the patient is in the Trendelenburg position, it is difficult to estimate the proper angle for trocar insertion.

Another problem is how to enter the abdomen after the resident has made two to three unsuccessful passes with the Veress needle. The Royal College in the United Kingdom suggests that, after two failed attempts to insert the Veress needle, an alternative such as Palmer's point or open technique should be used [9]. Three studies have shown that Veress insertion is successful 82–87% of the time after one attempt, 8–11% after two attempts, 2–4% after three attempts, and 0.7–3% after more than three attempts [14–16]. The Richardson study correlated injury increases with the number of attempts made [14].

The most reliable test for correct placement of the Veress needle is an initial peritoneal pressure of <10 mmHg, with evidence from three studies [14, 15, 17]. A Canadian survey reported that most gynecologists use the click sound test (82%) or Veress intraperitoneal pressure of 10 mmHg or less (74.3%) to ascertain correct needle placement [18]. The Royal College of Obstetrics and Gynecology in England also reach this conclusion [9].

A survey from the United Kingdom demonstrated that only 9% of gynecologists use Veress intraperitoneal pressure of 10 mmHg or less exclusively as a correct placement indicator, and an additional 62% used Veress intraperitoneal pressure in conjunction with other tests to gauge placement [3]. Moreover, even in the UK 44% of gynecologists use 25 mmHg of pneumoperitoneum exclusively [3]. Similarly, 45% of Canadian gynecologists demonstrated similar tendencies; 28.8% use 20–25 mmHg, and 16.2% use 16–19 mmHg [18].

In Canadian practice, surgeons hook up the gas and have it flowing while observing the pressure as the needle goes through the abdominal wall. Once it penetrates the peritoneum, the pressure drops to <6 mmHg in nearly all patients. In slightly obese patients the pressure can be 7, 8 or 9, but essentially never >10 mmHg. This is true whether the Veress is inserted at the umbilicus or the LUQ because it is exactly the same. Gas flow on low flow rate is limited by the size of the Veress needle, and the surgeon would never get more than 3.0 L/min in first access, although 1 L/min may be better during entry than 2 or 3 [18].

Anyway, trocar insertion into the umbilicus after creation of pneumoperitoneum was the standard method used for years. Although direct trocar insertion has been adopted by many surgeons, large enough studies have not been performed to determine whether this approach is as safe as insertion after pneumoperitoneum [19]. Direct insertion of the trocar was associated with fewer insufflation-related complications, it is faster than the Veress needle technique [20], and a meta-analysis did not show any meaningful differences from the perspective of significant complications [21].

Routinely the surgeon should look at the umbilical trocar site from below before assistants put the patient in the Trendelenburg position, because the surgeon may have penetrated the bowel through and through and not realize it, for lack of a good view.

Coming out, surgeon can look at as assistant withdraws the scope or move the scope to the inferior port to view the main trocar sheath. In all cases the abdomen should be inspected with a complete 360° rotation of the laparoscope. Adhesions immediately behind the entry site become obvious with this technique. When an adhesion is found adjacent to the laparoscope port, the surgeon can inspect the insertion site through one of the other ports.

Nevertheless, to decrease the risk of bowel injury at the umbilical entry site, some surgeons use the visceral slide test. It is quick and easy to perform in the office or the preoperative area. For this, the surgeon places an abdominal ultrasound (US) transducer over the umbilicus or the anticipated entry site and has the patient perform a big Valsalva maneuver, typically with a large breath. The surgeon then observes with US the motion of the bowel underneath (PUGSI test) [22].

The concept is if there is a significant sliding movement of the bowel with the Valsalva maneuver, the surgeon knows the bowel is not adherent directly underneath the probe. If the bowel wiggles in place without significant movement, it is possible there are adhesions in that region and the surgeon can choose an alternate entry site. Dr. Ceana Nezhat took the visceral slide step a step further with his PUGSI test: he reported on putting fluid in through a needle in the operating room with anesthesia, taking a large inspiration, and then observing the bowel's movement, subsequently moving to other sites until a safe entry location is indicated.

This maneuver also should be used in case of open laparoscopy, because the notion that the Hasson technique reduces the risk of bowel injury during laparoscopic access is incorrect. Various studies have reported the open access technique to be safer than the closed approach [23].

In contrast, other studies have shown the number of entry-related complications with the open technique to be significantly higher than with the closed entry technique [24]. This was confirmed by Sasmal et al., who found in 15,260 cases of laparoscopic cholecystectomy 63 cases of primary access-related complications with blind entry by Veress needle, for an overall incidence of 0.41%; major injuries in 11 cases included major vascular and visceral injuries, and minor injuries in 52 cases included omental and subcutaneous emphysema. For the closed method, the findings showed an overall incidence of 0.14% for primary access-related vascular injuries and 0.07% for visceral injuries. They concluded that primary access-related complications during laparoscopy are common and can prove to be fatal if not identified early. Sasmal et al. showed the same incidence of these injuries either in closed methods or in open methods, advising surgeons to beware of unrecognized bowel damages and the severe consequences they offer [25].

It is deemed empirically obvious that if a surgeon can get into bowel adherent to the anterior abdominal wall through a standard laparotomy incision, she or he can also do so through the "minilaparotomy" required for the Hasson technique. Furthermore, the reported incidence of intraabdominal adhesions after laparotomy ranges between 30% and 90% [26–28]. That means that the laparoscopy after a laparotomy exposes surgeon to further bowel damage for adhesions and this might encourage physicians to avoid laparoscopic surgery in these patients.

So, because the conventional umbilical approach can cause damage to adhesive organs, several closed alternative primary approaches to laparoscopic surgery have been introduced for use in patients with a history of laparotomy to avert damage to umbilical-adhesive organs [3, 9, 13, 20].

To estimate the incidence of complications arising during gynecologic laparoscopic surgery in patients who have undergone previous abdominal surgeries and to assess predictable factors associated with complications based on the characteristics of the previous laparotomy, Kumakiri et al. used a closed primary approach via either the ninth intercostal space or the posterior vaginal fornix to avert bowel injury in 307 patients with a history of laparotomy who underwent laparoscopic surgery in 7 years.

No complications developed during primary entry. Adhesiolysis was required in 195 areas of adhesion in 146 patients before laparoscopic surgery could proceed. These areas comprised 45 (14.7%) and 31 (10.1%) abdominal wall adhesions without and within the umbilicus, respectively, and 119 (38.8%) with intrapelvic adhesions. Complications in 41 patients (13.4%) included bowel damage ($n=5.35$), urinary system damage ($n=5.4$), and conversion to laparotomy because of technical difficulties ($n=5.2$). Overall, 38 complications were laparoscopically repaired, and one complication was repaired at minilaparotomy. Intrapelvic adhesions were found in all patients with complications, and adherent bowel was identified in 38 of these (92.7%). Their findings suggested that potential predictive factors of complications are a history of abdominal myomectomy and excisional endometriosis surgery performed because of intrapelvic adhesions [29].

A Reasoned Idea: Abdominal Entry Visualizing All Abdominal Layers

Over the past 30 years, the primary access-related complication rate has not decreased significantly despite improvement in technology and surgical skills. A part of the difficulty is in proper laparoscopic entry. One of the problems of bowel damage associated with laparoscopic blind access and with adhesions is the likelihood that it may not be immediately recognized and could present some time later, often after discharge from hospital. This potentially serious complication may require major abdominal reparative surgery and sometimes a temporary colostomy. It is essential, therefore, that women and attending staff understand that the recovery from laparoscopic procedures is usually rapid and, where this is not the case, that early diagnosis and treatment are essential and should involve senior medical staff.

The relative infrequency of these accidents prevents any individual laparoscopic surgeon from gaining a true appreciation of their importance or frequency. So, to exceed the contingency and to overcome the disadvantage of blind entry, a few years ago some surgeons begin to use a visual entry method that permits entry into the by direct vision trocars—single or multiple use—with a pneumoperitoneum, under optical vision, directly checking the abdominal layers, thus avoiding the blind introduction of the first trocar. Using the optical trocar, vital structures posterior to the peritoneum can be seen, even if sometimes they may be seen too late to avoid an injury.

This is the current trend followed by most laparoscopists, as the use of such tools enables entry with or without a pneumoperitoneum, with a Veress needle. It allows checking the entire procedure and recording on video acquisition systems, also for any possible medical-legal instances that may arise [3].

In the case of single-use trocars, the tools have a transparent sleeve, with a hollow mandrill, equipped with a transparent conical tip, or obturator, where the laparoscopic lens will be placed. The surgeon holds the trocar with the laparoscopic lens connected to the video recording system, in order to see the step-by-step procedure across the abdominal layers, and can stop in case of error or visceral adhesions to the peritoneum.

We began to use this method of entry in each patient in 2005, by a bladeless trocar with an optical viewing port (Endopath or Endopath Xcel; Ethicon Endo-Surgery, Cincinnati, OH, USA), and we called this procedure "Direct Optical Access" (or Direct Optical Entry) [30–33].

Fig. 5.1 At the beginning of laparoscopy, surgeon inserts a zero-degree laparoscope into the bladeless trocar's obturator and tests the light on the glove

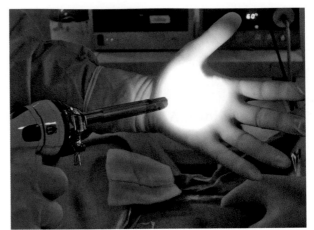

Direct Optical Access: Technique of Abdominal Entry

This technique was tested on a wide range of patients [30–33], comparing to Veress needle or open laparoscopy, and it is here described.

All laparoscopic procedures are performed under general anesthesia with endotracheal intubations. All patients are given a prophylactic dose of 2 g cefazolin IV, and an oral-gastric tube is also placed.

At the beginning of procedure, a zero-degree laparoscope is inserted into the obturator after the scope is dried with gauze because moisture in the obturator is hard to remove and results in poor visualization. The laparoscope is white balanced (focused on white gauze that is placed directly on the tip of the optical viewing obturator). Surgeons verify the lighted tip of trocars on the umbilicus (Fig. 5.1). The trocar is inserted into the abdomen under constant direct visualization using a 10-mm zero-degree laparoscope, trocar-assembled.

Surgeons lift the umbilicus (Fig. 5.2) to perform an intraumbilical incision (Fig. 5.3) with a small blade scalpel (about 11–15°) through the skin only, without fat dissection. The trocar with the scope through the obturator is placed in the incision (Fig. 5.4). At the beginning the trocars were without a handle (Endopath bladeless trocar), whereas successive new models had a handle (Endopath Xcel bladeless trocar). However, after incision, either the handle or the trocar is grasped by the surgeon (Fig. 5.5). The trocar is moved through the subcutaneous fat with a twisting motion, and a steady and gentle pressure is applied downward. This is done until the anterior rectus sheath is reached and identified; the applied pressure to the trocar is then released. The trocar is then moved with the same motion to traverse the next layer, the rectus abdomino muscle, and the pressure is applied and released again (Fig. 5.6). This procedure is repeated for all the other layers: the posterior rectus sheath, the preperitoneal fat, and the peritoneum until the peritoneal cavity is reached. The layers are continuously viewed by surgical staff and recorded on the monitor (Fig. 5.7).

Fig. 5.2 Before cutting the umbilical cutis and beginning entry to the abdomen, the surgeon lifts the umbilicus by two surgical forceps and elevates it

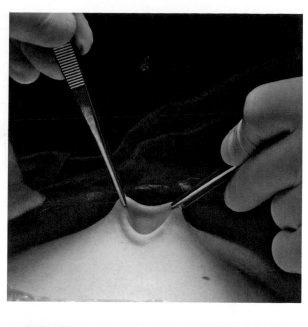

Fig. 5.3 To begin the laparoscopic entry, the surgeon makes an intraumbilical incision using a small blade scalpel (approximately 11–15°) through the skin only, without fat dissection

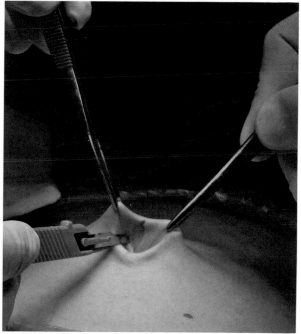

Fig. 5.4 The trocar lighted
tip with the laparoscope
through the obturator is
placed in the incision to
prepare the umbilical entry

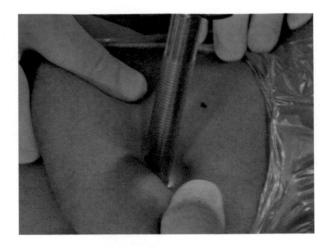

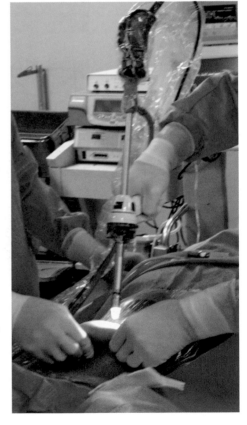

Fig. 5.5 After umbilical incision and trocar
lighted tip positioning on umbilical cutting,
both surgeons grab and elevate the abdomen
and the first surgeon grasps the handle of the
trocar and introduces it into the umbilical
incision. A few years ago the trocars were
without a handle (Endopath bladeless
trocar), whereas successively new models
have an handle (Endopath Xcel bladeless
trocar)

Fig. 5.6 The surgeon moves the trocar through the subcutaneous fat with a twisting motion, applying a steady and gentle pressure downward until the anterior rectus sheath is reached and identified. Then the surgeon moves the trocar with the same motion to traverse the next layer, the rectus abdominis muscle, and the pressure is applied and released again for all the other layers: the posterior rectus sheath, the preperitoneal fat, and the peritoneum until the peritoneal cavity is reached

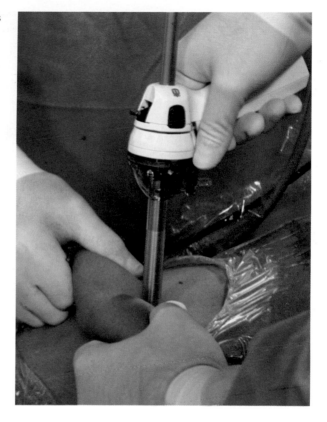

When the peritoneum is entered, the obturator is removed, the insufflation tubing is placed on the trocar and the low-flow CO_2 insufflation is started. The zero-degree laparoscope without the obturator is reinserted to check proper position of the trocar cannula and the entry site and adjacent viscera are inspected promptly, for continuing the operation (Fig. 5.8).

If the tip of the trocar cannula is found to be partially in the preperitoneal space, the insufflation is stopped; the zero-degree laparoscope is removed, reinserted in the obturator, and carefully advanced further using the same principles described above.

All data were recorded on the chart and the times were verified by the scrub nurse or technician, for an internal review and analysis of surgical staff. At the end of the laparoscopic procedure, the trocar is removed. The fascial defect does not need to be closed.

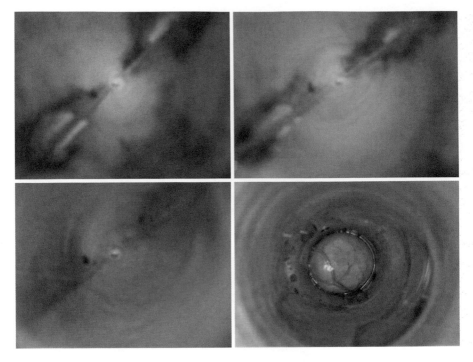

Fig. 5.7 The layers are continuously viewed by surgeons and recorded on the monitor

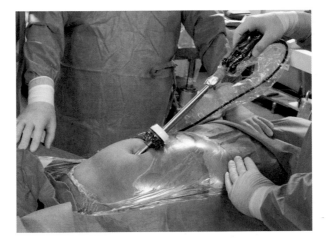

Fig. 5.8 After peritoneal and abdominal entry, the zero-degree laparoscope without the obturator is reinserted to check proper position of the trocar cannula, and pneumoperitoneum is immediately performed. The entry site and adjacent viscera are inspected promptly, before continuing the operation and positioning the ancillary trocars (the photo displays a moderately obese woman with a history of two previous median laparotomic operations)

Published Experiences on Direct Optical Entry

This technique was already tested in a large cohort of women: 368 patients by the same physicians in four studies and 196 women in another study (a total of 564). In the first investigation, 202 premenopausal patients homogeneous for age, parity, and BMI, undergoing laparoscopic surgery for simple ovarian cysts were prospectively randomly assigned to either open laparoscopy or Direct Optical Access (DOA).

The following parameters were compared: duration of access for entry into the abdomen, occurrence of vascular and/or bowel injury, and blood loss. No statistically significant differences were observed in the occurrence of major vascular and/or bowel injury between the two methods. However, time for establishment of abdominal entry was significantly reduced in the DOA group; so was the blood loss ($p < 0.05$). The visual entry system with the Direct Optical Access conferred a little statistical advantage over traditional Hasson entry, in terms of safety, minimal time saving, and in blood loss reduction, allowing a safe and fast visually-guided entry [30].

Then, in another paper, 186 postmenopausal women undergoing laparoscopic surgery for simple ovarian cysts were tested for laparoscopic access: 89 were assigned to direct optical access (DOA) (group I) and 97 to classical closed Veress needle approach plus trocar entry (group II). The compared parameters were: time needed for entry into the abdomen, occurrence of vascular and/or bowel injury, and blood loss. In the results no statistically significant differences were observed in the occurrence of major vascular and/or bowel injury ($p > 0.05$), whereas time for abdominal entry was significantly reduced in the DOA group, as well as the occurrence of minor vascular injuries ($p < 0.05$). Also in this comparison on the DOA and the Veress methods, the visual entry system offered a statistical advantage over the closed Veress needle approach, in terms of time saving and limiting minor vascular injuries, thus enabling a safe and fast visually-guided entry in postmenopausal subjects [31].

Another comparison involved 194 women: 93 assigned to direct optical access (DOA) entry (group I), and 101 to classical closed method by Veress needle and trocar entry (group II). All underwent laparoscopic surgery. No statistically significant differences were observed in the occurrence of blood loss and minor vascular injury between the two techniques; time for of abdominal entry, instead–-as well as minor bowel injuries—were significantly reduced in the DOA group. The results of this investigation still suggested that the visual entry system conferred a statistical advantage over a closed entry technique with Veress needle, in terms of time saving and the minor vascular injuries, thus enabling a safe and expeditious, visually-guided, entry for surgeons [32].

Nevertheless, authors analyzed the safety and the efficacy of a modified Direct Optical Entry (DOE) method versus the Hasson method by Open Laparoscopy (OL), in women with previous abdominopelvic surgery in a prospective case control study, on 168 women who underwent laparoscopic surgery: 86 were assigned to abdominal DOE (Group A) and 82 to OL (Group B). Statistical differences, in favor of the DOE group ($p < 0.01$), were found in duration of entry and blood loss. The vascular and bowel injuries in OL versus DOE were not statistically different.

Since obtaining access to the peritoneal cavity in laparoscopic surgery is a more difficult, time-consuming, and occasionally hazardous procedure in patients with previous abdominopelvic surgery, the authors of the study suggested that DOE was advantageous when compared with OL in terms of saving time enabling a safe and expeditious visually-guided entry for laparoscopy [33].

Rabl et al. examined the safety and efficacy of accessing the peritoneal cavity using an optical, bladeless trocar (Endopath bladeless trocar or Endopath Xcel; Ethicon Endo-Surgery Inc, Cincinnati, OH, USA) without previous pneumoperitoneum in 196 morbidly obese patients. The patients' characteristics and outcomes with consecutive and preferential use of an optical, bladeless, first trocar insertion without previous pneumoperitoneum in morbidly obese patients (body mass index >35 kg/m^2) were reviewed. No bowel or major abdominal vessel injuries occurred. In all, 98 patients (50%) had previous abdominal operations, most commonly a gynecologic lower abdominal procedure and in 32 patients (33%) who had a previous abdominal operation, authors found significant intra-abdominal adhesions that required laparoscopic adhesiolysis

In all, three patients had injuries related to direct optical entry: two had a superficial 1-cm laceration of the small bowel mesentery, and one had a laceration of a vessel in the greater omentum. In both patients with superficial small bowel mesenteric lacerations, a careful inspection of the adjacent small bowel and structures showed no other injuries. In the third patient, the greater omental vessel was ligated using a Harmonic Scalpel (Ethicon Endo-Surgery, USA). No hollow viscus, major vascular, or any other injury occurred. No local complications, such as bleeding, infection, or hernias occurred at the direct optical entry trocar site [34].

Discussion on Abdominal Entry Visualizing Systems

In such studies, no bowel or major vascular injury occurred, and no conversion to other techniques was necessary. In contrast to the Hasson technique, which is associated with problems such as losing CO_2 and potential for being a time-consuming procedure in obese people, Direct Optical Access or Entry is fast and does not have leakage of CO_2.

The laparoscopic entry in patients at high risk of abdominal wall adhesions can be fast and safe, so as the rate of complications that might occur during entry can be reduced by Direct Optical Access or Entry, respecting to Hasson' method. The results of investigation on Direct Optical Access in patients with previous abdominopelvic surgery, demonstrate some advantages of it over open laparoscopy: The Direct Optical Access provides a fast visual identification of the bowel during the insertion of the trocar and the entry injuries were numerically less in Direct Optical Access group. One of the supplemental advantages of Direct Optical Access over open laparoscopy is that, if an injury does occur, in most cases it could be recognized and managed appropriately [33].

Although Rabl found adhesions of the omentum and small bowel to the anterior abdominal wall due to previous lower abdominal operations in 33% of the patients, all these adhesions were in sites distant from the Direct Optical entrance [34]. The Direct Optical Access also provides immediate visualization during entry to the peritoneal cavity, and adhesions or adherent intra-abdominal organs may be identified before damage occurs [35].

Although others have reported using a direct visualization technique [35–40] their accounts differ from ours because they describe the optical trocar as being used after the pneumoperitoneum is created using a Veress needle [35–38] or after blunt dissection into the fascia and positioning two stay sutures in the anterior rectus sheath [37] or using the optical trocar in combination with a subcutaneous lifter [39].

Furthermore, a few studies have described the use of this technique in morbidly obese people [41–43]. Rosenthal et al. [42] reported their experience with Direct Optical entry and avoidance of fascial closure in 849 laparoscopic Roux-en-Y gastric bypasses in morbidly obese patients. Their study, like ours, reported no injuries to major vessels or bowel during insertion of the optical access trocar and reported a low risk of port-site hernias (0.2%) after a mean follow-up period of 10 months. Fascial closure can be a difficult and time-consuming procedure in obese people. The use of the bladeless blunt-tip trocar separates muscle and fascia rather than cutting it, which may help prevent trocar site hernia and abdominal wall vascular injury [44–46].

Berch et al. [43] also reported the same using the optical access trocar without a previous pneumoperitoneum in 327 obese patients. Their results showed no viscus or vascular injuries and no port-site hernias after a median follow-up period of 18 months. Similar to the Rabl study [34], 55% of their patients had previous abdominal operations.

Madan et al. [41] reported no bowel or vessel injury with the Direct Optical Access technique without previous pneumoperitoneum in 228 morbidly obese patients. In the last 50 patients, the mean recorded trocar-placement time was 25 s and insufflation time was 16 s. This shows that the Direct Optical Access technique permits fast entry into the peritoneal cavity even in morbidly obese patients.

Severe complications from using the Direct Optical Access technique have been described in one study [47] that reviewed three databases to identify possible complications. Of the 82 serious complications that were found, most were major vessel injuries (46.8%) and bowel injuries (30.4%). In all, four of these injuries resulted in death of the patients. All these complications happened during laparoscopy for general surgical and gynecologic procedures. However, an important limitation of that study was the lack of specific information about the total number of patients and other patients' characteristics; their risk factors, including whether they were obese, the exact technique that was used with the optical access trocar, or whether this technique was used appropriately.

After this literature appraisal, the results of present studies suggest that the Direct Optical Access technique represent, in a large cohort of patients (564), a safe and less time-consuming approach to abdominal entry, avoiding the risks of mini-laparotomy of blind or open laparoscopy. Based on the author's experiences and on literature reports, the Direct Optical entry could represent for surgeons a safe alternative approach to entry directly and safely in abdomen without creation of a pneumoperitoneum, where minor injuries cannot be immediately recognized in the classical closed method by Verres needle, since it requires a few minutes to produce an adequate pneumoperitoneum and to insert the trocar in the abdomen.

Nevertheless, the final decision as to which entry technique is to be routinely employed should be left to the surgeon, based on his/her personal experience and capability of swapping the laparoscopic access with another technique.

In the authors' opinion, the DOA approach should be recommended to young surgeons or trainees in the presence of resident and expert gynecologist supervision. The lack of feeling with closed-entry methods could be overcome with the help of a well- trained surgeon.

Conclusion

To minimize the possibility of complications, it is of utmost importance to closely follow all the above-described technical steps, including preparation of patient and of her/his bowel, location for trocar insertion, application of motions and pressure, and identification and visualization of all abdominal wall planes, among the other steps. Using an oral- or nasogastric tube would still be recommended to drain the stomach prior to access.

Another crucial aspect when using the Direct Optical Access technique without previous pneumoperitoneum is to communicate with the anesthesiologist to ascertain that the patient is completely paralyzed and have the bladder decompressed. Finally, small visual trocars and laparoscopes should be available for all at-risk cases, such as patients who have had one or more previous abdominal-pelvic procedures.

Although we acknowledge that no entry method is foolproof, authors have yet to experience an entry-related injury using the Direct Optical Access method [48, 49]. The results of this preliminary comparison of entry methods suggest that Direct Optical Access offers a small clinical advantage over other methods, in terms of saving time. Larger prospective studies with randomly assigned groups are needed to establish any significant differences between first entrance techniques.

References

1. Frishman G. Laparoscopic entry roundtable. J Minim Invasive Gynecol. 2009;16(4):400–7.
2. Sharp HT, Dodson MK, Draper ML, Watts DA, Doucette RC, Hurd WW. Complications associated with optical-access laparoscopic trocars. Obstet Gynecol. 2002;99:553–5.
3. Varma R, Gupta JK. Laparoscopic entry techniques: clinical guideline, national survey, and medicolegal ramifications. Surg Endosc. 2008;22(12):2686–97.
4. Ahmad G, Duffy JMN, Phillips K, Watson A. Laparoscopic entry techniques. Cochrane Database Syst Rev. 2008;16:CD006583.

5. Cakir TTD, Esmaeilzadem S, Atkan AO. Safe Veress needle insertion. J Hepatobiliary Pancreat Surg. 2006;13:225–7.
6. Shamiyeh A, Glaser K, Kratochwill H, Hörmandinger K, Fellner F, Wayand WU, et al. Lifting of the umbilicus for the installation of pneumoperitoneum with the Veress needle increased the distance to the retroperitoneal and intraperitoneal structures. Surg Endosc. 2009;23:313–7.
7. Roy GM, Bazzurini L, Solima E, Luciano AA. Safe technique for laparoscopic entry into the abdominal cavity. J Am Assoc Gynecol Laparosc. 2001;8(4):519–28.
8. Kaloo P, Cooper M, Molloy D. A survey of entry techniques and complications of members of the Australian Gynaecological Endoscopy Society. Aust N Z J Obstet Gynaecol. 2002;42:264–6.
9. RCOG Green-top Guideline. Preventing entry-related gynaecological laparoscopic injuries. 2008;49:1–10.
10. Hurd WH, Bude RO, DeLancey JO, Gauvin JM, Aisen AM. Abdominal wall characterization with magnetic resonance imaging and computed tomography. The effect of obesity on the laparoscopic approach. J Reprod Med. 1991;36:473–6.
11. Garry R. Towards evidence based laparoscopic entry techniques: clinical problems and dilemmas. Gynaecol Endosc. 1999;8:315–26.
12. Hurd WW, Bude RO, DeLancey JO, Pearl ML. The relationship of the umbilicus to the aortic bifurcation: implications for laparoscopic technique. Obstet Gynecol. 1992;80:48–51.
13. Granata M, Tsimpanakos I, Moeity F, Magos A. Are we underutilizing Palmer's point entry in gynecologic laparoscopy? Fertil Steril. 2010;94(7):2716–9.
14. Richardson R, Sutton CJG. Complications of first entry: a prospective laparoscopic audit. Gynaecol Endosc. 1999;8:327–34.
15. Vilos GA, Vilos AG. Safe laparoscopic entry guided by Veress needle CO_2 insufflation pressure. J Minim Invasive Gynecol. 2003;10:415–20.
16. Teoh BSR, Abbott J. An evaluation of four tests used to ascertain Veress needle placement at closed laparoscopy. J Minim Invasive Gynecol. 2005;12:153–8.
17. Azevedo JL, Guindalini RS, Sorbello AA, Silva CE, Azevedo OC, Aguiar Gda S, et al. Evaluation of the positioning of the tip of the Veress needle during creation of closed pneumoperitoneum in pigs. Acta Cir Bras. 2006;21:385–91.
18. Kroft J, Aneja A, Tyrwhitt J, Ternamian A. Laparoscopic peritoneal entry preferences among Canadian gynaecologists. J Obstet Gynaecol Can. 2009;31:641–8.
19. Altun H, Banli O, Kavlakoglu B, Kücükkayikci B, Kelesoglu C, Erez N. Comparison between direct trocar and Veress needle insertion in laparoscopic cholecystectomy. J Laparoendosc Adv Surg Tech A. 2007;17:709–12.
20. Vilos GA, Ternamian A, Dempster J, Laberge PY, The Society of Obstetricians and Gynecologists of Canada. Laparoscopic entry: a review of techniques, technologies, and complications. J Obstet Gynaecol Can. 2007;29(5):433–65.
21. Merlin TL, Hiller JE, Maddern GJ, Jamieson GG, Brown AR, Kolbe A. Systematic review of the safety and effectiveness of methods used to establish pneumoperitoneum in laparoscopic surgery. Br J Surg. 2003;90:668–79.
22. Nezhat C, Cho J, Morozov V, Yeung Jr P. Preoperative periumbilical ultrasound- guided saline infusion (PUGSI) as a tool in predicting obliterating subumbilical adhesions in laparoscopy. Fertil Steril. 2009;91(6):2714–9.
23. Bonjer HJ, Hazebrek EJ, Kazemier G, Giuffrida MC, Meijer WS, Lange JF. Open vs closed establishment of pneumoperitoneum in laparoscopic surgery. Br J Surg. 1997;84:599–602.
24. Jansen FW, Kolkman W, de Bakkum EA, Kroon CD, Trimbos-Kemper TC, Trimbos JB. Complications of laparoscopy: an inquiry about closed- versus open-entry technique. Am J Obstet Gynecol. 2004;190:634–8.
25. Sasmal PK, Tantia O, Jain M, Khanna S, Sen B. Primary access-related complications in laparoscopic cholecystectomy via the closed technique: experience of a single surgical team over more than 15 years. Surg Endosc. 2009;23(11):2407–15.
26. Brill AI, Nezhat F, Nezhat CH, Nezhat C. The incidence of adhesions after prior laparotomy: a laparoscopic appraisal. Obstet Gynecol. 1995;85:269–72.

27. Weibel MA, Majno G. Peritoneal adhesions and their relation to abdominal surgery: a post-mortem study. Am J Surg. 1973;126:345–53.
28. Szomstein S, Lo Menzo E, Simpfendorfer C, Zundel N, Rosenthal RJ. Laparoscopic lysis of adhesions. World J Surg. 2006;30:535–40.
29. Kumakiri J, Kikuchi I, Kitade M, Kuroda K, Matsuoka S, Tokita S, et al. Incidence of complications during gynecologic laparoscopic surgery in patients after previous laparotomy. J Minim Invasive Gynecol. 2010;17:480–6.
30. Tinelli A, Malvasi A, Hudelist G, Istre O, Keckstein J. Abdominal access in gynaecological laparoscopy: a comparison between direct optical and open access. J Laparoendosc Adv Surg Tech A. 2009;19:529–33.
31. Tinelli A, Malvasi A, Guido M, Istre O, Keckstein J, Mettler L. Initial laparoscopic access in postmenopausal women: a preliminary prospective study. Menopause. 2009;16:966–70.
32. Tinelli A, Malvasi A, Istre O, Keckstein J, Stark M, Mettler L. Abdominal access in gynaecological laparoscopy: a comparison between direct optical and blind closed access by Veress needle. Eur J Obstet Gynecol Reprod Biol. 2010;148:191–4.
33. Tinelli A, Malvasi A, Guido M, Tsin DA, Hudelist G, Stark M, Mettler L. Laparoscopic entry in women with previous abdomino-pelvic surgery. Surg Innov 2011; [Epub ahead of print].
34. Rabl C, Palazzo F, Aoki H, Campos GM. Initial laparoscopic access using an optical trocar without pneumoperitoneum is safe and effective in the morbidly obese. Surg Innov. 2008;15(2):126–31.
35. Swank DJ, Bonjer HJ, Jeekel J. Safe laparoscopic adhesiolysis with optical access trocar and ultrasonic dissection. A prospective study. Surg Endosc. 2002;16:1796–801.
36. McKernan JB, Finley CR. Experience with optical trocar in performing laparoscopic procedures. Surg Laparosc Endosc Percutan Tech. 2002;12:96–9.
37. Hallfeldt KK, Trupka A, Kalteis T, Stuetzle H. Safe creation of pneumoperitoneum using an optical trocar. Surg Endosc. 1999;13:306–7.
38. Jirecek S, Drager M, Leitich H, et al. Direct visual or blind insertion of the primary trocar. Surg Endosc. 2002;16:626–9.
39. Angelini L, Lirici MM, Papaspyropoulos V, Sossi FL. Combination of subcutaneous abdominal wall retraction and optical trocar to minimize pneumoperitoneum-related effects and needle and trocar injuries in laparoscopic surgery. Surg Endosc. 1997;11:1006–9.
40. String A, Berber E, Foroutani A, et al. Use of the optical access trocar for safe and rapid entry in various laparoscopic procedures. Surg Endosc. 2001;15:570–3.
41. Madan AK, Menachery S. Safety and efficacy of initial trocar placement in morbidly obese patients. Arch Surg. 2006;141:300–3.
42. Rosenthal RJ, Szomstein S, Kennedy CI, Zundel N. Direct visual insertion of primary trocar and avoidance of fascial closure with laparoscopic Roux-en-Y gastric bypass. Surg Endosc. 2007;21:124–8.
43. Berch BR, Torquati A, Lutfi RE, Richards WO. Experience with the optical access trocar for safe and rapid entry in the performance of laparoscopic gastric bypass. Surg Endosc. 2006;20:1238–41.
44. Liu CD, McFadden DW. Laparoscopic port sites do not require fascial closure when nonbladed trocars are used. Am Surg. 2000;66:853–4.
45. Shalhav AL, Barret E, Lifshitz DA, et al. Transperitoneal laparoscopic renal surgery using blunt 12-mm trocar without fascial closure. J Endourol. 2002;16:43–6.
46. Hamade AM, Issa ME, Haylett KR, Ammori BJ. Fixity of ports to the abdominal wall during laparoscopic surgery: a randomized comparison of cutting versus blunt trocars. Surg Endosc. 2007;21:965–9.
47. Sharp HT, Dodson MK, Draper ML, et al. Complications associated with optical-access laparoscopic trocars. Obstet Gynecol. 2002;99:553–5.
48. Tsin DA, Tinelli A, Malvasi A, Davila F, Jesus R, Castro-Perez R. Laparoscopy and natural orifice surgery: first entry safety surveillance step. JSLS. 2011;15(2):133-5.
49. Deffieux X, Ballester M, Collinet P, Fauconnier A, Pierre F. Risks associated with laparoscopic entry: guidelines for clinical practice from the French College of Gynaecologists and Obstetricians. Eur J Obstet Gynecol Reprod Biol. 2011;158(2):159-66

Chapter 6
Robotic-Assisted Surgery and Related Abdominal Entry

Crisitina Falavolti, Roberto Angioli, Patrizio Damiani, and Maurizio Buscarini

Introduction

Because laparoscopic surgery has revolutionized the concept of minimally invasive surgery for the last three decades [1], new equipment, cameras, and energy sources were developed that have enabled surgeons to perform more complex surgeries that were once only performed by laparotomies [1]. In the field of pelvic surgery, almost all types of cases now can be performed through a laparoscope, depending on the skill and experience of the surgeon and the availability of proper instrumentation [1]. Robotic-assisted surgery is one of the latest of the innovations in minimally invasive surgery. By the twentieth century, advances in task-specific surgical instrumentations, optics, and digital video equipment, as well as computer and robotic technology opened a new frontier for minimally invasive laparoscopic surgery. The recent introduction of advanced robotic devices, such as da Vinci surgical system, to the field of pelvic surgery has added new hope that operative times as well as the learning curve for minimally invasive surgery may be reduced. The surgeon now is able to operate, suture, and dissect with the facility of the human wrist and in addition, the superior three-dimensional view offered by this robotic system provides surgeons with an unprecedented view of the anatomy. The three-dimensional view is a significant advantage of the robotic surgical system that improves visualization and allows greater precision and accuracy. Furthermore, the surgeon seated at the surgical console performs the dissection with wristlike motions of the master controls, which provides finer, more delicate manipulation of tissue and facilitates procedures that are considered more difficult by conventional laparoscopy. The motions of the surgeon at the console unit are replicated by the robotic arms placed within the patient. During robotic

C. Falavolti (✉) • M. Buscarini
Division of Urology, Department of Urology, Campus Biomedico University, Rome, Italy

R. Angioli • P. Damiani
Division of Gynaecology, Department of Gynaecology,
Campus Biomedico University, Rome, Italy

A. Tinelli (ed.), *Laparoscopic Entry*,
DOI 10.1007/978-0-85729-980-2_6, © Springer-Verlag London Limited 2012

surgery, an assistant is available at the operating table. The assistant performs robot-related tasks, including alignment and exchange of robotic instruments, operative maneuvers with conventional instruments such as organ manipulation, tissue counter-traction, suction, and irrigation, and any necessary alterations in the position of the intrauterine manipulator. The presence of the scrubbed assistant is also crucial in the event that an emergency conversion to a laparotomy is required. Robotic technology is used mainly in pelvic surgery because the difficult access to the pelvic cavity is greatly facilitated by the use of robotic arms. In fact, a robot is used in both the urological and gynecological fields. More specifically, robotic-assisted surgery has been applied in many urological surgical procedures, such as for radical prostatectomy, partial nephrectomy, and cystectomy. In the same way, gynecological surgery has been improved by robotic-assisted surgery, both in the treatment of benign and malignant diseases. Robotic-assisted surgery is strictly linked to traditional laparoscopic techniques, with the advantages and disadvantages of minimally invasive surgery.

It has been shown that more than 50% of major laparoscopic complications occur during the first phase of laparoscopy—gaining access to the abdominal cavity [1, 2]. For this reason, robotic-assisted surgery requires safe abdominal access. Initial entry by trocar insertion is the most hazardous part of a laparoscopic procedure. The debate on methods and site of initial entry continues. Trocar insertion still accounts for 40% of laparoscopic complications and most of the fatalities [2, 3]. At least three different techniques are currently used to obtain laparoscopic and robotic access to the abdominal cavity: Verres needle, direct insertion, and the open technique. However, none of them entirely obviate the possibility of intraoperative complications caused by trocars and needles. The closed technique is probably the most widely used method. The peritoneal cavity is punctured blindly with the Verres needle, followed by insufflation of carbon dioxide. Thereafter, the first trocar, which is often placed near the umbilicus, is introduced blindly into the peritoneal cavity. Alternatively, the first trocar can be inserted blindly without prior creation of the pneumoperitoneum. In contrast, the open (Hasson) technique is characterized by the open introduction of the first trocar under direct vision. The pneumoperitoneum is subsequently established through the blunt-tipped trocar. Although the open technique is a very safe method to enter the peritoneal cavity, perforating lesions have also been described by different authors [4]. The technique of establishing pneumoperitoneum through the Veress needle is the most popular in urological and gynecological laparoscopy. Its wide application can be attributed to its traditional popularity and lack of evidence to suggest otherwise. General surgeons have embraced the open method of entry and suggest that it is safer than closed laparoscopy [5, 6].

Different studies failed to reveal any safety advantage of an open technique when compared with a closed method of entry, in terms of both visceral and major vascular injury. Major complications are very rare, accounting for 0.4 and 0.3/1,000. The vast majority of major vascular injuries occur during the set-up phase of laparoscopy (creation of the pneumoperitoneum, and installation of the trocars). The major vascular injury risk factors must be perfectly familiar to the surgeon so that the risk of accidents can be kept to a minimum. One of the risk factors in fact is the surgeon's lack of experience.

Installation for laparoscopy must be particularly careful both in very thin and in obese patients. In the first situation, the major vessels can be located <2.5 cm below the skin, which means an accident during installation of the P-needle is more likely. In the second situation, the surgeon needs to be thoroughly aware of the modifications to the anatomical relationships between the umbilicus and the aortic bifurcation in obese patients so as to avoid damaging the retroperitoneal vessels [7]. The most common major visceral structure damaged is the small bowel. Often, bowel injury is detected in patients with significant visceral adhesions. In the open technique, those injuries may be related to the lysis of intraabdominal adhesions and perforations with the instruments used to create the minilaparotomy. Moreover, prior abdominal surgery, which is often performed through a midline laparotomy, leads to adhesions of the small and large bowel to the anterior abdominal wall, and blind insertion may cause inadvertent perforation of the adjacent organs. In robotic surgery, the access of the principal trocar follows the traditional laparoscopic techniques described in the preceding. Port placements for other operative ports are chosen according to different surgical procedures and different corporeal districts involved. Those different approaches to the pelvic cavity are highlighted, comparing robotic abdominal entries between urological and gynecological surgeries.

Robotic-Assisted Laparoscopic Surgery in Urology

Urology is a dynamic surgical discipline that has undergone many developments and refinements over the past few decades. The advent of laparoscopic surgery was a major breakthrough in the urological landscape and provided a minimally invasive alternative to conventional open procedures [8]. The minimally invasive surgical landscape has changed markedly within the last half decade. This change has had a significant impact on patients, surgeons, and surgical trainees [9]. The decreased intraoperative estimated blood loss (EBL), shorter hospital stay, less postoperative pain, decreased medical complications, and quicker return to function makes laparoscopic urological surgery extremely appealing to physicians and patients alike [10]. Robotic surgery using the da Vinci surgical system (Intuitive Surgical, Sunnyvale, CA) is able to correct any tremor the surgeon may have. In addition, optimal port placement translates into noncollision of the robotic arms and can be instrumental in performing more precise surgery [11]. This, in conjunction with a 3D camera, allows for better preservation of critical anatomical structures, which translates into enhanced intraoperative and postoperative outcomes [12].

Robotic-Assisted Laparoscopic Radical Prostatectomy

Prostate cancer is a malignant tumor of cells from the prostate gland. It is the most common malignancy in U.S. men and the second leading cause of deaths from cancer after lung cancer. Generally it grows slowly and remains confined to the gland for many

Fig. 6.1 Port placement for robotic radical prostatectomy. *C* 12-mm robotic camera port; *1–2–3* 8-mm robotic working ports; *A₁* 10-mm assistant port; *A₂* 5-mm assistant port

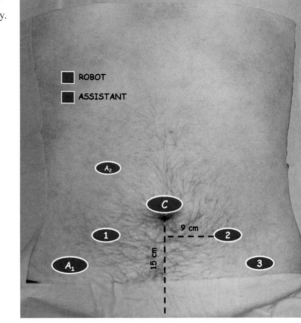

years. During this time, the tumor produces little or no symptoms or outward signs. Prostate cancer treatment often depends on the stage of the cancer. How fast the cancer grows and how different it is from surrounding tissue helps determine the stage. Treatment may include surgery, radiation therapy, chemotherapy or control of hormones that affect the cancer. Robot-assisted radical prostatectomy (RARP) is rapidly gaining acceptance in the urological community as a safe and efficacious treatment option for localized prostatic adenocarcinoma with comparable oncological outcomes to its open and laparoscopic counterparts. RARP also seemed to have decreased intraoperative estimated blood loss (EBL), risk of intraoperative transfusion, and anastomotic strictures in comparison with retropubic radical prostatectomy (RRP) [13, 14]. The small surgical incisions and minimally invasive approach may facilitate patient recovery and return to activity. In fact, RARP can be performed through a limited infraumbilical incision that limits postoperative pain. The patient should be placed into a slight Trendelenburg position to help lift the small intestine out of the pelvis. The Verres needle angle should be in the direction of the pelvis. Access to the pelvic cavity can be preperitoneal or transperitoneal. Five trocars are used for both the extraperitoneal and transperitoneal approaches and trocar placement does not differ. The preperitoneal approach has some advantages such as the decreased incidence of bowel injury, ileus, or urinoma formation. Intraabdominal access is obtained by either a Verres needle or Hasson technique. Once access is obtained, the abdomen is insufflated with CO_2 to 15 mmHg. Additional tanks of CO_2 gas should be available in the event of a long operation. The peripheral trocars are placed under direct visualization (Fig. 6.1).

A 12-mm trocar for the camera is introduced at the umbilicus at 15 cm superior to the pubic symphysis along the midline. For tall patients the distance from pubis to umbilicus has to be >15 cm. Two 8-mm trocars for the robotic arms are placed inferior and lateral to the umbilicus and 8-mm port above approximately 8–9 cm away and inferior to the camera port, and the third 8-mm robotic arm is placed 2 cm above and medial to the left iliac spine. For the assistant, a 10-mm trocar is introduced in the mirror image of the left the right iliac fossa, and a 5-mm trocar is placed slightly higher between the optic and right robotic trocar for suture introduction. It is very important to make sure that the fourth arm does not impede the third arm movement and that the second and the third arm do not collide with the camera. If there is a significant interference between robot arms and or assistant ports, adding another port in an appropriate position is recommended. In fact, many trocar configurations exist, with most variations resulting from surgeon preference, location of the first assistant, and the use of a three- or four-arm robotic technique.

Robotic-Assisted Laparoscopic Radical Cystectomy

Urothelial bladder cancer is the ninth most frequent cancer. Almost all urinary bladder tumors have a transitional cell histology in Europe and the United States. The excess risk of urinary bladder cancer is related to the amount of tobacco smoked, and the presence of blood in the urine is the principal outward sign. The probability of developing carcinoma of the bladder increases as an individual gets older. In older patients who are acceptable surgical candidates, it is imperative to use surgical techniques that will minimize stress inflicted to the body and allow for a smoother return to function. Robot-assisted radical cystectomy (RARC) offers an attractive minimally invasive alternative to the current gold standard of open radical cystectomy (ORC) for muscle-invasive bladder cancer and high-risk non–muscle-invasive disease [15]. The robotic-assisted radical cystectomy (RARC) has the potential advantages of less intraoperative blood loss, shorter hospital stay, less postoperative narcotic requirement, quicker return of bowel function, and earlier convalescence with an acceptable surgical learning curve for surgeons [16]; however, long operative times, significant fluid shifts, and postoperative morbidity approach that of the open technique. RARC is considered an evolving technique that affords patients and physicians alike an efficacious minimally invasive option in the treatment of bladder cancer [17]. It can provide a cost-effective alternative to ORC, with operative time and length of stay being the most critical cost determinants. Higher complication rates with ORC make total actual costs much higher than RARC [18].

During robotic surgery, the patient is positioned in exaggerated Trendelenburg position with the arms adducted and tucked at the sides. The port placement is very similar to the robotic prostatectomy setup. There are six ports, but they are shifted above approximately 3 cm. This position facilitates dissection of the urachus and proximal aortic, common iliac, and presacral lymph node tissues [19] (Fig. 6.2).

Fig. 6.2 Port placement for robotic radical cystectomy. *C* 12-mm robotic camera port ;*1–2–3* 8-mm robotic working ports; *A₁* 10-mm assistant port; *A₂* 5-mm assistant port

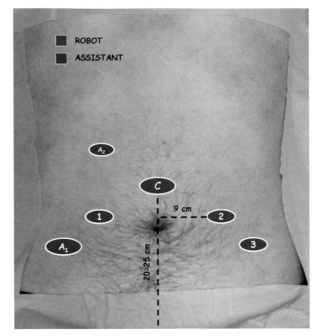

Robotic-Assisted Laparoscopic Renal Surgery

Partial Nephrectomy

The field of urology has embraced minimally invasive surgical procedures, from endoscopic to laparoscopic to robotic-assisted surgery [20]. Introduction of robotic assistants was proposed to increase the precision of movements within the operating field and was related to economic intentions [21]. Laparoscopic partial nephrectomy (LPN) is a minimally invasive technique that achieves comparable oncological and improved morbidity outcomes when compared with the open procedure. Robot-assisted partial nephrectomy (RAPN) overcomes many of the technical hurdles of the LPN and is now coming to the forefront for the minimally invasive surgical management of small renal masses (SRMs) [22]. Robotic surgery permits the reduction of intraoperative estimated blood loss (EBL) that has been shown to be an accurate predictor of early and late recovery of kidney function [23]. RAPN holds the promise of better long-term nephron preservation, and outcomes—including safety, functional results, and oncological control—continue to be reported as the technique emerges [24]. Indications for robotic-assisted

Fig. 6.3 Port placement for robotic partial nephrectomy (transperitoneal access). *C* 12-mm robotic camera port; *1–2* 8-mm robotic working ports; A_1 10-mm assistant port; A_2 5-mm assistant port

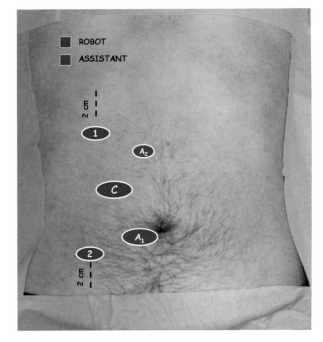

laparoscopic partial nephrectomy include exophytic renal lesions <4 cm, such as enhancing lesions or suspicious cystic renal lesions (Bosniak category III or IV).

Endophytic or central renal lesions are not recommended for robotic-assisted laparoscopic partial nephrectomy because they prove difficult to dissect while preserving hilar structures. Contraindications to robotic laparoscopic renal surgery include any pulmonary or cardiac conditions that would make it difficult for the patient to tolerate pneumoperitoneum.

The ports are placed in two different ways. The first is for transperitoneal partial nephrectomy, and the second is for retroperitoneal partial nephrectomy access. In transperitoneal access, after pneumoperitoneum established with Verres needle, a 12-mm periumbilical port is placed for the camera to visualize a hilar tumor. Ports may be shifted laterally and superiorly for upper pole tumors. Two 8-mm robotic instrument ports are placed approximately 8 cm from the camera in a wide V configuration centered on the renal tumor. These ports may be shifted laterally or superiorly for patients with a large body habitus or upper pole tumor location. A 12-mm assistant port is placed inferior to the camera port [25]. An optional 5-mm assistant port may be placed above the camera port if needed to retract the liver (Fig. 6.3).

For retroperitoneal access, a full flank position is used, the camera port is placed below the tip of the 12th rib, and the working ports are similarly placed for the transperitoneal approach (Fig. 6.4).

Fig. 6.4 Port placement for robotic partial nephrectomy (retroperitoneal access). *C* 12-mm robotic camera port; *1–2* 8-mm robotic working ports; A_1, 10-mm assistant port; A_2 5-mm assistant port

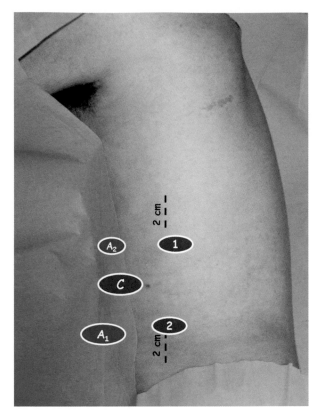

Pyeloplasty

Ureteropelvic junction (UPJ) obstruction is defined as an obstruction of the flow of urine from the renal pelvis to the proximal ureter. It is the most frequently observed cause of obstructive nephropathy in children. Congenital abnormalities are the most common cause of UPJ obstruction in young children, but adults may also present with obstruction after previous surgery or other disorders that can cause inflammation of the upper urinary tract. The most important symptoms are back pain, blood in the urine, kidney infection (pyelonephritis), and urinary tract infection (UTI). The treatment strategies for UPJ obstruction have seen a significant shift in the last several years. The introduction of the laparoscopic technique has allowed for reproducing the steps of the open dismembered pyeloplasty while avoiding a flank incision [26, 27]. Robotic-assisted pyeloplasty (RAP) can be offered as first-line treatment for primary or secondary ureteropelvic junction obstruction (UPJO). Indications for RAP are identical to those for open pyeloplasty [28]. However, in general, the widely accepted indications for selecting pyeloplasty over endopyelotomy are presence of anterior crossing vessels, grade 3–4 hydronephrosis, percent

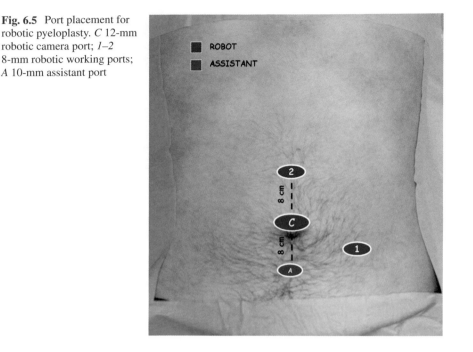

Fig. 6.5 Port placement for robotic pyeloplasty. *C* 12-mm robotic camera port; *1–2* 8-mm robotic working ports; *A* 10-mm assistant port

function of the affected kidney in the 15–25% range, and patients in whom primary endopyelotomy has failed. The patient is secured in the lateral decubitus position. The bed can be flexed to open the space between the iliac crest and costal margin. This facilitates movement of the bowel out of the surgical field. A 12-mm dilating trocar is placed at the umbilicus for the camera port, the two 8-mm working ports for the robotic arms are placed under laparoscopic control in a triangular fashion such that one is placed in the upper midline near the xiphoid process and the other is placed at the lateral border of the rectus inferior to the umbilicus. These ports are optimally placed by ensuring at least 8 cm between the camera port and each working port to avoid robotic arm collisions during the surgery. Many variations exist for the assistant port. Usually a 5-mm assistant port is placed infraumbilically along the midline and at least 8 cm away from the camera port (Fig. 6.5).

Robotic-Assisted Laparoscopic Adrenalectomy

Laparoscopic adrenalectomy (LA) has become the new standard of care for benign adrenal neoplasms and is being increasingly used for malignant disease. Robotic assistance (RA) offers unique advantages in visualizing and dissecting the adrenal gland, especially considering its challenging vasculature. Although LA remains the standard of care, RA is an excellent option in high-volume robotic centers from the standpoints of outcomes, feasibility, and cost [29]. Robotic adrenalectomy has been

Fig. 6.6 Port placement for robotic adrenalectomy. *C* 12-mm robotic camera port; *1–2–3* 8-mm robotic working ports; *A* 10-mm assistant port

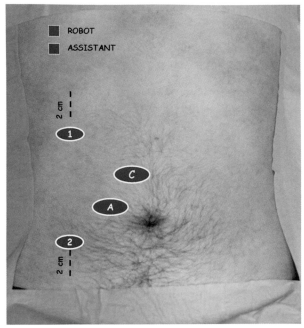

demonstrated to be a feasible minimally invasive approach. The patient is placed in the right lateral decubitus and slight Trendelenburg position. A transperitoneal approach is preferred. The access is possible via a Verres needle or with the open Hasson technique. For left-sided robotic adrenalectomy, three ports for the robotic arms (two robotic working ports and one camera port) are used plus an additional port for the bedside assistant. The 12-mm port is placed in the paramedian position halfway between the costal margin and umbilicus, two 8-mm robotic instruments are placed 2 cm inferior to the costal margin at the midaxillary line, and approximately 2 cm cephalad to the anterior superior iliac spine in the iliac fossa. A 10-mm port that is used for suction is placed superolateral to the umbilicus, and clip-applying devices are also placed by the assistant (Fig. 6.6).

Right-sided robotic adrenalectomy is typically performed via five ports, because an additional 5-mm port for the bedside assistant is required for liver retraction [30].

Robotic-Assisted Surgery in Gynecology

Robotic surgery mimics traditional surgical approaches to pelvic surgery when compared with conventional laparoscopy and recently has been associated with a shorter learning curve [31]. These advantages could potentially make it the ideal tool for performing complex oncological procedures, such as a radical hysterectomy, that require delicate dissection (cardinal ligament, ureter, and pelvic vessels) [32, 33] or relative simple gynecological procedures such as simple hysterectomy, multiple myomectomy, tubal surgery, severe endometriosis surgery, and other pathologies. The use of minimally invasive surgery for the treatment of gynecological cancer was first described in the early 1990s. These initial experiences demonstrated the safety and feasibility of minimally invasive surgery to treat these disorders [31–36]. In addition, it has been demonstrated that minimally invasive surgery is associated with less blood loss, shorter hospital stay, less postoperative pain, improved cosmesis, and a faster recovery when compared with traditional approaches [37–41]. In the gynecological literature, there are reports of robotic-assisted laparoscopy for simple hysterectomy [42–47], myomectomy, tubal reanastomosis [48, 49], sacral colpopexy [50], tubal ligation, salpingo-oophorectomy, ovarian cystectomy, and radical hysterectomy [51]. Yet despite these advantages, recent surveys of practicing gynecological oncologists revealed that most respondents believed minimally invasive surgery (conventional laparoscopy) had only a minimal role in the management of cervical cancer [52]. It is likely that well-known barriers to the use of advanced minimally invasive procedures, such as association with a long learning curve, lack of training, complexity of operations, limitation of technology and instrumentation, and the necessity of an expert assistant, were responsible for this sentiment. Recent advances in the field of minimally invasive surgery have focused on the incorporation of robotic technology for the treatment of gynecological malignancies. Since that time, a small number of investigators have reported a limited series documenting their experience with robotic surgery for the treatment of endometrial, ovarian, and cervical cancers [44, 53, 54].

Robotic-Assisted Laparoscopic Radical Hysterectomy and Pelvic Lymphadenectomy

Robotic-assisted laparoscopic radical hysterectomy is one of the most challenging laparoscopic procedures in gynecological oncology, requiring significant technical expertise and experience. The gynecological oncology community has been appropriately cautious in accepting laparoscopic procedures as a standard of care because of a lack of oncological outcome data. Many questions regarding the adequacy of the laparoscopic approach still remain. Data on specimen size, margin adequacy, and parametria appear to be equivalent [55]. With the follow-up data in some of the studies approaching or exceeding 5 years, some of these questions are being answered. In none of these studies does the recurrence rate in the laparoscopically or robotic-assisted managed patients exceed that of the patients who underwent an open procedure [56–60]. Robotic radical hysterectomy appears to be equivalent to total laparoscopic radical hysterectomy with respect to operative time, blood loss, hospital stay, and oncological outcome. However, the substantial magnification, dexterity, and flexibility combined with significant reduction in surgeon fatigue offered by the robotic system significantly simplify the most difficult stages of radical hysterectomy and pelvic lymphadenectomy [51]. The procedure was performed

Fig. 6.7 Port placement for robotic radical hysterectomy and pelvic lymphadenectomy. *C* 12-mm robotic camera port; *1–2–3* 8-mm robotic working ports; A_1 10-mm assistant port; A_2 5-mm assistant port

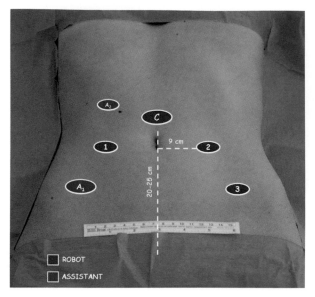

with the patient under general endotracheal anesthesia in the low dorsal and steep Trendelenburg position with adjustable Allen stirrups and lower extremity compression devices for deep venous thrombosis prophylaxis. Shoulder stops may be unwanted in order to avoid the risk of shoulder nerve injury associated with their use. A Foley catheter is inserted to drain the bladder. CO_2 insufflation is begun with a trocar and is continued to a pressure of 12 mmHg. Four ports are placed after the pneumoperitoneum is obtained. First, a 12-mm bladeless trocar is placed in the midline approximately 3 cm above the umbilicus under direct visualization. The abdomen must be fully insufflated before placement of additional trocars. Depending on the length of the patient's abdomen, this corresponds to approximately 20–27 cm superior to the pubic symphysis. Three working robotic arms are attached to 8-mm reusable trocars placed bilaterally, and ancillary 10-mm trocars are placed in the suprapubic region and the left or right upper quadrant. The robotic ports are placed 1–2 cm below and 8–10 cm lateral to the intraumbilical trocar and lateral to umbilicus and approximately 8–9 cm away and inferior to the camera port, so as to enable optimal movement of the robotic arm and minimize the risk of collision. The third robotic 8-mm port is placed at the level of the left iliac crest. The 10-mm assistant trocar is placed above the right iliac fossa. The three robotic arms are finally docked to the trocars (Fig. 6.7). Robotic-assisted hysterectomy has also provided a tool to overcome the surgical limitations seen with conventional laparoscopy in difficult cases in which variations in anatomy may limit laparoscopic techniques, such as pelvic adhesive disease with a scarred or obliterated anterior cul-de-sac [61].

Robotic-Assisted Laparoscopic Hysterectomy

Approximately 600,000 hysterectomies are performed annually in the United States, with the majority resulting from benign conditions [62–64]. Before the introduction of laparoscopic-assisted vaginal hysterectomy in the late 1980s, hysterectomies were approached by either a vaginal or abdominal route [65]. Since the 1990s, a definite trend toward laparoscopic hysterectomy has been seen. Despite the increasing acceptance of laparoscopy, hysterectomy via laparotomy remains the most common route. One explanation for this slow acceptance is the learning curve with conventional laparoscopy and its associated complications. Another has often been advanced pathology, such as pelvic adhesions, of which the scarred or obliterated anterior cul-de-sac is one example, in which the ability to complete a hysterectomy in a minimally invasive fashion is affected by the surgical anatomy field. This in turn is affected by the surgeon's skill level and the technical limitations of conventional laparoscopic instruments [66]. The use of robotic-assisted technology may provide a means to overcome both advanced pathology and the surgical limitations of conventional laparoscopy, by providing surgeons with improved dexterity and precision coupled with advanced imaging that allows for the completion of complex minimally invasive procedures in a fashion analogous to open surgery. The procedure is performed with the patient under general endotracheal anesthesia in the low dorsal and steep Trendelenburg position with adjustable Allen stirrups and lower extremity compression devices for deep venous thrombosis prophylaxis. Anti-skid measures should be incorporated at this time. The bladder is drained with a Foley catheter and the stomach is evacuated with a nasogastric tube. The pneumoperitoneum is obtained, followed by placement of either four or five trocars, depending on whether or not the patient-side cart has three or four robotic arms. A 12-mm port is placed either at or above the umbilicus, depending on the size of the uterus. This port accommodates the dual optical endoscope. As a general rule, at least a handbreadth distance, or approximately 8–10 cm between the endoscope and the top of an elevated uterus during manipulation, is necessary to allow for an adequate working distance between the endoscope and the uterine fundus. Two 8-mm ports that mount directly to the operating arms on the patient-side cart are placed in the left and right lower quadrants, respectively. As a general rule, these are located two finger-breadths from the anterior–superior iliac spines on a diagonal to the umbilicus. For larger uteri, these landmarks are moved further cephalad. A fourth port serves as an accessory port and can be placed between the camera port and either the left or right lower quadrant ports. This is typically a 10- to 12-mm port so as to facilitate the introduction of suture as well as instruments used for retraction, suction/irrigation, and specimen removal (Fig. 6.8). Once all desired ports are in place, the patient is placed in steep Trendelenburg. The patient-side cart with robotic arms is brought between the patient's legs and docked. Each port is attached to the assigned robotic arm, with the exception of the

Fig. 6.8 Port placement for robotic simple hysterectomy. *C* 12-mm robotic camera port; *1–2* 8-mm robotic working ports; *A* 10-mm assistant port

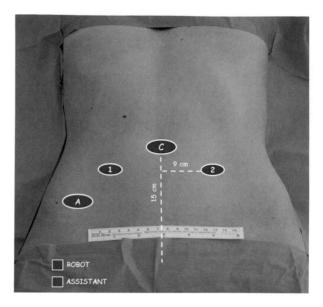

accessory port. With operative times approaching those of conventional laparoscopy, the robotic approach became more feasible for routine clinical use. Increased precision, 3D vision, and faster learning curves are possible advantages that might enable more providers to offer a laparoscopic approach to a broader patient population with more advanced pathology. This could ultimately lead to decreasing numbers of total abdominal hysterectomies. Minimal blood loss and fast recovery time are the major advantages of laparoscopic hysterectomy, not to mention excellent cosmetic results. Most women go home either the same or next day and are fully on their feet within a week or two.

Robotic-Assisted Laparoscopic Colposacropexy

More than 120,000 women have surgery for uterine and vaginal vault prolapse each year in the United States. Prolapse (or falling) of any pelvic floor organs (vagina, uterus, bladder, or rectum) occurs when the connective tissues or muscles in the body cavity are weak and cannot hold the pelvis in its natural position [67]. The weakening of connective tissues accelerates with age, after childbirth, with weight gain, and with strenuous physical labor. Women with pelvic organ prolapse typically have problems with urinary incontinence, vaginal ulceration, sexual dysfunction, and/or having a bowel movement. Sacrocolpopexy is a procedure to surgically correct vaginal vault prolapse in which mesh is used to hold the vagina in the correct anatomical position. This procedure can also be performed following a hysterectomy to treat uterine prolapse to provide long-term support of the vagina. Colposacropexy is the gold standard operation for repair of apical vaginal support defects. Laparoscopic

Fig. 6.9 Port placement for robotic colposacropexy. *C* 12-mm robotic camera port; *1–2–3* 8-mm robotic working ports; *A* 10-mm assistant port

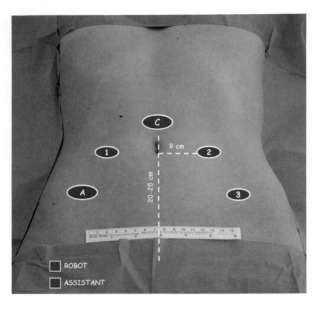

colposacropexy has become a substitute for open surgery in the treatment of pelvic organ prolapse. Although it is feasible to perform this operation using conventional laparoscopic techniques, a limited number of surgeons have mastered the advanced minimally invasive skills that are required. As for radical hysterectomy, a 12-mm bladeless trocar is placed in the midline approximately 3 cm above the umbilicus under direct visualization, and three working robotic arms are attached to 8-mm reusable trocars placed bilaterally, and ancillary 10-mm trocars are placed in the supra-pubic region and the left or right upper quadrant. The robotic ports are placed 1–2 cm below and 8–10 cm lateral to the intraumbilical trocar and lateral to umbilicus and approximately 8–9 cm away and inferior to the camera port. The right robotic port could also be placed parallel to the umbilicus port, in order to better reach the sacrum. The third robotic 8-mm port is placed at the level of the left iliac crest. The 10-mm assistant trocar is placed above the right iliac fossa (Fig. 6.9). Recent literature data suggest the feasibility and the safety of this surgical technique. Pending an evaluation on the long-term with larger series, it is possible to include robotic colpos-acropexy among the therapeutic options for symptomatic pelvic floor prolapse repair, considering this new surgical technique as a valid and feasible alternative [68].

Robotic-Assisted Laparoscopic Myomectomy

Leiomyoma is a benign smooth muscle neoplasm. It occurs mainly in women 40–50 years old. They can occur in any organs, but are more frequent in the uterus. uterine fibroids are leiomyomata of the uterine smooth muscle. Fibroids can have variable dimensions (a few to 10–15 cm) and can be single or multiple.

Fig. 6.10 Port placement for robotic myomectomy. *C* 12-mm robotic camera port; *1–2–3* 8-mm robotic working ports; *A₁* 10-mm assistant port

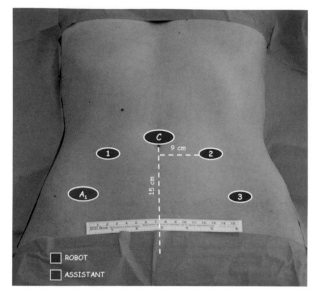

Often, fibroids are completely asymptomatic and the diagnosis is secondary to a gynecological visit or abdominal ultrasound. Sometimes they lead to excessive menstrual bleeding (menorrhagia), often cause anemia, and may lead to infertility or cause compression on other abdominal organs. Surgery is the right therapeutic choice for this frequent disease. Meticulous repair of the myometrium is essential for women considering pregnancy after laparoscopic myomectomy to minimize the risk of uterine rupture. When this surgery is performed via laparotomy, the defect is usually closed in layers. When the procedure is performed via laparoscopy, because of the limitations of fixed port placement, the repair is more likely to be completed using the bulk closure technique. The da Vinci robot enables 360° movement of the surgical head of the instrument. This enhanced surgical dexterity enables laparoscopic surgical closure of the uterine scar that can be done in layers and, therefore, better approximates that done via laparotomy [69]. The patient is placed in Trendelenburg. Peritoneal access is obtained using a 12-mm trocar placed inside or 2–5 cm above the umbilicus (10 cm from the top of the uterus). Two lateral 8-mm robotic ports are placed in the mid-axillary line 2 cm below the level of the umbilicus and separated by a minimum of 8 cm between port sites. An accessory port is placed 8 cm lateral to the right lateral port for suture removal, placement, irrigation, traction, and subsequent morcellation (Fig. 6.10). Robotic-assisted laparoscopic myomectomy presents operative and fertility outcome comparable with other traditional approaches, while ensuring a quicker surgical technique and better uterine closure.

Robotic-Assisted Laparoscopic Surgery for Benign Gynecological Disease

Many surgical procedures for benign gynecological disease are performed by minimally invasive surgery, such as asportation of adnexal cysts, asportation of moderate and severe endometriosis, infertility surgery, tubal surgery, reanastomosis, and supracervical hysterectomy. However, there are limitations to the procedures that can be performed by laparoscopy. Some procedures, such as a microsurgical anastomosis of the fallopian tubes or gradual and careful dissection of the cyst from the ovary wall, require extensive, precise microsurgical suturing techniques, which are difficult to achieve during conventional laparoscopy because the operator's hands are positioned far from the operative field. Traditional laparoscopy, however, is limited by a long learning curve, counterintuitive movements, two-dimensional views that limit depth perception, and ergonomic difficulty. Robotic-assisted laparoscopic surgery emerged, in part, to overcome these obstacles while maintaining the benefits of minimally invasive surgery.

The three-dimensional (3D) visual system in robot assisted surgery allows for improved spectral depth perception and its intuitive movements and articulating instruments allows for greater range of motion and filtration of any natural tremor of the surgeon [70–72]. The advantages of robotic-assisted procedures include intuitive movements, less physician fatigue, improved dexterity, and a shorter learning curve, bridging the gap from laparotomy to laparoscopic surgery [50]. These advantages permit more complex procedures to be performed endoscopically and even remotely. More advanced laparoscopic procedures, such as intracorporeal suturing and tying, and more precise excisions of various areas of the abdominal-pelvic cavity are possible. Use of robotic-assisted surgery for tubal reanastomosis, endometriosis, adnexal disease, and supracervical hysterectomy has been reported [50, 73–77]. In the field of gynecological surgeries, robotic-assisted laparoscopy seems to make the realization of minimally invasive surgery more possible. It could lead to a decrease of postsurgical adherences and therefore preserve the fertility of young patients. As in all laparoscopic procedures, patient positioning and port placement are vital. The procedure was conducted with the patient under general anesthesia in the supine position. A uterine manipulator was placed in the uterine cavity. Robotic surgery is performed with the patient in the dorsal lithotomy position on Allen stirrups. Preferably, all four robotic arms of the da Vinci patientside cart are employed. The camera port is always placed within the umbilicus. The three 8-mm da Vinci ports are positioned as follows: Port 1 is 8–10 cm to the right of the camera port, port 2 is 8–10 cm to the left of the camera port, and port 3 is 8–10 cm to the left of port 2. Ports 1 and 2 are safely located in an area of the abdominal wall that is between the epigastric vessels (superficial and inferior) and the superficial circumflex vessels, making injury of any of these vessels extremely unlikely. Port 3 is located in the left lateral portion of the anterior abdominal wall. In women with a smaller abdomen, it is necessary to slide port 3 about 15–30° caudal to port 2, while keeping the distance of 8–10 cm (Fig. 6.11).

Fig. 6.11 Port placement for robotic treatment of benign gynecological disease. *C* 12-mm robotic camera port; *1–2–3* 8-mm robotic working ports; *A* 5-mm assistant port

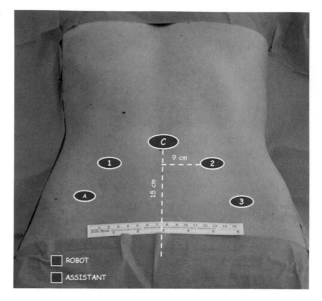

Optimal placement of robotic port 3 is undoubtedly the most challenging of the three 8-mm ports. Because of the obtrusive nature of the da Vinci patient-side cart, external interference between robotic arms 2 and 3 and between robotic arm 3 and the patient arm support systems (e.g., arm toboggans) is common during the learning curve of this operation. Moreover, internal interference between instruments in port 2 and port 3 is also possible, particularly if the degree of caudal shift of port 3 is excessive and the instrument crosses the pelvis transversely. Placement of the bedside surgical assistant port in robotic surgery has traditionally been high in the abdominal wall at either side of the umbilicus. However, it is strongly suggested that for most reproductive surgery applications, the assistant port must be placed in one of the lower quadrants. Such placement is based on considerations of patient safety, assistant safety, and surgical ergonomics. Reproductive microsurgery is suture intensive, and needle exchanges should never occur beyond the visual field of the console surgeon. In terms of assistant safety, placement of the assistant port as the most lateral port (instead of between the robotic camera arm and a robotic instrument arm) avoids the possibility that the assistant's hand could be caught between colliding robotic arms. Finally, placing the assistant port in the lower quadrant allows for an overall port configuration that is compatible with any advanced conventional laparoscopic maneuvers that may be needed during the case (approximating the "ultralateral" port placement previously described for conventional laparoscopy). The enabling nature of robotic technology makes tubal reanastomosis a perfect example of an operation that is more safely learned and performed robotically [78]. Robotic microsuturing can potentially be more reliable and precise than using hand-held instruments. This is especially true if the microsurgery must be performed with instruments controlled at a distance from the operative site, as in laparoscopic surgery. The robotic device functions safely without compromising sterility or interfering with nursing or anesthesia activities.

References

1. Chapron C, Dubuisson JB, Querleu D, Pierre F. Complications of laparoscopy: a prospective multicentre observational study. Br J Obstet Gynaecol. 1997;104(12):1419–20.
2. Fuller J, Ashar BS, Carey-Corrado J. Trocar-associated injuries and fatalities: an analysis of 1399 reports to the FDA. J Minim Invasive Gynecol. 2005;12:302–7.
3. Shirk GJ, Johns A, Redwine DB. Complications of laparoscopic surgery: how to avoid them and how to repair them. J Minim Invasive Gynecol. 2006;13(4):352–9.
4. Schäfer M, Lauper M, Krähenbühl L. Trocar and Verres needle injuries during laparoscopy. Surg Endosc. 2001;15(3):275–80.
5. Crist DW, Gadacz TR. Complications of laparoscopic surgery. Surg Clin North Am. 1993;73(2):265–89.
6. Wolfe BM, Gardiner BN, Leary BF, Frey CF. An analysis of complications. Gynaecological endoscopic cholecystectomy. An analysis of complications. Arch Surg 1991 Oct; 126(10): 1192-6.
7. Chapron CM, Pierre F, Lacroix S, Querleu D, Lansac J, Dubuisson JB. Major vascular injuries during gynecologic laparoscopy. J Am Coll Surg. 1997;185(5):461–5.
8. Hemal AK, Menon M. Laparoscopy, robot, telesurgery and urology: future perspective. J Postgrad Med. 2002;48:39–41.
9. Lee JY, Mucksavage P, Sundaram CP, McDougall EM. Best practices for robotic surgery training and credentialing. J Urol. 2011;185(4):1191–7.
10. Hemal AK, Menon M. Robotics in urology. Curr Opin Urol. 2004;14:89–93.
11. Hemal AK, Eun D, Tewari A, Menon M. Nuances in the optimum placement of ports in pelvic and upper urinary tract surgery using the da Vinci robot. Urol Clin North Am. 2004;31:683–92.
12. Menon M. Robot-assisted radical prostatectomy: is the dust settling? Eur Urol. 2011;59:7–9.
13. Coelho RF, Rocco B, Patel MB, Orvieto MA, Chauhan S, Ficarra V. Retropubic, laparoscopic, and robot-assisted radical prostatectomy: a critical review of outcomes reported by high-volume centers. J Endourol. 2010;24:2003–15.
14. Lowrance WT, Tarin TV, Shariat SF. Evidence-based comparison of robotic and open radical prostatectomy. ScientificWorldJournal. 2010;10:2228–37.
15. Richards KA, Hemal AK, Kader AK, Pettus JA. Robot assisted laparoscopic pelvic lymphadenectomy at the time of radical cystectomy rivals that of open surgery: single institution report. Urology. 2010;76:1400–4.
16. Richards KA, Kader K, Hemal AK. Robotic radical cystectomy: where are we today, where will we be tomorrow? ScientificWorldJournal. 2010;10:2215–27.
17. Babbar P, Hemal AK. Robot-assisted urologic surgery in 2010 - Advancements and future outlook. Urol Ann. 2011;3(1):1–7.
18. Martin AD, Nunez RN, Castle EP. Robot-assisted radical cystectomy versus open radical cystectomy: a complete cost analysis. Urology. 2011;77(3):621–5.
19. Fumo MJ, Badani KK, Menon M. Robotic radical cystectomy. In: Smith JA, Tewari AK, editors. Robotics in urologic surgery. Philadelphia: Saunders Elsevier; 2008.
20. McHone B, Jarrett TW, Pinto PA. Tips and tricks of laparoscopic partial nephrectomy. Minerva Urol Nefrol. 2010;62(3):273–81.
21. Poletajew S, Antoniewicz AA, Borówka A. Kidney removal: the past, presence, and perspectives: a historical review. Urol J. 2010;7(4):215–23.
22. Babbar P, Hemal AK. Robot-assisted partial nephrectomy: current status, techniques, and future directions. Int Urol Nephrol. 2011; [Epub ahead of print].
23. Colli J, Martin B, Purcell M, Kim YI, Busby EJ. Surgical factors affecting return of renal function after partial nephrectomy. Int Urol Nephrol. 2011;43(1):131–7.
24. Rogers C, Sukumar S, Gill IS. Robotic partial nephrectomy: the real benefit. Curr Opin Urol. 2011;21(1):60–4.
25. Rogers CG, Singh A, Blatt AM, Linehan WM, Pinto PA. Robotic partial nephrectomy for complex renal tumors: surgical technique. Eur Urol. 2008;53:514–23.
26. Kavoussi LR, Peters CA. Laparoscopic pyeloplasty. J Urol. 1996;150:1891–4.

27. Janetschek G, Peschel R, Bartasch G. Laparoscopic and retroperitoneoscopic kidney pyelo-plasty. Urologe A. 1996;35:202–7.
28. Stock JA, Esposito MP, Lovallo G. Robotic pyeloplasty. In: Stock JA, Esposito MP, Lantieri V, editors. Urologic robotic surgery. 1st ed. Totowa: Humana Press; 2008.
29. Bruhn AM, Hyams ES, Stifelman MD. Laparoscopic and robotic assisted adrenal surgery. Minerva Urol Nefrol. 2010;62(3):305–18.
30. Del Pizzo JJ. Miscellaneous adult robotic surgery. In: Smith JA, Tewari AK, editors. Robotics in urologic surgery. Philadelphia: Saunders Elsevier; 2008.
31. Hatch K, Hallum A, Surwit E, Childers J. The role of laparoscopy in gynaecologic oncology. Cancer. 1995;76:2113–6.
32. Nezhat CR, Burrell MO, Nezhat FR, Benigno BB, Welander CE. Laparoscopic radical hyster-ectomy with paraaortic and pelvic node dissection. Am J Obstet Gynecol. 1992;166(3):864–5.
33. Lowe MP, Bahador A, Muderspach LI, Burnett A, Santos L, Caffrey A, et al. Feasibility of laparoscopic extraperitoneal surgical staging for locally advanced cervical carcinoma in a gynecologic oncology fellowship training program. J Minim Invasive Gynecol. 2006;13(5): 391–7.
34. Childers J, Brzechffa P, Hatch K, Surwit E. Laparoscopically assisted surgical staging (LASS) of endometrial cancer. Gynecol Oncol. 1993;51:33–8.
35. Childers J, Surwit E. Combined laparoscopic and vaginal surgery for the management of two cases of stage I endometrial cancer. Gynecol Oncol. 1992;45:46–51.
36. Canis M, Mage G, Wattiez A, Pauly J, Manhes H, Bruhat M. Does endoscopic surgery have a role in radical surgery of cancer of the cervix uteri. J Gynecol Obstet Biol Reprod (Paris). 1990;19:921.
37. Abu-Rustum N, Gemignani M, Moore K, Sonoda Y, Venkatraman E, Brown C, et al. Total laparoscopic radical hysterectomy with pelvic lymphadenectomy using the argon-beam coag-ulator: pilot data and comparison to laparotomy. Gynecol Oncol. 2003;91:402–9.
38. Magrina J. Outcomes of laparoscopic treatment for endometrial cancer. Curr Opin Obstet Gynecol. 2005;17:343–6.
39. Magrina J, Mutone N, Weaver A, Magtibay P, Fowler R, Cornella J. Laparoscopic lymph-adenectomy and vaginal or laparoscopic hysterectomy with bilateral salpingo-oophorectomy for endometrial cancer: morbidity and survival. Am J Obstet Gynecol. 1999;181:376–81.
40. Gemignani M, Curtin J, Zelmanovich J, Patel D, Venkatraman E, Barakat R. Laparocopic-assisted vaginal hysterectomy for endometrial cancer: clinical outcomes and hospital charges. Gynecol Oncol. 1999;73:5–11.
41. Spirtos N, Schlaerth J, Gross G, Spirtos T, Schlaerth A, Ballon S. Cost and quality -of-life analysis of surgery for early endometrial cancer: laparotomy versus laparosocpy. Am J Obstet Gynecol 1996 Jun; 174(6):1795–9.
42. Reynolds RK, Advincula AP. Robot-assisted laparoscopic hysterectomy: technique and initial experience. Am J Surg. 2006;191:555–60.
43. Mettler L, Ibrahim M, Jonat W. One year of experience working with the aid of a robotic assis-tant (the voice-controlled optic holder AESOP) in gynaecological endoscopic surgery. Hum Reprod. 1998;13:2748–50.
44. Diaz-Arrastia C, Jurnalov C, Gomez G, Townsend Jr C. Laparoscopic hysterectomy using a computer-enhanced surgical robot. Surg Endosc. 2002;16:1271–3.
45. Advincula AP. Surgical techniques: robot-assisted laparoscopic hysterectomy with the da Vinci surgical system. Int J Med Robot. 2006;2:305–11.
46. Kho RM, Hilger WS, Hentz JG, Magtibay PM, Magrina JF. Robotic hysterectomy: technique and initial outcomes. Am J Obstet Gynecol. 2007;197:113. e1-4.
47. Payne TN, Dauterive FR. A comparison of total laparoscopic hysterectomy to robotically assisted hysterectomy: surgical outcomes in a community practice. J Minim Invasive Gynecol. 2008;15:286–91.
48. Rodgers AK, Goldberg JM, Hammel JP, Falcone T. Tubal anastomosis by robotic compared with outpatient minilaparotomy. Obstet Gynecol. 2007;109:1375–80.

49. Ferguson JL, Beste TM, Nelson KH, Daucher JA. Making the transition from standard gynecologic laparoscopy to robotic laparoscopy. JSLS. 2004;8:326–8.
50. Nezhat C, Saberi NS, Shahmohamady B, Nezhat F. Robotic assisted laparoscopy in gynecological surgery. JSLS. 2006;10:317–20.
51. Nezhat FR, Datta MS, Liu C, Chuang L, Zakashansky K. Robotic radical hysterectomy versus total laparoscopic radical hysterectomy with pelvic lymphadenectomy for treatment of early cervical cancer. JSLS. 2008;12:227–37.
52. Frumovitz M, Ramirez P, Greer M, Gregurich M, Wolf J, Bodurka D. Laparoscopic training and practice in gynecologic oncology among Society of Gynecologic Oncologists members and fellow-in-training. Gynecol Oncol. 2004;94:746–53.
53. Nezhat FR, Datta MS, Liu C, Chuang L, Zakashansky K. Robotic radical hysterectomy versus total laparoscopic hysterectomy with pelvic lymphadenectomy for treatment of early cervical cancer. JSLS. 2008;3:227–37.
54. Holloway RW, Brudie LA, Rakowski JA, Ahmad S. Robotic-assisted resection of liver and diaphragm recurrent ovarian carcinoma: description of technique. Gynecol Oncol. 2011;120:419–22.
55. Malzoni M, Malzoni C, Perone C, Rotondi M, Reich H. Total laparoscopic radical hysterectomy (type III) and pelvic lymphadenectomy. Eur J Gynaecol Oncol. 2004;25(4):525–7.
56. Jackson KS, Das N, Naik R, et al. Laparoscopically assisted radical vaginal hysterectomy vs. radical abdominal hysterectomy for cervical cancer: a match controlled study. Gynecol Oncol. 2004;95(3):655–61.
57. Pomel C, Atallah D, Le Bouedec G, Lopes AD, Godfrey KA, Hatem MH, et al. Laparoscopic radical hysterectomy for invasive cervical cancer: 8-year experience of a pilot study. Gynecol Oncol. 2003;91(3):534–9.
58. Malur S, Possover M, Schneider A. Laparoscopically assisted radical vaginal versus radical abdominal hysterectomy type II in patients with cervical cancer. Surg Endosc. 2001;15(3):289–92.
59. Ghezzi F, Cromi A, Ciravolo G, Volpi E, Uccella S, Rampinelli F, et al. Surgicopathologic outcome of laparoscopic versus open radical hysterectomy. Gynecol Oncol. 2007;106:502–6.
60. Li G, Yan X, Shang H, Wang G, Chen L, Han Y. A comparison of laparoscopic radical hysterectomy and pelvic lymphadenectomy and laparotomy in the treatment of Ib-IIa cervical cancer. Gynecol Oncol. 2007;105(1):176–80.
61. Advincula AP, Reynolds RK. The use of robot-assisted laparosocpic hysterectomy in the patient with a scarred or obliterated anterior cul-de-sac. JSLS. 2005;9:287–91.
62. Farquhar CM, Steiner CA. Hysterectomy rates in the United States, 1990–1997. Obstet Gynecol. 2002;99:229–34.
63. Wilcox LS, Koonin LM, Pokras R, et al. Hysterectomy in the United States, 1988–1990. Obstet Gynecol. 1994;83:549–55.
64. Lepine LA, Hillis SD, Marchbanks PA, Koonin LM, Morrow B, Kieke BA, et al. Hysterectomy surveillance—United States, 1980–1993. MMWR CDC Surveill Summ. 1997;46:1–15.
65. Reich H, Decaprio J, McGlynn F. Laparoscopic hysterectomy. J Gynecol Surg. 1989;5:213–6.
66. Wattiez A, Cohen SB, Selvaggi L. Laparoscopic hysterectomy. Curr Opin Obstet Gynecol. 2002;14:417–22.
67. Matthews CA. Robot-assisted laparoscopic colposacropexy and cervicosacropexy with the da Vinci surgical system. Surg Technol Int. 2010;20:232–8.
68. Moreno Sierra J, Galante Romo I, Ortiz Oshiro E, Núñez Mora C, Silmi Moyano A. Robotic assisted laparoscopic colposacropexy in the treatment of pelvic organ prolapse. Arch Esp Urol. 2007;60(4):481–8.
69. Ascher-Walsh CJ, Capes TL. Robot-assisted laparoscopic myomectomy is an improvement over laparotomy in women with a limited number of myomas. J Minim Invasive Gynecol. 2010;17(3):306–10.
70. Nezhat C, Lavie O, Lemyre M, Unal E, Nezhat CH, Nezhat F. Robot-assisted laparoscopic surgery in gynecology: scientific dream or reality? Fertil Steril. 2009;91:2620–2.

71. Falcone T, Goldberg JM. Robotics in gynecology. Surg Clin North Am. 2003;83:1483–9.
72. Degueldre M, Vandromme J, Huong PT, Cadiere GB. Robotically assisted laparoscopic micro-surgical tubal reanastomosis: a feasibility study. Fertil Steril. 2000;74:1020–3.
73. Falcone T, Goldberg JM, Margossian H, Stevens L. Robotic-assisted laparoscopic microsurgi-cal tubal anastomosis: a human pilot study. Fertil Steril. 2000;73:1040–2.
74. Field JB, Benoit MF, Dinh TA, Diaz-Arrastia C. Computer-enhanced robotic surgery in gyne-cologiconcology. Surg Endosc. 2007;21:244–6.
75. Goldberg JM, Falcone T. Laparoscopic microsurgical tubal anastomosis with and without robotic assistance. Hum Reprod. 2003;18:145–7.
76. Nezhat C, Lavie O, Hsu S, Watson J, Barnett O, Lemyre M. Robotic-assisted laparoscopic myomectomy compared with standard laparoscopic myomectomy: a retrospective matched control study. Fertil Steril. 2009;91:556–9.
77. Nezhat C, Lavie O, Lemyre M, Gemer O, Bhagan L. Laparoscopic hysterectomy with and without a robot: Stanford experience. JSLS. 2009;13:125–8.
78. Tinelli A, Malvasi A, Gustapane S, Buscarini M, Gill IS, Stark M, Nezhat FR, Mettler L. Robotic assisted surgery in gynecology: current insights and future perspectives. Recent Pat Biotechnol. 2011; [Epub ahead of print].

Chapter 7
Robotic-Assisted Surgery Entry in Gynecological Oncology

Farr R. Nezhat and Shao-Chun R. Chang-Jackson

Background

Laparoscopic surgery has profoundly revolutionized the concept of minimally invasive surgery in the last three decades [1]. Studies have clearly shown that laparoscopy has several advantages compared with laparotomy, including faster postoperative recuperation, shorter hospitalization course, cosmetic benefits, improved intraoperative visualization, decreased blood loss, and fewer complications [2, 3]. Despite these factors, several drawbacks exist with conventional laparoscopy. These include two-dimensional views, counterintuitive hand movements, a gradual learning curve, operator fatigue, and tremor amplification [4, 5]. Computer-enhanced telesurgery, called robotic-assisted surgery, is the latest innovation in the minimally invasive surgery field. It attempts to overcome the disadvantages of conventional laparoscopy by offering improved dexterity, coordination, and visualization, and decreasing surgeon fatigue [6].

F.R. Nezhat (✉)
Division of Gynecologic Oncology and Minimally Invasive Surgery, Department of Obstetrics and Gynecology, Columbia University, New York, NY, USA

Division of Gynecologic Oncology, Department of Obstetrics and Gynecology, St. Luke's-Roosevelt Medical Center, New York, NY, USA

S.-C.R. Chang-Jackson
Minimally Invasive Gynecologic Surgery, St. Luke's-Roosevelt Medical Center, New York, NY, USA

A. Tinelli (ed.), *Laparoscopic Entry*,
DOI 10.1007/978-0-85729-980-2_7, © Springer-Verlag London Limited 2012

119

Historical Perspective

Robotic surgery was first used in neurosurgery in 1985. The PUMA 560 was used for neurosurgical stereotactic maneuvers under computed tomography guidance [7]. Urology soon followed, in which the PROBOT was developed to aid in transurethral resection of the prostate through guidance from a preoperatively constructed three-dimensional image [8]. Orthopedic surgery also used a device called ROBODOC to assist in total hip replacement [9]. These predecessors incorporated the robot in a passive role in the operative field. Soon there developed a need for a surgical robot that could be actively controlled by the surgeon.

The current platform of robotic telepresence technology was developed from the collaborative efforts of the Stanford Research Institute, the United States Department of Defense, and the National Aeronautics and Space Administration [10]. Initial prototypes involved robotic arms that could be mounted on an armored vehicle to facilitate remote battlefield surgery.

One of the early predecessors and first applications of robotic-assisted technology to the field of gynecology was a voice-activated robotic arm known as Aesop (Computer Motion, Inc., Goleta, CA). The primary role of Aesop was to operate the camera during laparoscopic surgery. Another predecessor, Zeus (Computer Motion Inc.), involved a system with two "wristed" operating arms and a robotically controlled camera. The operative arms closely mimicked the movements of the human wrist and were controlled by the surgeon at a remote console [11].

Today, the da Vinci Surgical System (Intuitive Surgical, Sunnyvale, CA) is the only actively produced Food and Drug Administration–approved robotic surgical system incorporating an immersive telepresence environment. It has been incorporated into the gynecological armamentarium with increasing frequency. In benign gynecology, it has proved useful in performing intricate procedures in a minimally invasive fashion, such as myomectomies, tubal reanastomoses, complex hysterectomies, and treatment of extensive endometriosis and sacrocolpopexies.

In gynecological oncology, the robot has been increasingly used in a variety of applications, not only for radical hysterectomies in cervical cancer patients, but also for pelvic and paraaortic lymphadenectomies, trachelectomies, and ovarian transposition. In addition, it has been widely used in the management of endometrial and ovarian cancer.

Setup

The setup of the da Vinci Surgical System is based on the principle of robotic telepresence. The main surgeon is seated at a master console away from the operating table, remotely guiding the movements of a patient-side robotic device with a camera arm and two or three operative arms (Fig. 7.1a, b). The latest version, the da Vinci Si model, also supports an assistant surgeon's console. The master console contains two hand controls in which the surgeon's thumb and opposing finger operate the instruments and camera. Each of the hand controls allows complete freedom of upper limb movement in three dimensions, with each movement translated and downscaled into the motions of the robotic arms. The robotic arms are then connected to interchangeable "wristed" robotic instruments.

The master console also contains several foot pedals that are divided into main operational pedals (clutch and camera) and energy source pedals. The left side of the pedal platform contains the former: clutch, instrument switch, and camera motion. The right side of the pedal platform is dedicated to powering the energy sources employed by some of the robotic instruments. The clutch disengages the hand controls of the master console from the robotic arms of the patient-side cart. This allows for continuous optimal positioning of the surgeon's upper limbs during different stages of the operation. The other two left sided foot pedals are the camera motion pedal, allowing repositioning of the robotic camera arm while disengaging all other arms, and the switch pedal, allowing alternate use of two out of the three (or four as in the S and Si model) robotic instrument arms.

The patient is positioned in the modified dorsal lithotomy position with the legs in Allen stirrups to aid in placing a uterine manipulator or sponge stick. The arms

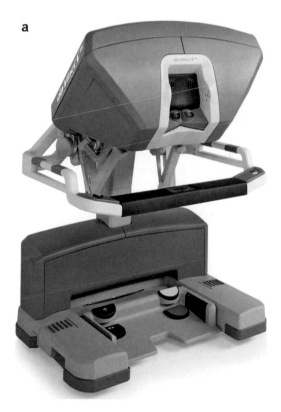

a

Fig. 7.1 Surgeon's console (**a**) and patient-side cart (**b**) (With permission from Intuitive Surgical, Inc, 2011)

b

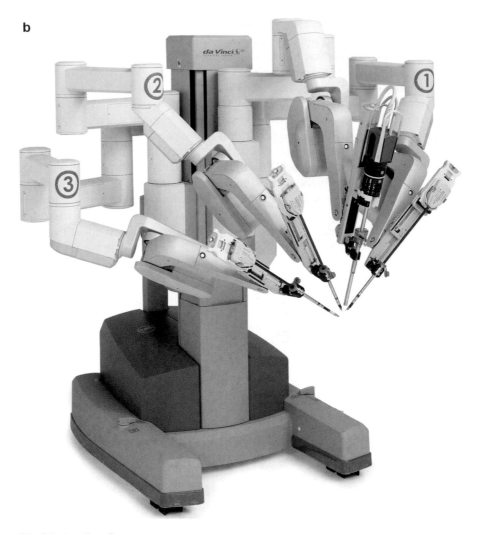

Fig. 7.1 (continued)

are usually tucked at the patient's sides to allow robot docking and bedside surgical assistance. Either the patient is strapped to the table or other anti-skid measures are employed to prevent patient movement during steep Trendelenburg positioning. A nasogastric or orogastric tube is usually placed to evacuate gastric contents, especially in cases of left upper quadrant entry.

The docking of the da Vinci patient cart is often the most cumbersome and precise part of the procedure. The side-docking method has been incorporated into gynecological surgery to aid in vaginal surgery, uterine manipulation, performing cystoscopy, or accessing the rectum. The parallel side-docking method has been used, in which the base of the patient-side cart is directly adjacent to the base of the operating table. The column of the patient-side cart is advanced to at least the level of the knee, if not more superior, to allow the camera port to be inserted through the umbilicus. It may be adjusted accordingly if the camera port is moved superiorly to accommodate upper abdominal procedures. The camera arm is then aligned to the midline of the patient. The remaining operative arms are attached systematically, with the numbers labeling the operative arms facing in the opposite direction of the side that the patient side-cart is situated.

Accurate port placement is essential in a robotic assisted procedure. If the robotic ports are placed incorrectly, either operative arm collision will occur or the wristed instruments will not achieve their full dexterity. The robotic endoscope enters the abdominal cavity through a 12-mm cannula placed at or above the umbilicus. Robotic instruments enter through 5- or 8-mm steel cannulas. The placement of the accessory ports varies with the type of procedure planned.

Procedures involving structures in the pelvic cavity, uteri <14 week size and pelvic lymphadenectomy have similar port placements (Fig. 7.2). A 12-mm port is first placed through the umbilicus for the robotic endoscope. Two 5- or 8-mm steel trocars are then placed 5 cm above and 1 cm medial to the anterior superior iliac crest. If the fourth robotic arm, which is available on the da Vinci *S* and Si systems, is used, the steel trocar can either be placed in the right or left lower quadrant, inferior and lateral to the other robotic instrument port, at least 10 cm apart. Such placement enables optimal movement of the robotic arms, minimizes the risk of collisions, and enables access to the pelvic floor. Robotic monopolar scissors and bipolar forceps may be placed through the bilateral lower quadrant trocars (Fig. 7.3). The electrosurgical scissors allow for dissection and resection, whereas the bipolar forceps are used for traction and electrodessication. A nonenergized instrument may be placed through the upper quadrant port such as forceps or a retractor. A 5- to 12-mm assistant port is also placed 1–2 cm above the camera port, between the camera port and one of the 8-mm trocars. Through this port, the assistant can introduce suture, instrumentation used for retraction, a suction/irrigator, vessel-sealing device, surgical clip applicator, or laparoscopic specimen bag.

For procedures extending above the pelvic brim such as sacrocolpopexies, uteri >14 weeks, paraaortic lymphadenectomy, or upper abdominal procedures, trocar placement must be modified, with the camera port placed approximately 5–8 cm above the umbilicus and the other trocars adjusted accordingly, based on the different camera port placement (Fig. 7.4).

Gynecological Oncology

Cervical Cancer

There is a rapidly growing body of literature for robotic procedures in treating cervical cancer, as there appears to be more of a need for complex and intricate procedures in the management of this malignancy. Robotic surgery specifically allows fine tissue dissection necessary in such procedures as ureterolysis and pelvic and paraaortic lymphadenectomy (Fig. 7.5a, b). Since Sert and Abeler reported the first

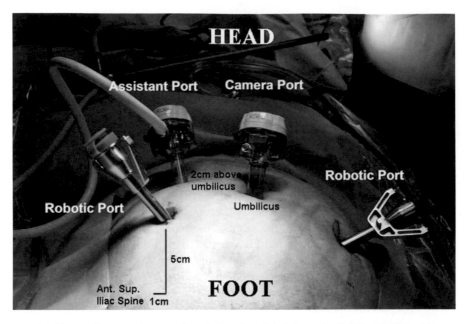

Fig. 7.2 Trocar placement for procedures below the pelvic brim and pelvic lymphadenectomy

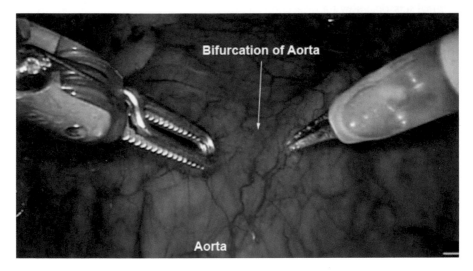

Fig. 7.3 Electrosurgical scissors and bipolar forceps, the common robotic instruments used for fine tissue manipulation and dissection

case of a robotic-assisted laparoscopic radical hysterectomy and pelvic lymph-adenectomy in 2006, there have been a number of articles published regarding robotic-assisted laparoscopic hysterectomy, pelvic and paraaortic lymphadenec-tomy, trachelectomy, parametrectomy, and ovarian transposition [12, 13].

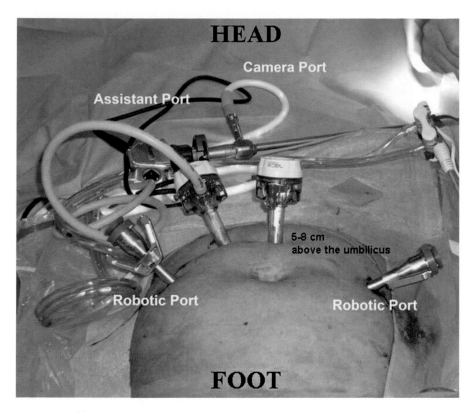

Fig. 7.4 Trocar placement for procedures above the pelvic brim and paraaortic lymphadenectomy

Sert and Abeler's procedure lasted 445 min, EBL was 200 mL and 22 lymph nodes were removed. No major complications were noted. In several case series describing robotic-assisted laparoscopic radical hysterectomy since then, the operative times have been between 355 and 390 min and average blood loss between 207 and 300 mL [14, 15].

Comparison with Laparoscopy and Laparotomy

When comparing robotic-assisted radical hysterectomy and pelvic lymphadenectomy with laparoscopic procedures, the results are either comparable or robotic procedures are found to be superior. Nezhat and co-workers found operative time, estimated blood loss, and hospital stay to be equivalent. Sert and Abeler have shown that robotic procedures are technically feasible and offer similar histopathological results, including number of lymph nodes, parametrial tissue, and vaginal cuff size. They also found that robotic-assisted laparoscopy was associated with decreased blood loss and shorter hospital recovery when compared with laparoscopy [16, 17].

When comparing robotic-assisted radical hysterectomy and pelvic lymphadenectomy to laparotomy, multiple studies have shown that robotic procedures are associated

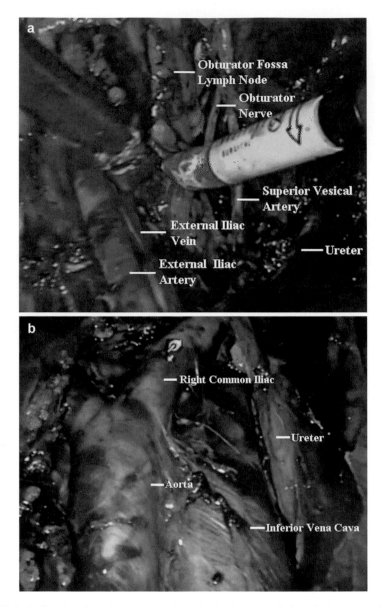

Fig. 7.5 Robotic pelvic lymphadenectomy (**a**) and robotic paraaortic lymphadenectomy (**b**)

with a lower incidence of complications, decreased blood loss, higher lymph node retrieval, shorter hospital recovery, and equivalent outcomes [18–22].

Robotic surgery used to treat cervical cancer is similar to laparoscopic surgery in the types of complications encountered. Cho and Nezhat reviewed the literature and noted that the most common complications occurring with robotic surgeries are lymphocysts/lymphoceles, pelvic infection and vaginal cuff complications. In comparison, procedures performed via laparotomy involve wound and gastrointestinal complications [13].

Fertility-Sparing Surgery

Robotic surgery has also been found to be useful in preserving fertility in early-stage cervical cancer patients. The dexterity and fine dissection achieved with the robot has been used successfully in performing radical trachelectomies [13]. There was also one case report describing the feasibility of using robotic technology for ovarian transposition [23]. The patient was a 32-year-old para 0 who had previously undergone a robotic-assisted hysterectomy and pelvic lymphadenectomy for treatment of Stage 1B1 squamous cell carcinoma of the cervix. After review of the final pathology, pelvic radiation was indicated. The patient underwent successful ovarian transposition to the bilateral pericolic gutters with the ovarian ligaments transfixed to the psoas muscles. No intraoperative or postoperative complications were noted.

Endometrial Cancer

Minimally invasive techniques have been used more frequently in the management of uterine malignancy. The Gynecologic Oncology Group has conducted a randomized prospective study comparing laparoscopy with laparotomy in the surgical treatment of uterine cancer (LAP2) and reported that laparoscopy is feasible and safe in terms of short-term outcomes and results in fewer complications and shorter hospital stay. They are continuing to collect data on long-term survival and recurrences in the two groups [24].

Comparison with Laparoscopy and Laparotomy

The majority of studies investigating robotic-assisted techniques and management of endometrial cancer have been case series, with more current studies evaluating the difference between laparoscopy and laparotomy [13]. When compared with laparotomy, robotic-assisted laparoscopic hysterectomy was associated with decreased blood loss (105 versus 241 mL), shorter hospital stay (1 versus 3.2 days), and fewer complications (3.6% versus 20.8%) [25]. In comparison with standard laparoscopy to treat early-stage endometrial cancer, robotic-assisted laparoscopy had significantly decreased median estimated blood loss (88 versus 200 mL), hospital stay (1 versus 2 days), operative time (242 versus 287 min), transfusion rate (3% versus 18%) and conversion to laparotomy (12% versus 26%) [25].

The most common complications noted with robotic surgery in treating endometrial cancer are conversion to laparotomy, vaginal cuff complications, and lymphocyst/

lymphocele complications. These are similar to the complications encountered with laparoscopic surgery. The unique complications affecting laparotomy procedures involve the incision and infectious issues [13].

Utility in the Morbidly Obese Patient

The robotic technique can also be useful in morbidly obese patients with endometrial cancer. As basal metabolic index increases in the morbidly obese patient, pathophysiological changes add complexity and risk to laparoscopic surgery. The aim of laparoscopic surgery in this patient population is to decrease surgical morbidity while also performing the procedure in the most thorough and efficient manner possible. Robotic-assisted surgery has made this goal feasible by giving the surgeon added dexterity and visualization, which is often difficult to achieve in obese patients secondary to the central fat distribution.

Studies have shown that when robotic surgery in obese patients is compared with laparoscopy, robotic surgeries have shorter operative times, less blood loss, and increased lymph node retrieval. When compared with laparotomy, robotic surgeries have decreased blood loss, hospitalization time, complication rate, and wound problems (Fig. 7.6) [13].

Ovarian Cancer

The data on the application of robotic technology for ovarian cancer staging is scant. There are only case reports or series in the literature documenting the experience with ovarian carcinoma and robotic-assisted laparoscopy [13]. Diaz-Arrastia et al., Kho et al., Lambaudie et al., Field et al., Veljovich et al., and Reynolds et al. all included ovarian cancer in their case series analysis, and reported anywhere from 1 to 64 patients, with no subgroup analysis specifically for ovarian cancer patients [20, 26–30]. The average operative time and blood loss was not specifically reported for the subset of ovarian cancer patients [13].

Advantages of Robotic Surgery

The development of surgical robotics is a dynamic process, a constant interplay between clinical need and technological capability [1]. As minimally invasive surgery becomes the standard rather than just a passing trend, robotic surgery will be used even more frequently. Robotic surgery has already overcome some of the limitations of conventional laparoscopy, such as the restricted degree of movement and the two-dimensional visual field. The robotic-assisted system also provides magnified stereovision, 7 degrees of freedom in the wristed instruments, and tremor [31].

Fig. 7.6 Well-healed trocar incision scars in a patient with BMI 50 and endometrial cancer, 2 months after robotic staging

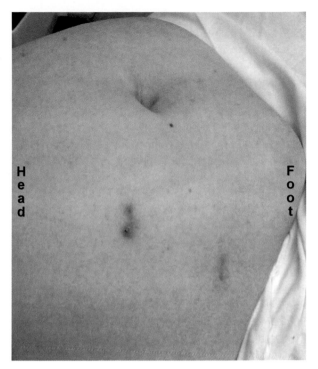

The improvement in surgeon ergonomics markedly decreases surgeon fatigue. These advantages over conventional laparoscopy may improve surgeon performance during complex suturing, tissue manipulation, and fine dissection that is necessary in complex gynecological oncology surgeries. In addition, unlike laparoscopy, robotics has the potential for telementoring and telesurgery. The first telesurgery, a robotic cholecystectomy, was performed in 2001, in which the patient was in France and the surgeon was in New York [32]. This may open the doors for future surgeries in areas in which experienced surgeons are limited. The remote console can also be modified into a teaching module where a primary surgeon can instruct a trainee.

Limitations of Robotic Surgery

However, there are several drawbacks of the present da Vinci Surgical System that deserve mention. One of these disadvantages is the lack of tactile feedback. This accounts for approximately 11% of ruptured suture materials [33]. The surgeon must also take care to avoid strangulation of tissue, which is of particular importance when performing total laparoscopic hysterectomy, during closure of the vaginal cuff. When using the fourth robotic arm, the surgeon must also be cognizant of the location of this operative arm, especially when it is away from the visual field. The surgical robotic arms may overlap, crushing vital structures. With the loss of haptic feedback, there may be delayed recognition of this injury. The loss of haptics can be overcome with more experience, training, and increasing vigilance of the surgical field.

The robotic three-dimensional visual system is designed in such a way currently that the surgeon may have tunnel vision when operating. The loss of peripheral vision may cause inadvertent injury. Again, increasing awareness of the entire surgical field will help overcome this limitation.

Another recently noted complication has been unintended monopolar thermal injury related to aberrant conduction of energy through the shaft of the robotic shears. To avoid this complication, the surgeon must take particular care to avoid contact of vital structures to any area but the intended operative tip of the instrument.

Seamon and co-workers demonstrated that more conversions are expected during the initial transition to robotics; beyond the 65th percentile of procedures, no conversions were seen [34]. Secondly, the high cost of the system is often a deterrent. The substantial financial cost of robotics compared with conventional laparoscopy causes practical barriers to its use. The average unit costs about two million dollars, with the instruments averaging $2,000 per 10 uses. There are scant data regarding the financial impact of the robot, although Bell et al. reported that laparotomy procedures were costlier than robotic procedures because of the increased length of hospital stay [35]. As robotic technology becomes more familiar and prevalent, the cost of supplies and equipment may decrease.

Robotic surgery can improve the learning curve of surgeons attempting to learn advanced laparoscopy techniques compared with the learning curve for standard laparoscopy [36]. However, extreme care must be taken regarding the conclusions that are drawn from some studies examining robotic surgery. There is a distinction that must be made between surgeons that have been trained in conventional laparoscopy first and then make the transition to robotic surgery. These surgeons already have the fundamental skills enabling them to handle robotic technology easier. This can lead to improved outcomes over a gynecological oncologist who does not have the same experience. Therefore, it is misleading to state that robotics is better than laparoscopy overall, unless specific circumstances or individuals specify otherwise. Caution must be taken in advocating robot technology as being superior to the traditional methods without examining the data critically.

The Future

Robotics presents a new paradigm in the field of minimally invasive surgery, but like any novel technology, it has its advantages and limitations. The initial experiences with case series and cohort studies appear promising, but with the lack of randomized prospective studies, there continues to be the need for further research in this field. In terms of gynecological oncology procedures, long-term outcome studies comparing robotic, laparoscopic, and laparotomy approaches also need to be evaluated. In the modern era of minimally invasive techniques, current developments in surgical robotics represent only the initial attempts to simplify complex laparoscopic procedures. Much research is still needed to fully appreciate the potential of robotics in the operating arena and adequately train the surgeons of the future.

References

1. Nezhat C, Nezhat F, Nezhat CH. Nezhat's operative gynecologic laparoscopy with hysteroscopy. New York: Cambridge University Press; 2008.
2. Paraiso MF, Walters MD, Rackley RR, Melek S, Hugney C. Laparoscopic and abdominal sacral colpopexies: a comparative cohort study. Am J Obstet Gynecol. 2005;192:1752–8.
3. Mais V, Ajossa S, Guerriero S, Mascia M, Solla E, Melis GB. Laparoscopic versus abdominal myomectomy: a prospective, randomized trial to evaluate benefits in early outcome. Am J Obstet Gynecol. 1996;174:654–8.
4. Stylopoulos N, Rattner D. Robotics and ergonomics. Surg Clin North Am. 2003;83:1321–37.
5. Desimone CP, Ueland FR. Gynecologic laparoscopy. Surg Clin North Am. 2008;88:319–41.
6. Nezhat C, Saberi NS, Shahmohamady B, Nezhat F. Robotic-assisted laparoscopy in gynecological surgery. JSLS. 2006;10:317–20.
7. Kwoh YS, Hou J, Jonckheere EA, Hayati S. A robot with improved absolute positioning accuracy for CT guided stereotactic brain surgery. IEEE Trans Biomed Eng. 1988;35:153–60.
8. Davies BL, Hibberd RD, Coptcoat MJ, Wickham JE. A surgeon robot prostatectomy: a laboratory evaluation. J Med Eng Technol. 1989;13:273–7.
9. Bauer A, Borner M, Lahmer A. Clinical experience with a medical robotic system for total hip replacement. In: Nolte LP, Ganz R, editors. Computer assisted orthopedic surgery. Bern: Hogrefe & Huber; 1999. p. 128–33.
10. Satava RM. Robotic surgery: from past to future–a personal journey. Surg Clin North Am. 2003;83:1491–500.
11. Advincula AP, Song A. The role of robotic surgery in gynecology. Curr Opin Obstet Gynecol. 2007;19:331–6.
12. Sert BM, Abeler VM. Robotic-assisted laparoscopic radical hysterectomy (Piver type III) with pelvic node dissection—case report. Eur J Gynaecol Oncol. 2006;27:531–3.
13. Cho JE, Nezhat FR. Robotics and gynecologic oncology: review of the literature. J Minim Invasive Gynecol. 2009;16:669–81.
14. Kim YT, Kim SW, Hyung WJ, Lee SJ, Nam EJ, Lee WJ. Robotic radical hysterectomy with pelvic lymphadenectomy for cervical carcinoma: a pilot study. Gynecol Oncol. 2008;108:312–6.
15. Fanning J, Fenton B, Purohit M. Robotic radical hysterectomy. Am J Obstet Gynecol. 2008;198:649. e1-4.
16. Sert BM, Abeler VM. Robotic radical hysterectomy in early-stage cervical carcinoma patients, comparing results with total laparoscopic radical hysterectomy cases. The future is now? Int J Med Robot. 2007;3:224–8.
17. Nezhat FR, Datta MS, Liu C, Chuang L, Zakashansky K. Robotic radical hysterectomy versus total laparoscopic radical hysterectomy with pelvic lymphadenectomy for treatment of early cervical cancer. JSLS. 2008;12:227–37.
18. Zakashansky K, Chuang L, Gretz H, Nagarsheth NP, Rahaman J, Nezhat FR. A case-controlled study of total laparoscopic radical hysterectomy with pelvic lymphadenectomy versus radical abdominal hysterectomy in a fellowship training program. Int J Gynecol Cancer. 2007;17:1075–82.
19. Boggess J, Gehrig P, Cantrell L, et al. A case control study of robotic assisted type III radical hysterectomy with pelvic lymph node dissection compared with open radical hysterectomy. Am J Obstet Gynecol. 2008;19:357–9.
20. Lambaudie E, Houvenaeghel G, Walz J, et al. Robot- assisted laparoscopy in gynecologic oncology. Surg Endosc. 2008;22:2743–7.
21. Ko EM, Muto MG, Berkowitz RS, Felmate CM. Robotic versus open radical hysterectomy: a comparative study at a single institution. Gynecol Oncol. 2008;111:425–30.

22. Magrina JF, Kho RM, Weaver AL, Montero RP, Magtibay PM. Robotic radical hysterectomy: comparison with laparoscopy and laparotomy. Gynecol Oncol. 2008;109:86–91.
23. Molpus KL, Wedergren JS, Carlson MA. Robotically assisted endoscopic ovarian transposition. JSLS. 2003;7:59–62.
24. Walker JL, Piedmonte MR, Spirtos NM, et al. Laparoscopy compared with laparotomy for comprehensive surgical staging of uterine cancer: gynecologic oncology group study LAP2. J Clin Oncol. 2009;27:5331–6.
25. DeNardis SA, Holloway RW, Bigsby GE, Pikaart DP, Ahmad S, Finkler NJ. Robotically assisted laparoscopic hysterectomy versus total abdominal hysterectomy and lymphadenectomy for endometrial cancer. Gynecol Oncol. 2008;111:412–7.
26. Diaz-Arrastia C, Jurnalov C, Gomez G, Townsend Jr C. Laparoscopic hysterectomy using a computer-enhanced surgical robot. Surg Endosc. 2002;16:1271–3.
27. Kho RM, Hilger WS, Hentz JG, Magtibay PM, Magrina JF. Robotic hysterectomy: technique and initial outcomes. Am J Obstet Gynecol. 2007;197:113. e1-4.
28. Field JB, Benoit MF, Dinh TA, Diaz-Arrastia C. Computer-enhanced robotic surgery in gynecologic oncology. Surg Endosc. 2007;21:244–6.
29. Veljovich DS, Paley PJ, Drescher CW, Everett EN, Shah C, Peters 3rd WA. Robotic surgery in gynecologic oncology: program initiation and outcomes after the first year with comparison with laparotomy for endometrial cancer staging. Am J Obstet Gynecol. 2008;198:679. e1-9; discussion 679. e9-10.
30. Reynolds RK, Burke WM, Advincula AP. Preliminary experience with robot-assisted laparoscopic staging of gynecologic malignancies. JSLS. 2005;9:149–58.
31. Marchal F, Rauch P, Vandromme J, Laurent I, Lobontiu A, Ahcel B, et al. Telerobotic-assisted laparoscopic hysterectomy for benign and oncologic pathologies: initial clinical experience with 30 patients. Surg Endosc. 2005;19:826–31.
32. Marescaux J, Leroy J, Gagner M, et al. Transatlantic robot-assisted telesurgery. Nature. 2001;413:379–80.
33. Degueldre M, Vandromme J, Huong PT, Cadière GB. Robotically assisted laparoscopic microsurgical tubal reanastomosis: a feasibility study. Fertil Steril. 2000;74:1020–3.
34. Seamon LG, Bryant SA, Rheaume PS, et al. Comprehensive surgical staging for endometrial cancer in obese patients: comparing robotics and laparotomy. Obstet Gynecol. 2009;114: 16–21.
35. Bell MC, Torgerson J, Seshadri-Kreaden U, Suttle AW, Hunt S. Comparison of outcomes and cost for endometrial cancer staging via traditional laparotomy, standard laparoscopy and robotic techniques. Gynecol Oncol. 2008;111:407–11.
36. Cho JE, Shamshirsaz AH, Nezhat C, Nezhat C, Nezhat F. New technologies for reproductive medicine: laparoscopy, endoscopy, robotic surgery and gynecology. A review of the literature. Minerva Ginecol. 2010;62:137–67.

Chapter 8
Single-Access Surgery: Less Is More?

Tahar Benhidjeb, Michael Stark, Jakob R. Izbicki, and Oliver Mann

Background

Laparoscopic surgery achieved high standards during the twentieth century. It is associated with lower morbidity, less pain, faster recovery, and a shorter hospital stay than open surgery. Is it, despite this achievement, still possible to make abdominal surgery simpler and safer, because it is the goal of every surgeon to minimize patient morbidity while maximizing the beneficial outcomes of the planned procedure? Most of the discomfort and complications associated with open and laparoscopic surgery are caused by the abdominal incisions: The longer is the incision, the stronger is the pain intensity and the higher is the risk for wound infection and hernia. To avoid this, it is necessary to perform surgical procedures without cutting the surface of the body and use natural openings as an entry to the abdomen or other parts of the body. Theoretical advantages of this natural orifice surgery (NOS) include less invasiveness by eliminating abdominal incisions, postoperative abdominal wall pain, wound infection, and hernia. Anthony Kalloo was the first to report an experimental transgastric peritoneoscopy [1]. When the gastroenterologists reached the intraperitoneal cavity through the wall of the stomach, the term *natural orifice transluminal endoscopic surgery* (NOTES) was

T. Benhidjeb (✉)
Department of General, Visceral and Thoracic Surgery, University Medical Center
Hamburg-Eppendorf, Hamburg, Germany

The New European Surgical Academy (NESA), Berlin, Germany

M. Stark
The New European Surgical Academy (NESA), Berlin, Germany

The USP Hospital Palmaplanas of Mallorca, Mallorca, Spain

J.R. Izbicki • O. Mann
Department of General, Visceral and Thoracic Surgery, University Medical Center
Hamburg-Eppendorf, Hamburg, Germany

A. Tinelli (ed.), *Laparoscopic Entry*,
DOI 10.1007/978-0-85729-980-2_8, © Springer-Verlag London Limited 2012

introduced to describe procedures performed through natural body openings. As soon as other body openings became the target, this term became irrelevant because the vagina, for example, cannot be described as a lumen. The acronym NOS is therefore more appropriate and includes also the transgastric approach [2]. Parallel to the American Natural Orifice Surgery Consortium for Assessment and Research (NOSCAR) group, the New European Surgical Academy (NESA) established in Berlin on June 23, 2006 the first European-based NOS working group [3, 4]. During the first meeting the NOS concept and published experimental achievements have been presented and discussed and the pharmacological and physiological challenges concerning the transgastric and transvaginal approach have been considered. The NOS working group decided to focus on the use of the transvaginal approach in women because the Douglas pouch offers relatively easy and safe access to the peritoneal cavity (see further details in Chap. 13). This was also the preferred approach for many other authors to perform the first cholecystectomy or appendicectomy using the hybrid technique [5–7]. However, the NOSCAR group and very few other authors got involved with the transgastric route, which turned out to be a technical challenge, because current flexible endoscopes and instruments are quite restricted in design and too unstable in the peritoneal cavity [8]. The ability to manipulate, cut, and sew tissue is especially challenging when working through the gastrointestinal tract, which is both long and flexible, and is only possible with new technologies. Considering these limitations, some authors switched to transumbilical access and simply called it embryonic natural orifice transumbilical endoscopic surgery (eNOTES) [9–11] or natural orifice transumbilical surgery (NOTUS) [12], with the embryonic notation referring to the umbilical opening in utero. Other names include the single laparoscopic port procedure (SLAPP) [13], single port laparoscopic surgery (SPLS) [14], single-port laparoscopy (SPL) [15], and single laparoscopic incision transabdominal (SLIT) surgery [16]. Endoscopic surgery through the umbilicus is another option when trying to obtain the same cosmetic results. Interestingly, most authors who reported on their experience with single-access surgery claimed to be the first to describe this "new" technique.

History

The idea of single-access surgery through a single dedicated port is not new because it was introduced and practiced by the Austrian endoscopic surgeon Wittmoser in the 1960s for operative thoracoscopic interventions on the autonomic nervous system. He performed a sympathectomy at the sudomotor and vasomotor fibres of the thoracal sympathetic ganglions by means of endoscopy for the upper extremity. For the lower extremity the endoscopic approach became possible with development of the new method of retroperitoneoscopy. Here the endoscope is put in position and the retroperitoneal cavity is inflated with CO_2 until the lumbale ganglions, on the right side between the psoas and vena cava and on the left between the psoas and aorta, are easily accessible [17, 18]. Wheeless is credited with performing the first single-incision tubal ligation, in 1969 [19]. In the 1990s, Pelosi et al. presented may be the first performances of laparoscopic hysterectomy with bilateral salpingo-oophorectomy and appendectomy using a single umbilical puncture. The surgical outcomes demonstrated that the single-puncture technique is a safe and effective procedure [20, 21]. Probably the first reported cases of single-access laparoscopic cholecystectomy were published in 1997, when Navarra et al. described a series of 30 cases performed with two 10-mm trocars placed via a single umbilical incision. The gallbladder was retracted using three traction sutures through the abdominal wall. Even cholangiography was achieved successfully in eight cases [22]. Esposito et al. performed one-trocar appendectomy in 25 patients, positioning only one trocar infraumbilically with the use of a 10-mm operative telescope. The appendix is identified, dissected when necessary, grasped laparoscopically with a 450-mm operative atraumatic instrument introduced through the operative channel of the laparoscope, and then exteriorized through the umbilical cannula. The appendectomy was performed using traditional method outside the abdominal cavity. There was no intraoperative or perioperative mortality or morbidity. The mean overall hospitalization time was 2 days (1–4 days). At a maximal follow-up of 20 months the children have no clinical problems nor any visible scar related to the laparoscopic appendectomy. In conclusion, the author considered the one-trocar appendectomy an appropriate alternative procedure to other techniques of laparoscopic appendectomy [23]. Piskun et al. described in 1999 a technique that uses two transumbilical trocars and two transabdominal gallbladder stay sutures and does not require abdominal wall incisions outside the umbilicus [24]. This method was used in 10 patients without complications such as wound infection. Kagaya et al. reported in 2001 on a "Twin-Port" system that allows a 5-mm camera and a forceps to be inserted through a single port for the laparoscopic cholecystectomy procedure. An infraumbilical incision of approximately 10 mm was made to insert the "Twin-Port." After pneumoperitoneum was performed, a 5-mm camera and grasper were inserted to expose the gallbladder. A 5-mm trocar was inserted approximately 1 cm below the xiphoid process, and laparoscopic cholecystectomy was performed via two ports. The gallbladder was removed through the opened "Twin-Port." This method was performed in 40 patients without acute inflammatory gallbladder disease [25].

All of these procedures did not gain popularity because of difficulties such as lack of triangulation, counterintuitive movement secondary to crossing of instruments, clashing of instruments, challenging visualization secondary to an in-line view, and difficulty retracting with flexible instruments owing to force dissipation. Because of these limitations, the initial dissemination of single-access surgery was slow and followed by a long-lasting dwindling of interest. Later, the technically challenging aspect of NOS, particularly the transgastric approach was the main reason for the renaissance of single-access surgery that is nothing else than a "reduced" form of laparoscopic surgery without any relation to NOS, because the umbilicus is not an orifice, but a defect that has been completely closed at birth. Nonetheless, this precise anatomical fact did not bar some authors from doing a "cross-fertilization" by still claiming that the umbilicus is an embryonic orifice and resulting in acronyms, such as eNOTES [9–11, 26] or NOTUS [12]. By now most authors consider single-access surgery as a bridge between traditional laparoscopic surgery and NOS.

Table 8.1 Acronyms associated with single access surgery

eNOTES (embryonic NOTES)
uNOTES (umbilical NOTES)
TUES (TransUmbilical Endoscopic Surgery)
TULA (TransUmbilical Laparoscopic Assisted)
NOTUS (Natural Orifice TransUmbilical Surgery)
OPUS (One Port Umbilical Surgery)
LESS (Laparo-Endoscopic Single-Site Surgery)
SPL (Single Port Laparoscopy)
SPLS (Single Port Laparoscopic Surgery)
SPA (Single Port Access)
SPAS (Single Port Access Surgery)
SLAPP (Single Laparoscopic Port Procedure)
SLIT (Single Laparoscopic Incision Transabdominal Surgery)
SIL (Single Incision Laparoscopy)
SILS (Single Incision Laparoscopic Surgery)
SSL (Single-Site Laparoscopy)
SIMPLE (Single Incision Multi-Port Laparo-Endoscopic surgery)
PSPA (Pure Single Port Access)
TUOL (transumbilical open laparoscopy)
VSUS (Visibly Scarless Urologic Surgery)

Nomenclature

The "re-launch" of single-access surgery has been marred by the lack of an agreed scientific nomenclature, with a resulting profusion of terms/acronyms, none of which are semantically accurate [27]. In the meantime, more than 20 acronyms describing single-access surgery have been reported (Table 8.1).

Taking this into consideration, defined terminology is a primary prerequisite for allowing a comprehensive flow of information among specialists and specialties. Informal discussions among thought leaders and interested specialists have indicated the need for an umbrella group that would lend direction to the rational development of single-access surgery and serve as its driving force [28]. To this end, the Laparoendoscopic Single-Site Surgery Consortium for Assessment and Research (LESSCAR) was formed to serve as an international multidisciplinary ad hoc organization to advance the field of single-access surgery in a cohesive and responsible manner. The primary goal of LESSCAR is to develop the necessary techniques and technology to standardize the clinical outcomes of single-access surgery. The recently published white paper was the result of deliberations that took place during the inaugural meeting of LESSCAR in Cleveland, OH, in July 2008 [28]. To select the most appropriate name/designation for this field, LESSCAR thought the selected name should accurately encompass the following broad concepts: (1) a single entry port; (2) applicability to multiple locations (abdomen, pelvis, thorax); (3) laparoscopic, endoscopic, or robotic surgery; (4) umbilical or extra-umbilical access; (5) an intraluminal and transluminal (percutaneous single-port access) approach; and (6) a broad reach so as to be inclusive, not exclusive. After extensive deliberations, LESSCAR unanimously concluded that the term laparoendoscopic single-site (LESS) surgery most accurately conveys the broad philosophical and practical aspects of the field [28]. To convey all procedural details clearly and fully, all scientific publications on LESS would require a mandatory descriptive second line that succinctly provides all relevant information at the very outset, such as single incision length and location (abdominal [umbilical or extra-umbilical], thoracic, or pelvic); approach (transperitoneal, retroperitoneal, percutaneous intraluminal, or transluminal); number and type of ports used; type of surgery (laparoscopic, endoscopic, or robotic); type of laparoscope used (straight or flexible); type of instruments used (straight, curved, bent, articulating, or flexible); and whether any ancillary instrumentation is used [28]. Parallel to these activities, the industry has begun to adopt and trademark nomenclature of its own. Covidien, Inc. has been calling this technique single-incision laparoscopic surgery (SILS), and Ethicon EndoSurgery, Inc. has proposed the name single-site laparoscopy (SSL). Karl Storz refers to this technique with the new brand name Single Portal (S-PORTAL). It does embrace both single site as well as single port access, catching the similarities, a single portal of entry for the camera and instrumentation. It does not matter where this portal is sited or created; S-PORTAL covers natural as well as surgically created access points. Regardless of the final name that emerges, the current lack of consistent nomenclature has led both industry and individuals to trademark names that will apparently be used for what may be economic gain in the future. In contrast, LESSCAR is undertaking efforts to secure trademark protection for the acronym LESSCAR with the aim not to restrict its use, but rather to ensure that it can be used freely by all individuals, organizations, and institutions that wish to conduct research and use single-access procedures. It is possible that the term's use might be restricted if a for-profit organization were to acquire trademark privileges [28].

Rationale

Single-access surgery is an extension of traditional multi-incision laparoscopic surgery in the quest for reduction of surgical trauma and residual scarring to the patient. The main point for reducing the number of incisions should not only be the esthetic advantage, but also lowered incision risks of the triad "pain, infection, hernia." This leads to the question whether it is realistic to expect such benefits by performing one single incision of at least 20 mm length, located at the umbilicus in almost all cases.

Incisional pain after laparoscopic surgery has been found to dominate over visceral and shoulder pain in both incidence and intensity in the first postoperative week. The findings of a systematic review comparing the effects of minilaparoscopic and conventional laparoscopic cholecystectomy on patient outcomes suggest that reducing the size of trocar incision results in some limited improvements in surgical outcomes [29]. Interestingly, although reduced incisional pain is one of the main points of the rationale for undertaking minilaparoscopic cholecystectomy, only 5 out of 13 studies in the review appeared to have assessed this specifically. Of these, three studies reported reduced pain with minilaparoscopic cholecystectomy [29]. In this systematic review the size of minilaparoscopic instruments used was 2–5 mm, which might tend to result in less pain. Thus, it is barely conceivable that an incision of >20 mm may result in reduced pain intensity.

One of the most frequent causes of morbidity after laparoscopic surgery is wound infection [30], although it is significantly lower than conventional open surgery [31]. Laparoscopic surgery is associated with smaller wounds and minimal tissue damage and, therefore, presumably lowers risk of wound infection (<6%) [32, 33]. The umbilicus has been blamed to be the source of wound infection in the umbilical trocar site, whereas the other trocar sites are usually free from infection [34]. The reason for this is the umbilicus itself, which is an area rich in bacteria. Other reasons seem to be the smaller diameter of the other trocars and the umbilical site being mostly the site for retrieval of specimens [32]. Beside the discomfort that represents omphalitis for the patient, it is a risk factor for the development of incisional umbilical hernia above all.

The true incidence of late-onset port site hernias is difficult to accurately determine because patients may be asymptomatic or lost to follow-up. The reported overall incidence of this phenomenon is 0.65–2.8% in laparoscopic gastrointestinal surgery [35–37]. The risk factors for development of hernia are among others the trocar diameter, and the site of the port. There is a direct correlation between trocar size and the subsequent development of a port site hernia. It is reported that 86.3% of hernias occur in ports of 10 mm or greater diameter and 2.7% in ports <8 mm [37]. In addition, the location of ports is critical to prevent subsequent herniation. The most common site of port site hernias is the umbilical or paraumbilical region (93.7% of port site hernias in post-laparoscopic cholecystectomy) [38]. There is an inherent anatomical weakness in this area because of its embryological function. Traditionally, large ports are inserted here via the Hasson technique to facilitate the introduction of the laparoscope and often retrieval of specimens. This further weakens the integrity of the single layer of fascia at the linea alba [37].

In single-access surgery the 20-mm incision is performed exactly through the anatomical weakness of the umbilicus, which is also used to extract a specimen, such as gallbladder or appendix. Moreover, in most cases it is necessary to enlarge the incision up to 30 mm so as to be able to retrieve a larger specimen, such as colon, kidney, or uterus. Consequently, postoperative hernia formation in single-access surgery will occur at least as often as in traditional laparoscopic surgery.

Devices

The fundamental idea of single-access surgery is to have all of the laparoscopic working ports entering the abdominal wall through the same incision. Multi-lumen ports specifically developed for a single incision approach allow the insertion and interchange of several instruments through a single port while pneumoperitoneum is maintained. The real challenge of this kind of surgery is that it imposes major ergonomic restrictions and limitations such that the level of difficulty in the execution of surgical interventions is much higher with this approach and require extreme dexterity and skill on the part of the surgeon. The ergonomic limitations, which restrict operative maneuverability, are the consequence of both the reduced operating work space imposed by the port (port instrument crowding) and the current generation of straight laparoscopic instruments. Further difficulties include the conflict between the operative instruments, and the camera, the smaller degree of instrument triangulation compared with that of conventional laparoscopic surgery, and the maintenance of pneumoperitoneum. As a result of the limited space with using only a single incision, it is difficult for both the surgeon and the assistant to work in the area.

A wide variety of single-access surgery procedures and platforms have been reported in both the homemade and industry-designed literature. They can be categorized as specialized multilumen ports, angled, and articulating instruments. The following reviews the different industry-designed access platforms that are currently available.

Industry-Designed Access Platforms

TriPort and QuadPort

The TriPort (Olympus Medical, Tokyo, Japan) was the first available access system approved by the U.S. Food and Drug Administration (FDA). The TriPort (Fig. 8.1a, b) and QuadPort (Fig. 8.2) are multichannel ports that allow three or four instruments, respectively, to be inserted [39]. The device is composed of a body wall retractor component and a valve component composed of an elastomeric material that allows instrument passage. The TriPort contains one 12-mm and two 5-mm valves, whereas the QuadPort consists of one 5-mm, one 12-mm, and two 10-mm valves for instrument insertion. In addition, each port also contains an additional insufflation valve and valve for smoke evacuation. To maintain pneumoperitoneum, the ports contain a gelatin material. The TriPort can be deployed in incisions from 12 to 25 mm. A sheath is placed through the fascial opening, and the peritoneal surface of this sheath has a self-expanding ring, allowing the TriPort to remain inside the peritoneum. Because the sheath is adjustable in size, the outer component of the port can be placed snugly against the skin regardless of the abdominal wall thickness. The TriPort is introduced into the abdomen through the fascial defect via an introducer device [40]. Instruments require lubrication to pass through the ports without unnecessary drag. Iodine solution works well because it lubricates but does not coat the laparoscope with material such as a viscous lubricant that obscures the view. The design allows usage in patients with varying abdominal wall thicknesses (up to 10 cm). The presence of valves as opposed to trocars helps to diminish external clashing of instruments. Furthermore, the low profile of the valves allows for curved instruments to be inserted into the abdomen easily [39]. The disadvantages of the TriPort include the relative need for umbilical placement. It may be difficult to pass the introducer through a fascial defect not located at the umbilicus because cephalad distraction of the umbilical stalk allows a 45° angle of approach. This also can be limiting because the target tissue may be too far away for roticulating instruments [40].

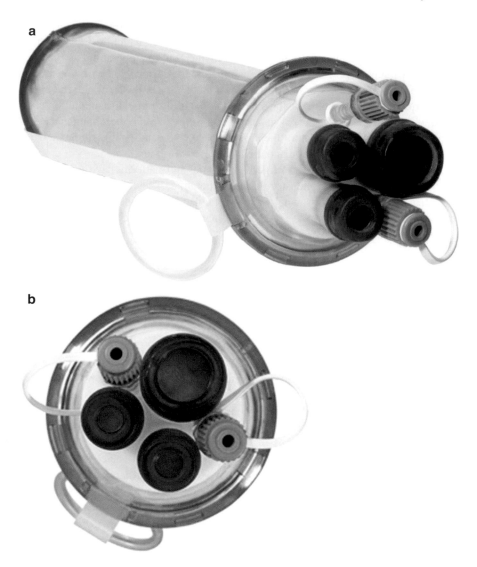

Fig. 8.1 (a, b) TriPort (Courtesy of Olympus Medical, Tokyo, Japan)

SILS Port

The SILS port (Covidien, Inc. Norwalk, CT) is a foam port that, once inserted into the abdominal wall, conforms to the incision size to prevent insufflate leakage (Fig. 8.3a–d). Insertion requires an incision of at least 2 cm. Preplaced spaces within the foam can accommodate either 5- or 12-mm trocars. This allows considerable flexibility in trocar arrangement without resulting in loss of pneumoperitoneum. Because of its foam design, use of this port in obese patients is restrictive

Fig. 8.2 QuadPort (Courtesy
of Olympus Medical, Tokyo,
Japan)

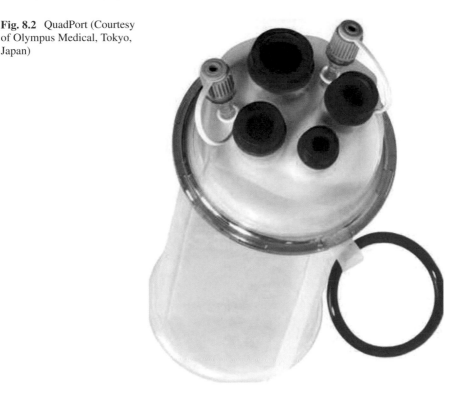

secondary to the increased abdominal wall thickness [39]. Burgos et al. [41]
described their initial experience with the SILS port in performing laparoscopic
prostatectomy. They compared their experience with their previous experience
with the TriPort and noted that the SILS port was easier to place, had less leakage
of pneumoperitoneum and, if required, was easier to reinsert. Conversely, they
noted that less clashing of instruments occurred secondary to the absence of trocars with the TriPort.

Single Site Laparoscopy Access System

The Single Site Laparoscopy (SSL) Access System (Ethicon Endo-Surgery,
Cincinnati, OH) consists of a fixed length wound retractor (available in 2 or 4 cm),
a retractor attachment ring, and a low-profile seal cap (Fig. 8.4). The cap includes
access for two 5-mm and one 15-mm instruments [39]. A 2- to 2.5-cm incision is
required to gain access to the peritoneal cavity. Because of the design of the seal,
trocars are not required, which should decrease the amount of clashing. Furthermore,

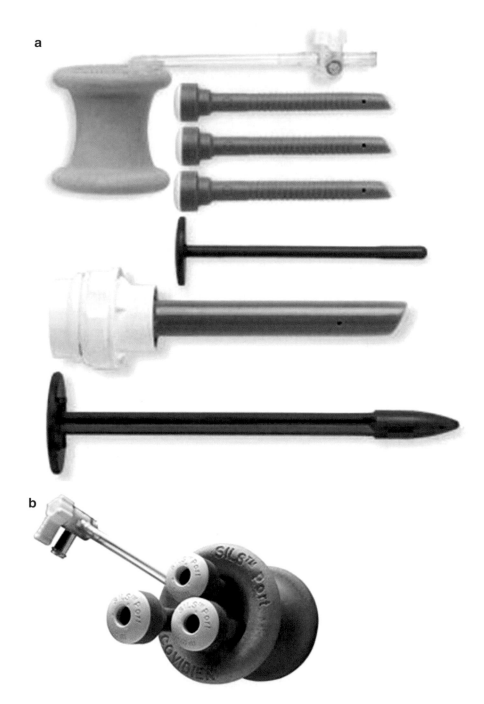

Fig. 8.3 (**a**) SILS Port system (Courtesy of Covidien, Inc. Norwalk, CT). (**b**) SILS Port with inserted trocars (Courtesy of Covidien, Inc.). (**c**) SILS Port in situ (Courtesy of Covidien, Inc.). (**d**) SILS Port in situ with inserted instruments (Courtesy of Covidien, Inc.)

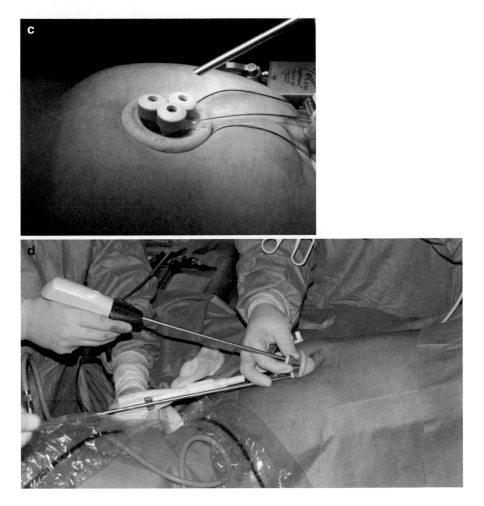

Fig. 8.3 (continued)

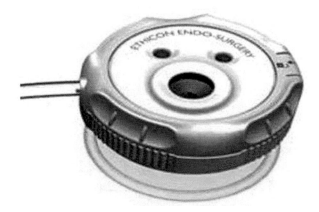

Fig. 8.4 Single site
laparoscopy access system
(Courtesy of Ethicon
Endo-Surgery, Cincinnati,
OH)

the seal cap is capable of rotating 360°, theoretically allowing reorientation of instruments throughout the procedure. The seal cap is removable, allowing easier specimen removal. The authors have no experience using this system. Lim et al. reported their experience using the SSL Access System for performing right hemicolectomy. They reported several advantages, including use of a wide range of instruments secondary to the low-profile seal cap. Furthermore, they state that, at the end of the procedure, the retractor component served as a wound protector during specimen retrieval [39].

X-CONE

X-CONE (Karl Storz, Tuttlingen, Germany), the first and actually only reusable and stable access for transumbilical laparoscopy, offers maximum instrument mobility with minimal access diameter (Fig. 8.5a–c). It is constructed from flaccid polymers and stainless steel. It features a very simple design, a sophisticated and safe and comfortable introduction technique as well as high stability and secure hold in the tissue. However, its centerpiece is the newly designed, X-CONE seal, which centrally stabilizes the telescope while offering full lateral range of motion for the working instruments, rather than fixing them at a pivot point like other sealing systems. Because of its slender design, X-CONE is especially suited for reconstructive procedures. To insert the X-CONE, a mini-laparotomy is performed at the umbilicus using an approximately 2.5-cm long incision and subsequent digital exploration. Afterward, the atraumatic X-CONE halves are successively inserted in a similar manner as retractors and joined to form a sealing cone using a simple pivoting movement. The X-CONE seal is snapped on to seal and protect the assembly against inadvertent loosening. Furthermore, the X-CONE seal permits a particularly flexible use of the instruments while ensuring that all familiar features are still offered. For example, the 5-mm telescope can be switched to one of the working channels, and instruments up to 12.5 mm in size (clip applicator, stapler, etc.) can be inserted via the central port. In combination with X-CONE, special curved instruments permit adequate triangulation, a good overview of the site and exact manipulation both inside and outside of the body. The use of a long telescope creates room for an ergonomic overall setup. The system is fully compatible with three-chip HD cameras and permits optimal image display. Important advantages of this platform compared with the other commercially available ports are the reusability and the ease and rapidity of insertion.

ENDOCONE for Single Portal Laparoscopic Surgery

The ENDOCONE system (Karl Storz, Tuttlingen, Germany), was designed as a holistic solution to enable instrument triangulation, albeit reduced from the ideal 60–30°

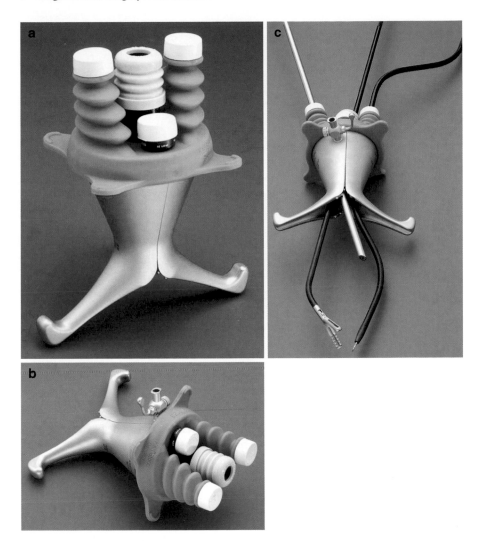

Fig. 8.5 (**a**) X-CONE (Courtesy of Karl Storz, Tuttlingen, Germany). (**b**) X-CONE(Courtesy of Karl Storz). (**c**) X-CONE with inserted angled instruments (Courtesy of Karl Storz)

because of the imposed restricted space imposed by the access port (Fig. 8.6a, b). To achieve this, the shape of the port is complex and consists of a proximal section (cone) leading to a short cylindrical section for negotiation through the abdominal wall and having an outer diameter of 35 mm. This cylindrical section has a protruding rim feature of sufficient width that aids insertion of the ENDOCONE (by a clockwise movement) and ensures secure retention within the abdominal wall. The special features of the port include (1) ease of insertion and extraction; (2) effective hold on and sealing of the abdominal wall permitting sustained pneumoperitoneum; (3) a novel

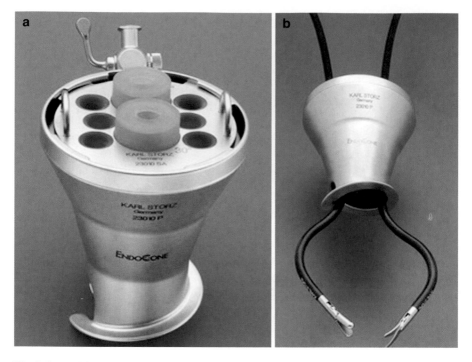

Fig. 8.6 (**a**) ENDOCONE (Courtesy of Karl Storz, Tuttlingen, Germany). (**b**) ENDOCONE with inserted angled instruments (Courtesy of Karl Storz)

patented multivalve seal cap or bulkhead, which provides protected specimen extraction when detached, and enables insertion of several instruments in addition to a 5-mm forward viewing or oblique laparoscope; (4) valves in seal cap admit up to eight instruments of 3-, 5-, and 10-mm diameter; (5) integral insufflations port; and (6) its own dedicated first-generation of proximally deviating (to increase operative space between the two hands of the surgeon) curved coaxial instruments. The ENDOCONE is inserted though a 35-mm incision along the lower margin of the umbilical pit. After mobilization and proximal lifting of the umbilicus, the linea alba is incised over a distance of 30 mm and the peritoneum opened to enable corkscrew insertion of the ENDOCONE using a clockwise movement. Thereafter the abdomen is insufflated through the dedicated insufflations point on the port and the instruments inserted.

GelPOINT

The GelPOINT (Applied Medical, Rancho Santa Margarita, CA) features a GelSeal (Applied Medical) gelatin platform for port placement; an Alexis (Applied Medical) wound retractor for fixation to the abdominal wall; self-retaining, low-profile trocars; and a built-in valve for insufflations (Fig. 8.7a, b). Although similar to the GelPort

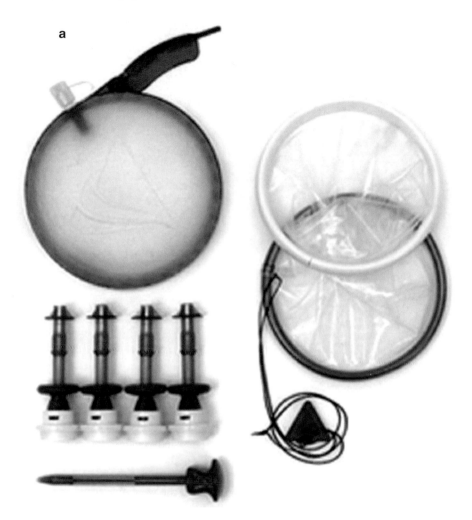

Fig. 8.7 (**a**) GelPOINT port system (Courtesy of Applied Medical, Rancho Santa Margarita, CA). (**b**) GelPOINT port system with inserted trocars (Courtesy of Applied Medical)

Fig. 8.7 (continued) **b**

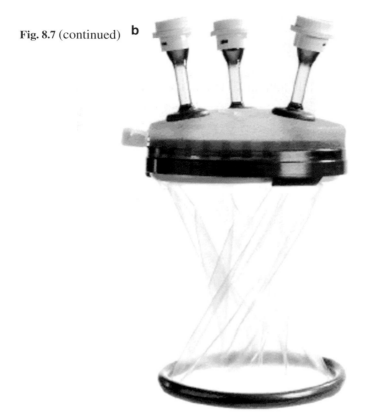

(Applied Medical), which is popular in hand-assisted laparoscopic surgery, the GelPOINT has several important distinctions. It is smaller and does not contain a perforation within the gel cap. An insufflation port is located on the side of the device, thus reducing instrument clashing, and a suture attached to the wound protection apparatus allows for easier platform removal. Potential advantages compared with other platforms may include adaptation to different trocar configurations (a limitless number and size of trocars can be inserted), a larger outer working profile providing less external clashing, and the ability to accommodate to different abdominal wall thicknesses [39].

SPIDER

The Single Port Instrument Delivery Extended Reach (SPIDER; TransEnterix, Inc., Durham, NC) consists of a retractable sheath, two laterally placed instrument delivery tubes that can operate in three dimensions, and two rigid channels (Fig. 8.8). A docking device that serves to attach the SPIDER to the operating table is available separately. This platform differs from the other commercially available devices in that it is able to provide intraabdominal triangulation of instruments. Furthermore, crossing of instruments is not required, and therefore, the right hand controls the

Fig. 8.8 Single Port
Instrument Delivery
Extended Reach=SPIDER
(Courtesy of TransEnterix,
Inc., Durham, NC)

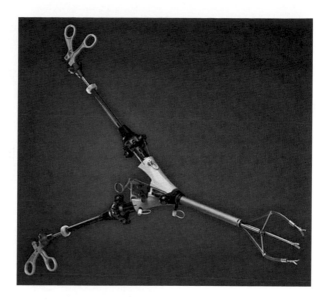

right instrument and vice versa. The device also contains additional ports for insufflation and smoke evacuation. This device is smaller than other access platforms, and therefore may minimize fascial dissection (a 1.8-cm facial incision is required). It also provides articulation of instruments, which is useful, yet may limit retraction of tissues because of force dissipation. The device has been FDA approved [39].

Uni-X

The Uni-X single-port laparoscopic device, recently acquired from Pnavel Systems (Pnavel Systems, Morganville, NJ), is a system that looks like a cow's udder with a design allowing the simultaneous use of three 5-mm laparoscopic instruments through a single fascial incision (Fig. 8.9). The device is funnel shaped, which allows for a wide range of motion because the length of the tunnel through which an instrument can pass is shorter than a standard laparoscopic trocar. The Uni-X system also has a port to allow abdominal insufflation. Fascial fixation sutures are necessary to maintain the device in its position, and accompanying curved laparoscopic instruments are available that may be helpful when multiple instruments are operated through a single incision [40].

OCTO Port

The OCTO Port (Dalim Surgnet, Seoul, South Korea) has not been approved for use in North America, but has received approval in Europe (Fig. 8.10). It consists of an inferior base plate that sits under the skin edge in the peritoneum, an external disc with self retractor, and a detachable transparent silicone cover. It is capable of holding

Fig. 8.9 Uni-X (Courtesy of
Pnavel Systems, Morganville,
NJ)

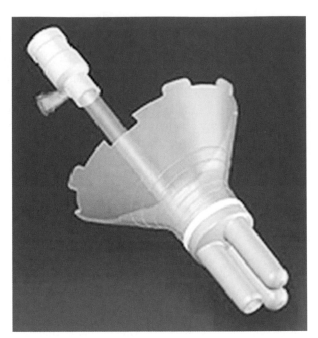

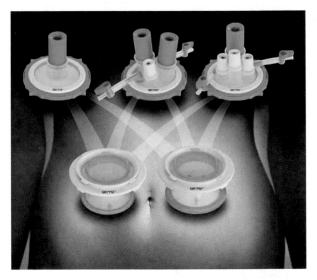

Fig. 8.10 OCTO Port
Modular Laparoscopy System
(Courtesy of Dalim Surgnet,
Seoul, South Korea)

one to four working channels. A separate port is available for smoke evacuation. The cover is easy to remove, thus allowing easy specimen extraction, and is easy to change during the procedure, providing flexibility in terms of the number of instruments that can be used. The cannulas are of different heights, which reduces external clashing of instruments [39].

AirSeal

An access port called AirSeal (SurgiQuest, Orange, CT) involves a technology disruptive to the typical trocar concept. All traditional laparoscopic ports use a mechanical barrier to maintain pneumoperitoneum while allowing instrument passage and limited specimen extraction through their lumen. AirSeal ports do not use a mechanical barrier, but rather a pressure barrier that well exceeds the pneumoperitoneum (Fig. 8.11a). This pressure barrier can be conceptualized as similar to the air curtain blowing down from the ceiling at the entrance of many operating suites. The barrier is created by gas pumped through openings within the housing of the port, creating turbulence that can be regulated and exceeding the pressure of the pneumoperitoneum, thus preventing gas loss, even when instruments and specimens are passed through its lumen. It uses a combination air pump and specialized tubing, with a

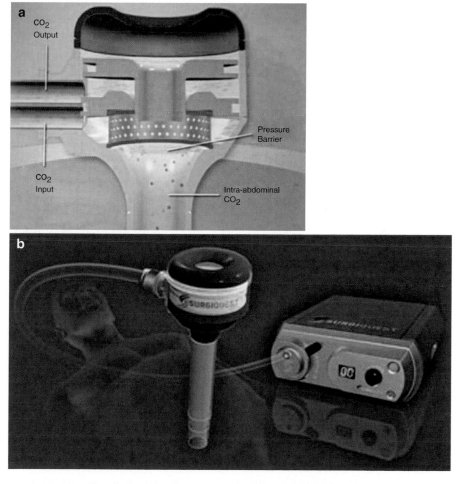

Fig. 8.11 (**a**) AirSeal with pressure barrier to maintain the desired intraabdominal pressure (Courtesy of SurgiQuest, Orange, CT). (**b**) AirSeal with air pump (Courtesy of SurgiQuest)

filter serving to recirculate and filter the carbon dioxide used to create the pneumo-peritoneum (Fig. 8.11b) [39]. AirSeal allows for the passage of multiple or odd-shaped instruments, extracorporeal knot tying without gas loss, and enhanced specimen extraction. The pressure barrier also reduces friction, particularly notice-able with laparoscopic stapling devices. Additionally, it is capable of maintaining operative exposure during suctioning and provides automatic smoke evacuation and filtration. The lack of a mechanical barrier makes it possible to have ports of differ-ent shapes and sizes and has the potential for inclusion with overtubes to maintain regulated insufflation for endoscopic procedures. A 12-mm AirSeal port is FDA approved and currently available on a limited basis in the United States. One down-side of the AirSeal port is the noise associated with the pressure barrier, which is comparable with opening the valve of a standard laparoscopy port [39].

The expense of single-access surgery is a significant issue that may lessen its dissemination. Many centers that perform a high volume of single-access surgeries have chosen to work with a homemade port design, or simply make multiple facial incisions through one larger skin incision. Homemade single ports tend to be made from readily available material in the operating room. One simple and low-cost approach consists of the use of three standard laparoscopic trocars through a single skin incision with multiple fascial puncture sites.

Angled and Articulating Instruments

The ability to triangulate and grasp tissues firmly enough to allow traction and countertraction for exposure and dissection is a basic requirement of surgery. One technical challenge of single-access surgery is limited triangulation and retraction of tissues because of confinement of optics and working instruments to a single axis. The industry is proposing solutions to many of these problems through the development of special curved instruments, and next-generation flexible, articulat-ing, or motorized instruments.

The use of coaxial proximally deviating instruments allows the surgeon to achieve acceptable triangulation, which is not possible with other devices for single port surgery, especially when straight instruments are used. Indeed, according to the specific procedures and situations as well as surgeon's preferences, a combination of curved and straight shaft may be the correct choice (Fig. 8.12). The curvature can also be used to arch over foreground structures to reach the desired anatomical structure, lift and tent tissues, and obtain triangulation and the back of the curvature for atraumatic blunt dissection of tissue planes.

Although almost all angled instruments are reusable, all actually available articulating and flexible instruments are disposable and undergoing continuous design improvements. Articulating instruments include Roticulator (Covidien, Inc. Norwalk, CT), Real Hand (Novare Surgical Systems, Cupertino, CA), Thermaseal (Novare Surgical Systems), Autonomy Laparo-Angle, and endoshears (Cambridge Endo, Framingham, MA).

Covidien, Inc. has a line of instruments that can be articulated and rotated. Their Roticulator line includes a dissector, grasper, and scissors (Fig. 8.13a, b). All three

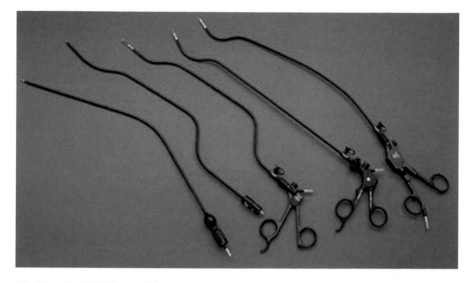

Fig. 8.12 S-PORTAL curved instruments (Courtesy of Karl Storz, Tuttlingen, Germany)

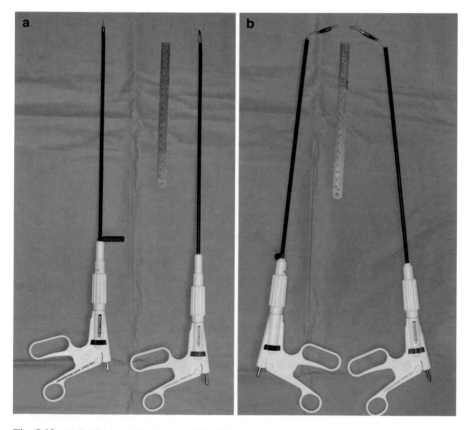

Fig. 8.13 (**a**) Roticulator (Courtesy of Covidien, Inc., Norwalk, CT). (**b**) Roticulator extending the distal part (Courtesy of Covidien, Inc.)

instruments have zero to 80° articulation at the distal end of the shaft. They function by extending the distal part of the instrument shaft beyond its outer sheath. The extended portion is bent, and the more it is extended, the closer it is to 80° articulation. This creates difficulty in performing tasks that require fine motor control, particularly at full articulation. The instruments also have integrated monopolar electrocautery connectors [40].

Novare Surgical Systems, Inc. manufactures the RealHand instrument line. These instruments articulate similar to a human wrist. The surgeon articulates the handle against the fulcrum of the port, and the distal shaft of the instrument articulates in a mirror image fashion using cables that connect the handle to the distal shaft. The multiple degrees of freedom make fine dissection and cutting more feasible than with the Covidien articulating instruments (Fig. 8.14). The RealHand instrument line also is quite broad, including 11 different types of instrument tips. One of these tips is shaped like a curved dissector, but is also capable of cutting and sealing tissue. The Thermaseal 5-mm instrument (Novare Surgical Systems) uses a separate energy source and heats tissue by increasing temperature without an electrical current, using a process the manufacturer terms *thermal ligation* [40].

Cambridge Endo manufactures instruments similar to those in the Novare instrument line. There are four different types of tips, including a needle driver, dissector, scissors, and a monopolar hook. A tissue grasper should be available in the near future. Although some features are different, the basic premise is the same in that the surgeon's hand articulates the distal shaft using the port as a fulcrum [40].

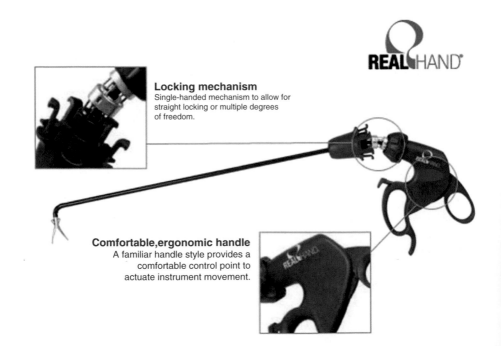

Locking mechanism
Single-handed mechanism to allow for straight locking or multiple degrees of freedom.

REAL HAND

Comfortable,ergonomic handle
A familiar handle style provides a comfortable control point to actuate instrument movement.

Fig. 8.14 RealHand technology (Courtesy of Novare Surgical Systems, Inc. Cupertino, CA)

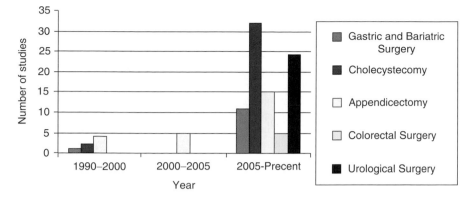

Fig. 8.15 Distribution of single-incision laparoscopic surgery (SILS) studies during the past two decades (Ahmed et al. [26]. Reprinted with permission from Springer Science + Business Media)

Application and Results in Abdominal and Pelvic Surgery

Ahmed et al. recently published the first systematic review collating the evidence on single-access surgery in general surgery, urology, and gynecology [26]. This study was performed according to guidelines from the preferred reporting items for systematic reviews and metaanalyses (PRISMA) [42]. For this, a broad search of the English language literature was performed in October 2009 using the Medline (1950 to date), EMBASE (1980 to date), and PsychINFO (1966 to date) databases. The Cochrane database and Database of Abstracts of Reviews of Effectiveness (DARE) were also reviewed. The research until October 2009 used *single-incision laparoscopic surgery* and related terms as keywords. References from retrieved articles were reviewed to broaden the search. Case reports, case series, and empirical studies that reported procedural outcomes, technical and clinical challenges, and training issues related to single-access surgery in adult abdominal and pelvic surgery were included in the review. Letters, bulletins, and comments were excluded. Number of patients, type of instruments, operative time, blood loss, conversion rate, length of hospital stay, length of follow-up evaluation, and complications were extracted from the reviewed items. The review included 102 studies classified as level 4 evidence according to the Oxford Centre for Evidence-Based Medicine [43]. Most of these studies investigated single-access surgery in cholecystectomy ($n = 34$), appendectomy ($n = 24$), and nephrectomy ($n = 17$) (Fig. 8.15, Table 8.2).

A total of 34 studies reported experiences of SILS *cholecystectomy*, with study populations ranging from 1 to 297 patients in each study. Conventional ports and 5-mm instruments were used most often. Overall, the mean operating time ranged from 30 to 143 min, and blood loss was minimal. The rate of conversion to conventional laparoscopy ranged from 0% to 24%, but only five patients required open surgery. The mean hospital stay ranged from 0 to 4.4 days. The most commonly reported complication was bile leak, with incidences ranging from 0% to 7% [26].

A total of 24 studies investigated the feasibility of SILS *appendectomy* in study populations ranging from 1 to 200 patients. Most surgeons used conventional ports

Table 8.2 Identified current single access surgery procedures [39]

High-volume procedures	Intermediate-volume procedures	Low-volume procedures
Cholecystectomy	Adrenalectomy	Bariatric procedures
Appendectomy	Splenectomy	Myomectomy
Inguinal hernia repair	Hysterectomy	Prostate resection
Oopherectomy	Pelvic organ prolapse	Cystectomy
Salpingectomy	Donor nephrectomy	Partial nephrectomy
Endometriosis surgery	Ureteral re-implant	Retroperitoneal lymph dissect
Tubal ligation	Ileal interposition	Esophageal myotomy
Pyeloplasty	Radical nephrectomy	Distal pancreatectomy
Simple nephrectomy	Small bowel resection	
Renal cyst decortication	Fundoplication	
Ablative renal surgery		
Pelvic lymphadenectomy		
Nephrectomy		
Gastric banding		
Colon resection		

with a variety of different-sized instruments. Overall, the mean operating time ranged from 15 to 88 min. The use of additional ports ranged from 0% to 41%, and the rate of conversion to open appendectomy ranged from 0% to 21%. The hospital stay was 1–7 days. The most common complications were wound infection (range, 0–14%) and intraabdominal abscess (0–7%).

In *gastric surgery*, 11 studies reported outcomes for gastrostomy, gastric banding, and sleeve gastrectomy. The number of patients in each of the three case series ranged from 5 to 22. There were relatively few complications and conversions to conventional laparoscopic or open surgery [26].

There are only few reported papers on single access *colorectal* surgery, most of them being case reports or small patient series. A total of six studies, with study populations ranging from 10 to 36 patients in each study, demonstrated the feasibility and safety of this approach in benign and malignant colorectal tumors as well [44–47]. As an alternative to the standard laparoscopic procedure, single-incision laparoscopic sigmoidectomy via the umbilicus is technically feasible (Fig. 8.16a, b). Single access intestinal resection and anastomosis remain technically challenging even for skilled laparoscopic surgeons. Safe anastomosis and a safe method for specimen removal have impeded the development of SILS in colorectal surgery.

Single-access surgery has been adopted for a wide variety of *urological* procedures along the entire renal tract system. Although 24 studies have reported outcomes for these procedures, the number of patients in each study has been small (range, 1–17). The outcomes of single access nephrectomy were reported in 17 studies. The mean operating time ranged from 90 to 420 min. The mean blood loss ranged from 10 to 420 mL, and the mean length of hospital stay was <3 days in all the studies. The most commonly reported complication was parenchymal bleeding, but this was limited to single cases in four studies. No cases required open surgery,

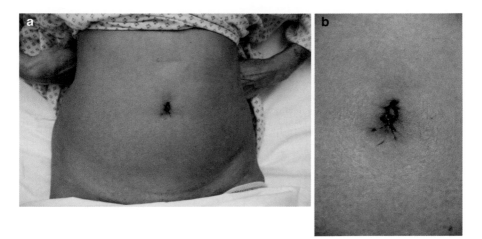

Fig. 8.16 (**a**) Single access transumbilical sigmoid resection for diverticulitis. (**b**) Single access transumbilical sigmoid resection for diverticulitis

but the rate of conversion to conventional laparoscopic surgery ranged from 0% to 33%. Several case series have demonstrated feasibility, a low conversion rate, and a low complication rate for single-access surgery in other urological procedures. However, none of the studies involved more than six patients except for an isolated study investigating outcomes for 15 patients undergoing pyeloplasty [26].

Single-access surgery has been used in *gynecology* as early as 1969, when a laparoscopic tubal ligation was described by Wheeless [19]. Wheeless later reported on 3,600 patients, 2,600 of whom had a one-incision tubal ligation [48].

Park et al. recently reported their initial experience with single access *gynecological* surgeries [49]. In this prospective single-center study, 200 patients underwent single access gynecological surgery (105 total hysterectomies; 11 subtotal hysterectomies; 43 oophorectomies; 31 ovarian cystectomies; five salpingectomies; two myomectomies; and three adhesiolysis only). The median age and body mass index were 45.5 years and 22.9 kg/m², respectively. Single-access surgery was successfully completed in 187 patients without the need for ancillary ports (93.5%). Two patients required a conventional multiport, and nine needed one additional port. Two patients were converted to a laparotomy. One intraoperative and five postoperative complications occurred. The complication rate was 3.2% (6/187). The median operative time was 120 min (54–250) for a total hysterectomy, 180 (150–345) for a subtotal hysterectomy, 60 (27–245) for an oophorectomy, 105 (50–185) for a cystectomy, and 60 (30–115) for a salpingectomy [49]. Single-access surgery is safe and feasible for gynecological indications. However, this prospective observational case series did not show superiority of single-access surgery over conventional laparoscopic procedures.

Jung et al. recently published a randomized prospective study aiming to compare single access hysterectomy and four-port total laparoscopic hysterectomy in terms of postoperative pain. The study enrolled 68 patients who were randomly assigned to one of two groups. Four patients in the single access group were converted to other laparoscopic approaches. The two study groups did not differ in terms of patient demographics and surgical outcomes. Postoperative pain scores, measured using a visual analog scale, did not differ between the two groups. However, significantly higher total requests for analgesics were observed in the single access group (11.3 ± 4.1 versus 7.7 ± 2.7; $p = 0.001$). Compared with four-port total laparoscopic hysterectomy, single access hysterectomy is a feasible approach with comparable operative outcomes. However, reduction of postoperative pain is not evident with this method [50].

Conclusion

The concept of performing laparoscopic surgery via a single incision regardless of the technique is rapidly gaining traction among patients, surgeons, and industry. Although numerous ports (each with its inherent advantages and disadvantages) exist, at present no clear-cut advantage of one port over another has been established. Barring randomized evaluation with appropriate comparative variables, surgeon and institutional preference likely will determine platform selection clinically. At present, the major advantage of single-access surgery is improved cosmetics without visible abdominal scars (Fig. 8.16a, b). Other theoretical and potential benefits include probably shorter operative time, lower costs, and a shortened time to full physical recovery. Multicenter, randomized, prospective studies are needed to compare short- and long-term outcome measures against those of conventional laparoscopic surgery. At this, primary points should be pain, wound infection, hernia, and cosmetics, wherein patient's safety, reliability, and the seriousness of scientific conduct are mandatory.

References

1. Kalloo AN, Singh VK, Jagannath SB, et al. Flexible transgastric peritoneoscopy: a novel approach to diagnostic and therapeutic interventions in the peritoneal cavity. Gastrointest Endosc. 2004;60:114–7.
2. Stark M, Benhidjeb T. Transcolonic endoscopic cholecystectomy: a NOTES survival study in a porcine model. Gastrointest Endosc. 2007;66:208–9.
3. Rattner D, Kalloo A. ASGE/SAGES working group on natural orifice transluminal endoscopic surgery. Surg Endosc. 2006;20:329–33.
4. Stark M, Benhidjeb T. Natural orifice surgery: transdouglas surgery—a new concept. JSLS. 2008;12:295–8.
5. Zorrón R, Filgueiras M, Maggioni LC, et al. NOTES transvaginal cholecystectomy: report of the first case. Surg Innov. 2007;14:279–83.
6. Bessler M, Stevens PD, Milone L, et al. Transvaginal laparoscopically assisted endoscopic cholecystectomy: a hybrid approach to natural orifice surgery. Gastrointest Endosc. 2007;66:1243–5.
7. Marescaux J, Dallemagne B, Perretta S, et al. Surgery without scars: report of transluminal cholecystectomy in a human being. Arch Surg. 2007;142:823–6; discussion 826–27.

8. Swanstrom LL, Whiteford M, Khajanchee Y. Developing essential tools to enable transgastric surgery. Surg Endosc. 2008;22:600–4.
9. Gill IS, Canes D, Aron M, Haber GP, Goldfarb DA, Flechner S, et al. Single-port transumbilical (E-NOTES) donor nephrectomy. J Urol. 2008;180:637–41; discussion 641.
10. Canes D, Desai MM, Aron M, Haber GP, Goel RK, Stein RJ, et al. Transumbilical single-port surgery: evolution and current status. Eur Urol. 2008;54:1020–9.
11. Desai MM, Stein R, Rao P, Canes D, Aron M, Rao PP, et al. Embryonic natural orifice transumbilical endoscopic surgery (E-NOTES) for advanced reconstruction: initial experience. Urology. 2009;73:182–7.
12. Nguyen NT, Reavis KM, Hinojosa MW, Smith BR, Wilson SE. Laparoscopic transumbilical cholecystectomy without visible abdominal scars. J Gastrointest Surg. 2009;13:1125–8.
13. Rao P, Rao S, Rané A, Bondaio F, Rao P. Evaluation of the R-port for single laparoscopic port procedures (SLAPP): a study of 20 cases. Surg Endosc. 2008;22 Suppl 1:S279.
14. Remzi FH, Kirat HT, Kaouk JH, Geisler DP. Single-port laparoscopy in colorectal surgery. Colorectal Dis. 2008;10:823–6.
15. Kaouk JH, Goel RK, Haber GP, Crouzet S, Desai MM, Gill IS. Single-port laparoscopic radical prostatectomy. Urology. 2008;72:1190–3.
16. Nguyen NT, Hinojosa MW, Smith BR, Reavis KM. Single laparoscopic incision transabdominal (SLIT) surgery-adjustable gastric banding: a novel minimally invasive surgical approach. Obes Surg. 2008;18:1628–31.
17. Wittmoser R. Thorakoskopische operationen am mediastinalen vagus. Langenbecks Arch Klin Chir. 1957;287:230–3.
18. Wittmoser R. Endoskopische sympathicotomie bei hyperhidrosis und raynaud-syndrom. Langenbecks Arch Chir. 1973;334:971–2.
19. Wheeless CR. A rapid, inexpensive, and effective method of surgical sterilization by laparoscopy. J Reprod Med. 1969;5:255.
20. Pelosi MA. Laparoscopic hysterectomy with bilateral salpingo-oophorectomy using a single umbilical puncture. N J Med. 1991;88:721–6.
21. Pelosi MA, Pelosi 3rd MA. Laparoscopic appendectomy using a single umbilical puncture (minilaparoscopy). J Reprod Med. 1992;37:588–94.
22. Navarra G, Pozza E, Occhionorelli S, Carcoforo P, Donini I. One-wound laparoscopic cholecystectomy. Br J Surg. 1997;84:695.
23. Esposito C. One-trocar appendectomy in pediatric surgery. Surg Endosc. 1998;12:177–8.
24. Piskun G. Transumbilical laparoscopic cholecystectomy utilizes no incisions outside the umbilicus. J Laparoendosc Adv Surg Tech A. 1999;9:361–4.
25. Kagaya T. Laparoscopic cholecystectomy via two ports using the "Twin-Port" system. J Hepatobiliary Pancreat Surg. 2001;8:76–80.
26. Ahmed K, Wang TT, Patel VM, Nagpal K, Clark J, Ali M, et al. The role of single-incision laparoscopic surgery in abdominal and pelvic surgery: a systematic review. Surg Endosc. 2011;25:378–96.
27. Box G, Averch T, Cadeddu J, Cherullo E, Clayman R, Desai M, et al. Nomenclature of Natural Orifice Transluminal Endoscopic Surgery (NOTES) and Laparoendoscopic Single-Site Surgery (LESS) procedures in urology. J Endourol. 2008;22:2575–81.
28. Gill IS, Advincula AP, Aron M, Caddedu J, Canes D, Curcillo 2nd PG, et al. Consensus statement of the consortium for laparoendoscopic single-site surgery. Surg Endosc. 2010;24:762.
29. McCloy R, Randall D, Schug SA, Kehlet H, Simanski C, Bonnet F, et al. Is smaller necessarily better? A systematic review comparing the effects of minilaparoscopic and conventional laparoscopic cholecystectomy on patient outcomes. Surg Endosc. 2008;22:2541–53.
30. Hasson HM, Rotman C, Rana N, et al. Open laparoscopy: 29 year experience. Obstet Gynecol. 2000;96:763–6.
31. Gaynes RP, Culver DH, Horan TC, et al. Surgical site infection rates in the United States, 1992–1998: the National Nosocomial Infections Surveillance System basic SSI risk index. Clin Infect Dis. 2001;33 Suppl 2:S69–77.
32. Hamzaoglu I, Baca B, Böler DE, Polat E, Özer Y. Is umbilical flora responsible for wound infection after laparoscopic surgery? Surg Laparosc Endosc Percutan Tech. 2004;14:263–7.

33. Schwenk W, Haase O, Neudecker JJ, Müller JM. Short term benefits for laparoscopic colorectal resection. Cochrane Database Syst Rev. 2005;3:CD003145.
34. Voitk AJ, Tsao SG. The umbilicus in laparoscopic surgery. Surg Endosc. 2001;15:878–81.
35. Bowrey DJ, Blom D, Crookes PF, et al. Risk factors and the prevalence of trocar site herniation after laparoscopic fundoplication. Surg Endosc. 2001;15:663–6.
36. Susmallian S, Ezri T, Charuzi I. Laparoscopic repair of access port site hernia after Lap-Band system implantation. Obes Surg. 2002;12:682–4.
37. Barry M, Winter C. Laparoscopic port site hernias: any port in a storm or a storm in any port? Ann Surg. 2008;248:687–8.
38. Nassar AH, Ashkar KA, Rashed AA, et al. Laparoscopic cholecystectomy and the umbilicus. Br J Surg. 1997;84:630–3.
39. Khanna R, White MA, Autorino R, Laydner HK, Isac W, Yang B, et al. Selection of a port for use in laparoendoscopic single-site surgery. Curr Urol Rep. 2011;12(2):94–9.
40. Romanelli JR, Earle DB. Single-port laparoscopic surgery: an overview. Surg Endosc. 2009;23:1419–27.
41. Burgos JB, Flores JA, de la Vega JS, et al. Early experience in laparoscopic radical prostatectomy using the laparoscopic device for umbilical access SILS port. Actas Urol Esp. 2010;34:495–9.
42. Liberati A, Altman DG, Tetzlaff J, Mulrow C, Gøtzsche PC, Ioannidis JP, et al. The PRISMA statement for reporting systematic reviews and metaanalyses of studies that evaluate health care interventions: explanation and elaboration. BMJ. 2009;339:b2700.
43. EBM Oxford centre for evidence-based medicine 2009. www.cebm.net/levels_of_evidence.
44. Boni L, Dionigi G, Cassinotti E, Di Giuseppe M, Diurni M, Rausei S, et al. Single incision laparoscopic right colectomy. Surg Endosc. 2010;24:3233–6.
45. Ramos-Valadez DI, Patel CB, Ragupathi M, Bartley Pickron T, Haas EM. Single-incision laparoscopic right hemicolectomy: safety and feasibility in a series of consecutive cases. Surg Endosc. 2010;24:2613–6.
46. Vestweber B, Alfes A, Paul C, Haaf F, Vestweber KH. Single-incision laparoscopic surgery: a promising approach to sigmoidectomy for diverticular disease. Surg Endosc. 2010;24:3225–8.
47. Gash KJ, Goede AC, Chambers W, Greenslade GL, Dixon AR. Laparoendoscopic single-site surgery is feasible in complex colorectal resections and could enable day case colectomy. Surg Endosc. 2011;25:835–40.
48. Wheeless Jr CR, Thompson BH. Laparoscopic sterilization. Review of 3600 cases. Obstet Gynecol. 1973;42:751–8.
49. Park HS, Kim TJ, Song T, Kim MK, Lee YY, Choi CH, et al. Single-port access (SPA) laparoscopic surgery in gynecology: a surgeon's experience with an initial 200 cases. Eur J Obstet Gynecol Reprod Biol. 2011;154:81–4.
50. Jung YW, Lee M, Yim GW, Lee SH, Paek JH, Kwon HY, et al. A randomized prospective study of single-port and four-port approaches for hysterectomy in terms of postoperative pain. Surg Endosc. 2011;25(8):2462–9. doi:10.1007/s00464-010-1567-z.

Chapter 9
Reduced Port Surgery: Single Port Access to the Abdominal and Pelvic Cavity

Paul G. Curcillo II, Stephanie A. King, and Erica R. Podolsky

Introduction

The true definition of a "dilemma" is the presence of "two truths." It does not always mean a person must choose between the alternatives, but at times face the dilemma that he or she needs to accept both truths, although one may not be a desirable as the other. This very idea of accepting a desirable path along with a not so desirable path is faced by surgeons and their patients every day. As we look to offer patients treatment and potential cure of their disease, we also offer the unfortunate truth that along with the desired path of improving their condition they will certainly experience "the pain" that we inflict upon them.

As one looks over the past century of surgical treatment of disease, many operative procedures have not changed in their basic principles of technique. A gallbladder has always been removed by retracting the fundus high, manipulating the infundibulum to aid in exposing the critical areas, and dissecting the cystic duct and artery. Detachment from the liver bed then completes the procedure. Likewise, a hysterectomy and

---

Authors' Note Over the past several years, a number of approaches to this new platform of Single Port surgery have arisen. These techniques can be found throughout the literature, and, although we will discuss some of these techniques, this chapter will primarily focus on the development of Single Port Access as a philosophy one needs to ponder as they venture into this field on their own. With regard to terminology and acronyms, we will compare and contrast a few of these, but given that the most common term used during presentations and discussions is "Single Port," we will try to be consistent and keep to that term as part of the Reduced Port Surgical Field we see developing.

P.G. Curcillo II(✉) • S.A. King
Department of Surgical Oncology, Fox Chase Cancer Center, Philadelphia, PA, USA

E.R. Podolsky
Department of Surgery, College of Medicine, Drexel University,
Philadelphia, PA, USA

A. Tinelli (ed.), *Laparoscopic Entry*,
DOI 10.1007/978-0-85729-980-2_9, © Springer-Verlag London Limited 2012

oophorectomy have always involved identification of the attachments and blood supply, identification and protection of the ureter, control of the vasculature, elevation of a bladder flap, and finally removal of the cervix with closure of the vaginal cuff. Although we have seen advances in instrumentation, vessel sealing techniques, and cauterization, none of these have truly affected the pain that accompanies the surgery we perform. Advancements in anesthesia have clearly helped with intraoperative pain and postoperative discomfort, but the real driving force from a surgeon's standpoint to improve pain has been to continually strive to decrease the amount of trauma we inflict upon the body in terms of incision size. The appearance of laparoscopy has clearly aided us in this quest. We have seen patients tolerate the surgery better, recover faster, and experience a decrease in the pain and discomfort of subsequent issues that develop with time associated with large incisions (i.e., wound infections and hernias). Although it would seem that we have reached the point where we offer same day surgery, discharge of patients with simple oral pain medication, and minimal scarring, we are now embarking on taking this to a new level. Initially thought to be the surgery of tomorrow, NOTES (Natural Orifice Transluminal Endoscopic Surgery) brought the concept of elimination of incisions entirely and the potential for elimination of general anesthesia. Not easily practiced by most surgeons, many were on the sidelines, awaiting something else into which they could delve. However, with the appearance of Single Port Access surgery [1, 2], there has clearly been a new excitement in surgery. Further reduction in the number and size of scars has allowed many surgeons to enter and participate in this new trend of further minimizing the pain we offer, and aiming for the goal of eliminating the "dilemma" of surgical treatment.

Single Port Access Surgery: A New Approach to an Old Idea

Over the past 4 years approaching laparoscopy through a single incision has brought with it a new approach to advancing surgery. Initially presented as a well thought out, stepwise approach to improving our technique of laparoscopy, we have now seen a new pattern of acquisition of new surgical techniques by surgeons. Thus, a few words on the true initial development of Single Port Surgery are warranted in order to aid surgeons in advancing to the next level in their own practices.

Single Port Access Surgery: Initial Reports

Laparoscopy is not nearly as new as many believe it to be. Some of the first laparoscopic procedures were done through a single hole, as the main desire was simply aiding in diagnosis of intraabdominal disease [3]. Obviously, the advent of improved radiologic techniques has eliminated many diagnostic laparoscopies in favor of totally painless, noninvasive, and nearly risk free imaging techniques. Although not a general surgery tool, single port laparoscopy has been used by gynecologist for

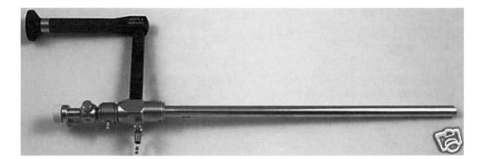

Fig. 9.1 Operative laparoscope

simple procedures beyond diagnosis such as tubal ligations or endometrial ablations with an operative laparoscope (Fig. 9.1). Ultimately, applying these ideas of single incisions for laparoscopy, Pelosi went on to describe not only gynecological procedures [4] but appendectomy [5] as well through one laparoscopic incision. Although a wonderful idea and proven approach, the devices were simple, and technically not all surgeons could apply this approach. As laparoscopy grew through the nineties, most surgeons seemed comfortable with four small holes as compared with the standard large incisions, and there was not much enthusiasm to make the already newly acquired, albeit difficult technique of laparoscopy, any more difficult. In 1997, Navarra [6] applied this concept to the cholecystectomy by using a single incision through the umbilicus and placing several needles through the abdominal wall to aid in retraction. Although not truly "single port" because he used strategically placed needles through extra umbilical sites, this was perhaps the first real application of "reduced port surgery" as a new concept to improve what we do every day. Over the next few years, as other surgeons began using and promoting Navarra's concept, Navarra, himself, raised a number of concerns regarding safety and applicability as well as costs [7]. Interestingly enough, following the introduction of Single Port Access in the spring of 2007 by Curcillo and King, this same path has been once again revisited. An explosion of papers and reports of techniques and devices has filled our literature and meetings, but again, the question of applicably, costs, and safety have been repeatedly raised by Curcillo and King [8–11]. As we move forward with surgical technique, one must remember that with each advancement we have to ensure safe adoption and practice of new techniques, with an eye to the costs creating a stable foundation for adoption. Simply reporting novel ideas and technique and then considering the costs later in development as we move forward will prevent real evolution of techniques. Although several authors had reported reduction in port sites in laparoscopic cholecystectomy [12, 13], again we did not see any real traction in the application of these techniques in a widespread fashion. Most surgeons seemed content with four 5-mm holes as opposed to the larger incisions previously being used for open surgery. This group saw laparoscopy as so much better, perhaps there was no great desire to make what seemed to be small improvements by elimination or downsizing of further port sites. Although reports of large series of minilaparoscopy proved the technique safe and effective [14], even this seemingly small step was not readily adopted. Thus, we seemed to be stagnating; awaiting something.

Single Port Access: Development

The first two steps that contributed to the development of Single Port Access were the development of the two ports, single stitch technique of ventral hernia repair and the serendipitous downstaging of port sites in a laparoscopic cholecystectomy in 2006. The two port hernia repair clearly offered the benefit of fewer port sites, but ventral hernia surgery did not require as many steps and details as a cholecystectomy or colon resection. With regard to gynecology, the operative laparoscope, although useful for simple procedures, was difficult to apply to more complex procedures and was not readily applied routinely. As it was becoming apparent in the development of Single port Access that we could begin applying the one port of entry approach to multiple procedures, applying it to cholecystectomies was simply a matter of time. Initially, placement of more than one trocar through a single port of entry was done in gastrostomy tubes and with the use of articulating instruments [15]. Concurrently, the elimination of the subxiphoid port in cholecystectomies demonstrated that we could do multiple procedures through a single port of entry with multiple trocars. This allowed us to progress from four incisions down to three incisions; subsequently two incisions, and ultimately down to Single Port Access Surgery. Very early on, SPA surgery was focused on minimizing instruments in order to minimize the number of trocars we required. The first SPA cholecystectomies were performed using two instruments rather than three, as has been proven safe in obtaining the critical view [16] of the cystic duct region. In addition, the use of new instruments (articulating) was thought to be the facilitating factor in the performance of surgery through one port of entry. As we reviewed our early experience of fewer than 25 cases, we found two questions arose. We were doing the same safe operations we were doing before, and were we developing a technique that could be readily applied by our colleagues. It was these questions that gave rise to the concept of Single Port Access surgery as a platform and ultimately Reduce Report Surgery as a future.

Single Port Access: Focus on Instruments or Technique?

Demonstrating a new technique with a new instrument carried with it the responsibly of the surgeon developing or testing it to consider all aspects of advancement of new techniques. The question is not solely "can we use this instrument?" but rather "should we use this instrument or platform?" Single Port Access was developed based on the concept of "e-SPA" (Fig. 9.2) [8]. The important elements of development of a new platform were defined and answered before proceeding fur-

Fig. 9.2 e-SPA

e-SPA

- *Evolution of a procedure*

- *Evidence for a procedure*

- *Effects on the patient from a procedure*

- *Ergonomics - effects on us from a procedure*

- *Energy sources and their effects*

- *Economics of a procedure*

- *Environmental effects of a procedure*

- *Education of a procedure*

ther in order to ensure we maintained safety and efficacy without increasing costs, and we attempted to maintain an educational perspective for both practicing surgeons and training residents and fellows. If a technique revolves around instrumentation, we have found that with each difficulty encountered or hurdle approached, oftentimes another device or instrument becomes the answer. This "dependent progression of devices" can oftentimes increase not only costs, but also raise the bar in terms of difficulty in education and adoption of the technique. In the first reports of SPA Surgery [17–19], the question was raised regarding the critical view and the costs of the instruments. As Single Port progressed, the foundation for development became a focus on the steps of the procedure and the best way to handle each through a single port of entry. With the critical view of the cystic duct the gold standard of safety in laparoscopic cholecystectomy, the initial technique was questioned because only two instruments were being used when tradition and safety demanded three. Initial evaluation allowed the addition of the third instrument rather than moving forward with only two [10]. With respects to work within gynecology, it was clear that one of the most important tools in the procedure was the tissue sealing device. As the important devices on the market were straight and rigid, it seemed only to make sense that all the instruments used be rigid, otherwise delivery of the rigid instrument across the vessel would be limited if articulation was required to dissect it out. Within months of initial development, cholecystectomies and hysterectomies were routinely being done single port with straight rigid instruments and technical aspects of dissection mirroring standard multiport laparoscopic procedures.

Single Port Access: The Access

Since the beginnings of Single Port surgery, one of the most common misconceptions has been that a "single access" device was necessary to perform single port surgery. Even as Single Port Access was beginning in 2007, the earliest concerns over development were the lack of a device that seemed to be the "Holy Grail" of single port surgery.

However, it became apparent quite early on, that a number of procedures could easily be performed using multiple trocars through a single skin incision [15, 16]. By opening up the area under the skin and fat and exposing a larger area of fascia, it became apparent that multiple trocars could be placed within the same skin incision and, ultimately, single port surgery could in fact mimic multiport laparoscopy [20]. This new type of access through the abdominal wall allowed surgeons to migrate from four port sites to one, using the same number of instruments for each procedure. Very early on, it was evident that the technique was not only possible, but trainable and reproducible by other surgeons as well. The driving force over the next few years was a corporate push to promote single port access devices, despite the fact that for the added expense, no benefits other than cosmesis were being produced. Interestingly enough, these devices actually became more and more restrictive, because now the instruments needed to be placed through very small incisions, rather than spreading them out through separate fascial defects within the same skin incision. This resulted in the concept of "pseudo triangulation" being created by using yet more instrumentation in terms of articulating and roticulating instrumentation. Despite the fact that the articulating instruments were already proving more difficult to adapt, they were seeing use rise to help compensate for the lack of triangulation and separation of the instruments.

Single Port Surgery: Classifications

As with most new concepts and techniques, we began to see a divide develop in the approaches, and separate philosophies arose within this field while still in its infancy. Single Port Access (SPA) surgery has grown to include all procedures and has offered the ability to do new procedures without the additional costs, both economical and ecological, of new added disposable instruments. Multiple trocars through a separate port of entry has proven itself a readily adapted technique, offering the benefit of "independence of motion" of the instruments and the minimization of elastic recoil (i.e., the force against which our hands and forearms needs to work within a single port device). The issue of specimen extraction continues to be a bit more difficult in Single Port Access, as multiple small holes need to be converted to a single hole in order to remove large specimens. Further, once the specimen is out, the larger facial defect needs to be closed, and then access regained in order to explore the abdominal cavity. The Single Port Device techniques (SILS™, LESS), have developed as techniques that revolve around an access device that allows the instruments to be placed through a single device within one large fascial defect. Resulting in an easier technique to remove large specimens and reinsert the access device for re-exploration, these devices have gained traction with large organ removal. However, given that all the instruments are entering through a single device, they necessarily affect each other's movements, resulting in loss of independence of motion and increased elastic recoil, thus increasing the force against which we need to work with both our forearms and hands [21].

Fig. 9.3 SPA circle of entry

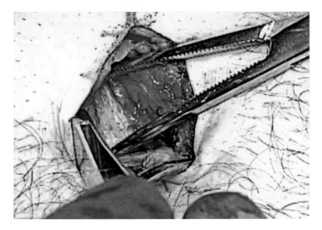

Single Port Access: Versatility

Every surgeon performs each procedure in almost a uniform method along with his colleagues throughout the world. At the same time, each surgeon likes to modify the procedure somewhat. Access has offered that possibility. Accessing the abdominal cavity in virtually the same way as multiport laparoscopy, single port access allows each surgeon to modify which trocar is used for retraction and which trocar is used for dissection. In addition, because there are no "fixed" number if entry sites as with the single port devices, more or less instruments can be inserted. Given that only 5mm fascial defects have been created, we have not lost the benefits of single port surgery in that we don't finish with one large defect (> 2cm) along with multiple smaller defects as well.

Single Port Access Surgery: The Technique

In reality, Single Port Access surgery is simply a replication of multiport laparoscopy. Access to the abdominal wall is virtually the same for both. The SPA surgery technique [20] is performed just as with standard laparoscopy. Initially, the abdomen is entered in the preferred technique of the surgeon. A small skin incision is made, and the abdomen is then entered in the open technique or with the Veress needle. Once insufflated, the abdomen can be entered with a 5-mm trocar and explored. Once the environment is deemed accessible for SPA surgery, subsequent trocars can be place by raising flaps of the soft tissue and skin off the fascia, creating the SPA entry circle through which the instruments are placed (Fig. 9.3). It is an important property of laparoscopy that modifications can be made as necessary. From the very beginning of the procedure, the surgeon can determine whether or not single port is possible and can use alternative sites of port entry through the abdominal wall. As no large initial incision is being made, a conversion to multiport surgery is easily made without any sacrifices or unnecessary large defects in the fascia. It is

Fig. 9.4 "Spread" afforded
by angling the tips of the
trocars outward prior to
inserting them into the
abdominal wall

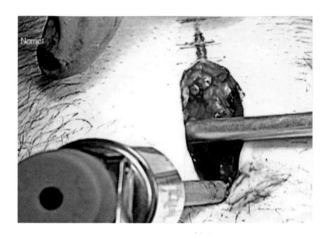

Fig. 9.5 Triangulation
(interior abdominal wall)

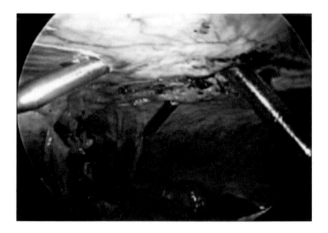

important to maximize the space utilized within the "circle of entry." Placing the
trocars close together limits the triangulation one can obtain from the "spread"
afforded by angling the tips of the trocars outward before inserting them into the
abdominal wall (Fig. 9.4). This outer spread (trocars positioned approx. 3–4 cm
apart) translates into the triangulation afforded at the abdominal wall (Fig. 9.5) on
the inside of the abdominal cavity, thus facilitating dissection and retraction.
The most important property of Single Port surgery is the ability to utilize an adequate number of instruments to perform the desired procedure. In gallbladder surgery, this translates into being able to perform a single port cholecystectomy much
the same way as a multiport cholecystectomy, in that four instruments can be placed
thought the central fascial defect, thus mimicking the standard multiport laparoscopic procedure. This is important in being able to preserve basic principles such
as the critical view in dissection of the cystic duct area in cholecystectomy. There is

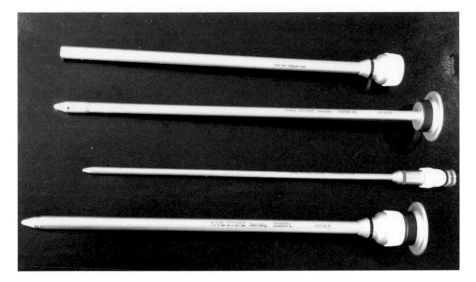

Fig. 9.6   Very low profile trocars/Sleeves

virtually no limitation in the number of trocars placed, as others can be added in other positions within the same defect, or remote sites can be utilized.

Single Port Access: The Right Tools for the Job

Whenever one tries a new procedure or technique, it is often best not to make it more difficult than it already is. The right instruments need to be used, and the right technique needs to be applied. Anything else, and one is setting themselves up for failure. Although the right tools for the Single Port Surgery are standard instruments and trocars already in most operating rooms, unlike the single port device techniques, there are specific properties of the trocars that need to be adhered to in order to facilitate the technique. Given the small amount of real estate present in the operative area, the "virtual cylinder" limits the size of the trocar head that should be used in single port access surgery. Generally, *very low profile* trocars with head sizes <2 cm are necessary, with newer *sleeves* further reducing the heads (Fig. 9.6). In addition, the shaft themselves need to be thin and have limited threading so as to minimize the potential of air leak from trocar sites enlarging into one another. The SPA technique has allowed the surgeon to maintain use of standard rigid instrumentation as with multiport laparoscopy, allowing control of costs, and avoiding the use of more difficult to learn instruments. However, as an occasional articulating instrument may be necessary, it is advised to learn to use these novel devices during multiport procedures to minimize the learning curve during single port procedures.

Single Port Access: Adopting It into Your Practice

Given that nothing special is needed to perform single port access surgery, it actually can be readily adopted by most surgeons. However, the best approach is to focus on a stepwise progression rather than leaping directly to single port. Begin by eliminating one port step at a time. In the same vein, one should also move from simple procedures to more complex ones in a stepwise fashion. Should new instruments be found that may or may not enhance single port procedures, it is best to learn them during multiport procedures and then adapt them to single port access when comfortable. Lastly, patience is the most important step in adoption. A new angle of view is being introduced. This will result in slower dissection while the surgeon develops a "sense" of this inline view. The camera can no longer be moved to another area for visualization, so only one view is afforded throughout the case. Introducing instruments is also a bit more cumbersome in the beginning. Bringing the instruments in alongside the camera is a new perspective we must develop as we move away from the triangulated insertion of multiport laparoscopy.

Single Port Surgery: The First Step to More Access Sites

Just as a stepwise progression to single port surgery will require a few extra port sites in the beginning; these additional port sites also offer the safe approach to single port surgery. In fact, the concept of reducing port sites needs to be complimented by the concept of reducing port site lengths. Just as one hole is better than four, a 2- or 3-mm hole is better than a 5. In this approach, perhaps the better procedure will be a Single Port Access surgery with one or two needle-scopic instruments being included as well (Fig. 9.7). Although a single hole is not the end result, a safer procedure may result with one main operative entry site and a separate 2-mm hole or transvaginal trocar (Fig. 9.8) placed to facilitate dissection and retraction. It is with this platform of Reduced Port Surgery that we will see a combination of a Single Port surgery, minilaparoscopy, and NOTES procedures combining to push forward the next approach to laparoscopy.

Fig. 9.7 Needlescopic
instruments

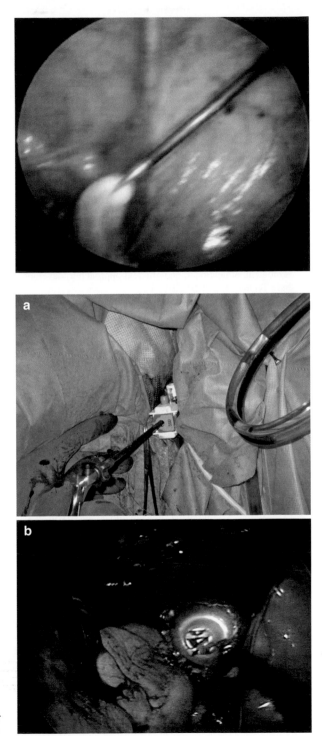

Fig. 9.8 Transvaginal trocar
exterior (**a**) and interior (**b**)

References

1. Rao PP, Bhagwat SM, Rane A, Rao PP. The feasibility of single port laparoscopic cholecystectomy: a pilot study of 20 cases. HPB. 2008;10(5):336–40.
2. Curcillo PG, Podolsky ER, Rottman SJ. Single port access (SPA): cholecystectomy. Gastroenterology. 2008;134(4):A-858.
3. Schollmeyer T, Soyinka AS, Schollmeyer M, Meinhold-Heerlein I. Georg Kelling (1866–1945): the root of modern day minimal invasive surgery. A forgotten legend? Arch Gynecol Obstet. 2007;276(5):505–9.
4. Pelosi MA, Pelosi 3rd MA. Laparoscopic hysterectomy with bilateral salpingo-oophorectomy using a single umbilical puncture. N J Med. 1991;88(10):721–6.
5. Pelosi MA, Pelosi 3rd MA. Laparoscopic appendectomy using a single umbilical puncture (minilaparoscopy). J Reprod Med. 1992;37(7):588–94.
6. Navarra G, Pozza E, Occhionorelli S, Carcoforo P, Donini I. One-wound laparoscopic cholecystectomy. Br J Surg. 1997;84:695.
7. Navarra G, Ascanelli S, Sortini D, Soliani G, Pozza E, Carcoforo P. Laparoscopic transabdominal suspension sutures. Surg Endosc. 2002;16(9):1378.
8. Podolsky ER, St John-Dillon L, King SA, Curcillo PG. Reduced port surgery: an economical, ecological, educational, and efficient approach to development of single port access surgery. Surg Technol Int. 2010;20:41–6.
9. Podolsky ER, Curcillo PG. Single port access surgery: evaluation of access platforms, versatility and fascial defects. Surg Endosc. 2010;24:S639. doi:10.1007/s00464-010-0972-7.
10. Podolsky ER, Curcillo PG. Reduced-port surgery: preservation of the critical view in single-port-access cholecystectomy. Surg Endosc. 2010;24(12):3038–43.
11. Podolsky ER, Curcillo PG. A comparison of independence of motion in single port access techniques. Surg Endosc. 2010;24:S499. doi:10.1007/s00268-011-1099.
12. Slim K, Pezet D, Stencl Jr J, Lechner C, Le Roux S, Lointier P, et al. Laparoscopic cholecystectomy: an original three-trocar technique. World J Surg. 1995;19(3):394–7.
13. Mori T, Ikeda Y, Okamoto K, Sakata K, Ideguchi K, Nakagawa K, et al. A new technique for two-trocar laparoscopic cholecystectomy. Surg Endosc. 2002;16(4):589–91.
14. Sarli L, Iusco D, Gobbi S, Porrini C, Ferro M, Roncoroni L. Randomized clinical trial of laparoscopic cholecystectomy performed with mini-instruments. Br J Surg. 2003;90(11):1345–8.
15. Podolsky ER, Rottman SJ, Curcillo 2nd PG. Single port access (SPA) gastrostomy tube in patients unable to receive percutaneous endoscopic gastrostomy placement. Surg Endosc. 2009;23(5):1142–5.
16. Podolsky ER, Rottman SJ, Poblete H, King SA, Curcillo PG. Single port access (SPA) cholecystectomy: a completely transumbilical approach. J Laparoendosc Adv Surg Tech A. 2009;19(2):219–22.
17. Podolsky ER, Rottman SJ, Curcillo 2nd PG. Single port access (SPA) cholecystectomy: two year follow-up. JSLS. 2009;13(4):528–35.
18. Romanelli JR, Roshek 3rd TB, Lynn DC, Earle DB. Single-port laparoscopic cholecystectomy: initial experience. Surg Endosc. 2010;24(6):1374–9.
19. Gumbs AA, Milone L, Sinha P, Bessler M. Totally transumbilical laparoscopic cholecystectomy. J Gastrointest Surg. 2009;13(3):533–4.
20. Wu AS, Podolsky ER, King SA, Curcillo 2nd PG. Single port access (SPA) technique: video summary. Surg Endosc. 2010;24(6):1473.
21. Curcillo PG, Podolsky ER, King SA – The Road to Reduced Port Surgery: From Single Big Incisions to Single Small Incisions, and Beyond. World J Surg. 2011 Jul;35(7):1526-31. DOI 10.1007/s00268-011-1099-2

Chapter 10
The Evolution of Minimally Invasive Gynecological Surgery: Gas-Less Laparoscopic Inspection and Single Hole Surgery (GLISHS)

Nicola Gasbarro, Maurizio Brusati, Pietro Lupo, Sandro Gerli, and Gian Carlo Di Renzo

In memory of a special man, skilled doctor and a brilliant inventor, Dr. Pietro Lupo. We miss you so much and you will always be in our hearts. Nicola and all your true and sincere friends.

Introduction

In the last two decades, laparoscopy has become the standard treatment for many gynecological conditions. However, one major obstacle to the more widespread application of endoscopic procedures has been the limitations encountered with conventional laparoscopy. These include poor surgeon ergonomics, counterintuitive hand movement owing to undesirable long instruments, limited degrees of instrument motion within the body, and maintenance of CO_2 pneumoperitoneum. Another major obstacle has been the rising cost of laparoscopic surgery, which always employs new and expensive tools to improve the safety and execution of operations.

In the same years, open surgery has developed the minilaparotomy approach, and procedures such as the mini-laparomyomectomy and mini-laparohysterectomy have well-established advantages over the same laparoscopic operations. These include a shorter duration of surgery, fewer technical difficulties, and less cost. However, minilaparotomy surgery is a challenge in obese patients or when the uterus is much enlarged.

In an attempt to overcome the obstacles of both techniques, we developed a new minimally invasive surgical approach that combines gas-less laparoscopic inspection of

N. Gasbarro (✉)
Unit of Obstetrics and Gynecology, Santa Maria delle Grazie Hospital, Pozzuoli (Na), Italy

M. Brusati • P. Lupo
Unit of Obstetrics and Gynecology, General Hospital of Chivasso, Turin, Italy

S. Gerli • G.C. Di Renzo
Department of Obstetrics and Gynecology, University of Perugia, Perugia, Italy

A. Tinelli (ed.), *Laparoscopic Entry*,
DOI 10.1007/978-0-85729-980-2_10, © Springer-Verlag London Limited 2012

the surgical site and exteriorization through the same tiny incision of the pathological organ that is operated on by conventional instruments and open abdominal technique.

This section describes the principles and practice of the procedure named Gas-less Laparoscopic Inspection and Single Hole Surgery (GLISHS).

Why Gas-Less?

Gas-less laparoscopy means laparoscopy without pneumoperitoneum, in which abdominal distention is created and maintained by the mechanical elevation and suspension of the anterior abdominal wall through various devices.

The advantages of the gas-less approach are both technical and physiopatho-logical. Regarding the physiopathological aspects, note that the CO_2 pneumoperi-toneum required for conventional laparoscopic procedures may negatively affect the cardiopulmonary system [1, 2, 3, 4, 5, 6, 7, 8, 9], acid-base balance [10, 11, 12], the immunitary system [13, 14, 15], and fetal-maternal circulation [16, 17, 18, 19, 20] (Table 10.1).

These physiological changes are well tolerated in healthy patients, but may result in life-threatening cardiac arrhythmia, myocardial infarction, cardiac failure, or pul-monary insufficiency in case of older and higher-risk patients and longer operations. [21, 22, 23, 24, 25, 26, 27] A further problem of CO_2 laparoscopy is possible con-tamination of the carbon dioxide with latex dust from the hose system, which jeop-ardizes sensitized patients. [28] To complete the picture, various animal studies suggest that CO_2 insufflation promotes intraperitoneal dissemination and implanta-tion of tumor cells. [29, 30, 31, 32, 33, 34, 35, 36, 37] Theoretically, the CO_2 pneu-moperitoneum might promote tumor spreading in two ways. First, it can be hypothesized that abdominal insufflation causes turbulence, displacing tumor cells,

Table 10.1 Physiological changes associated with CO_2 pneumoperitoneum

Cardiopulmonary system	Acid-base balance	Endocrine and immunitary system	Pregnancy	Cancer
↓ Venous return	↑ CO_2 pulmonary artery	↑ Norepinephrine	↓ Fetal-maternal circulation	Intra-abdominal tumor spreading?
↓ Cardiac output	↑ CO_2 end-tidal	↑ Endothelin	Fetal acidosis ?	
↑ Mean arterial pressure		↓ Macrophages and granulocytes phagocytosis		
↑ Pulmonary artery pressure				
↑ Pulmonary vascular resistance				

Table 10.2 Technical advantages of gas-less laparoscopy

1. It allows use of umbilical access for the simultaneous insertion of the endoscope and surgical instruments, conventional or laparoscopic
2. It allows retrieval of gross surgical specimens through the same primary access
3. It allows performance of selected operations, such as tubal pregnancies and removal of pedunculated myomas, without ancillary trocars or with only one trocar
4. It works better than conventional laparoscopy in conjunction with vaginal surgery, such as laparoscopically assisted vaginal hysterectomy
5. If the laparoscopic approach fails, it can still support a minilaparotomic procedure
6. There are no limits to the use of conventional suction devices when a prompt evacuation of massive hemoperitoneum is needed
7. It can be performed under regional anesthesia

and that the leakage of CO_2 alongside trocars causes a high local gas flow at the port sites (chimney effect) responsible for the abdominal wall metastases reported in consequence of laparoscopic procedures (port site metastases). [38, 39, 40, 41, 42, 43, 44, 45, 46, 47, 48, 49, 50, 51, 52, 53, 54, 55, 56, 57, 58] Second, CO_2 produces severe acidosis of the peritoneal surface, favoring peritoneal tumor cell adhesion. [59, 60, 61, 62] Gas-less laparoscopy avoids all of the possible complications and side effects caused by carbon dioxide. [63, 64, 65, 66]

Apart from these physiopathological aspects, the laparoscopy with pneumoperitoneum exhibits many technical disadvantages related to the maintenance of a closed working cavity to prevent gas leakage. [67, 68, 69] Indeed, if gas leakage is no longer a problem, the umbilical opening can simultaneously give access to the endoscope and surgical instruments, laparoscopic as well as conventional. [70, 71] Moreover, by this way gross surgical specimens can be removed easily. In this manner, selected operations, such as tubal pregnancies and removal of pedunculated myomas or endometriosis electrocoagulation can be performed with only one trocar or without ancillary trocars altogether. [72] For the same reason, in more complex operations umbilical access may overcome the suprapubic trocar. The technique also works better than conventional laparoscopy in conjunction with vaginal surgery, as in laparoscopically assisted vaginal hysterectomy, or in support of a minilaparotomic procedure when the laparoscopic approach fails or appears contraindicated. [70, 73] Furthermore, there is no limit to the use of aspirator devices that otherwise could collapse the insufflated peritoneal cavity, when a prompt evacuation of a severe hemoperitoneum is needed. Finally, the gas-less approach allows endoscopic surgery to be carried out under spinal anesthesia or peridural anesthesia, which would be problematic under the pneumoperitoneum because of high intraabdominal pressure and the resulting pain and diaphragmatic compression [74] (Table 10.2).

For the same reason, patients operated on without the use of gas only occasionally complain about mild postoperative shoulder pain, whereas patients who have undergone pneumoperitoneum sometimes experience medium strong pain in the neck or shoulder region for up to 5 days. [75, 76]

Brief History of Gas-Less Laparoscopy [68, 77, 72, 78, 73]

A physician named Bertram Bernheim is credited with the first documented gas-less laparoscopy at Johns Hopkins Hospital, Baltimore, MD. This report from 1911 describes the use of a proctoscope and an ordinary light for illumination to view the abdominal viscera: He named the procedure "organoscopy." However, the advantages of the gas-less technique wouldn't become evident until the late 1980s, when pioneering endoscopic surgeons Kurt Semm, Erich Muhe, and Philippe Mouret popularized laparoscopic operations.

In 1977, Michel Mintz, in reviewing the data from about 100,000 laparoscopic procedures performed in France, came to the conclusion that "the brief period of gaseous insufflation is the most dangerous stage." In 1985, Muhe himself, after the first six laparoscopic cholecystectomies, changed the technique, eliminating the pneumoperitoneum.

Since then, a number of devices have been conceived for the mechanical suspension of the abdominal wall in the gas-less laparoscopy. When using some devices an initial or permanent low pressure pneumoperitoneum is needed, whereas other devices can be applied in isopneumic conditions, without pneumoperitoneum (Table 10.3).

Basically, two systems of abdominal lift have been proposed. In the extraperitoneal system, such as the Hashimoto's device and the Laparotenser, the abdominal wall is suspended by means of metal wires inserted into the subcutaneous fat of the

Table 10.3 Gas-Less devices

Initial or permanent low-pressure pneumoperitoneum required	Isopneumic conditions
Abdominal Cavity Expander-System (ACE-WISAP, Semm 1991)	Nagai's device (1993)
T Shaped fan (Gazayerli, 1991)	Hashimoto's device (1993)
Suspendor 3-X (Mouret, 1991)	Laparolift - Laparofan (Chin, 1993)
Coathanger (Maher, 1992)	Laparotenser (Lucini, 1994)
U-Shaped Retractor (Kitano, 1992)	Abdolift (Kruschinski, 1996)
Winch-Retractor (Araki, 1993)	Variolift (Kruschinski, 1997)
Sling (Banting, 1993)	Gaslup (Gasbarro-Lupo, 1999)
Spreading Trocars (Dragojevic, 1994)	
Peritoneal Cavity Augmentation (PCA, Schaller 1994)	
Pelvi-Snake (Volz, 1996)	

abdominal wall; whereas the intraperitoneal systems, such as the Pelvi-snake and Laparolift, are placed under the abdominal wall through an umbilical incision.

We have a preference for intraperitoneal devices because they elevate the abdominal wall to a greater extent than extraperitoneal devices. In fact, as the subcutaneous tissue is not firmly attached to the other layers of the abdominal wall, the peritoneal elevation created by the extraperitoneal systems is smaller and therefore visualization worse.

It has to be admitted that all gas-less systems share the drawback of compromised visibility. They elevate the lower abdomen as a truncated pyramid rather than elevating the entire abdomen as a dome as with pneumoperitoneum (the so-called tent effect). Because the upper abdomen is not elevated, there is less space for the bowel to occupy. Consequently, exposing the cul-de-sac and ovarian fossae can result in difficulty owing to the presence of bowel. A steeper Trendelenburg position can obviate this problem.

In our experience, the Laparolift-Airlift device (Origin Medsystems, Menlo Park, CA) is among the ones that offer lesser tent effect, and we used it until 1998. It consists of an adjustable arm that is attached to the side of the operating table. The surgeon can raise and lower it electronically. The arm is connected to the airlift, a disposable sterile balloon retractor that is inserted flat through the umbilical incision. After entering the peritoneal space, the balloon is deployed by means of an inflation bulb and attached to the Laparolift arm. The maximum lifting force of about 13 kg is equivalent to a pneumoperitoneum pressure of 15 mmHg. Unfortunately, this device cannot be applied when there are adhesions in the midabdominal region, and the procedure has to be converted to a pneumoperitoneum.

The Gaslup System

To overcome these difficulties we developed a new intraperitoneal, isopneumic system, the GasLup system (Fig. 10.1a). [79]

The device consists of three small retractors that are individually inserted into the abdominal cavity through an umbilical incision (Fig. 10.1b) about 15 mm in length and positioned under the abdominal wall at 3, 9, and 12 o'clock. This ensures, similar to the pneumoperitoneum, the opening up of the reservoir for intestinal loops in the upper abdomen, which enhances visibility in the pelvis.

Moreover, when adhesions are encountered the retractors can be differently arranged and only two retractors can be used in case of expanded adhesions. An adapter allows the connection of the retractors to a horizontal arm that in turn is supported by a vertical sliding arm attached to the side of the operating table and sterilely draped (Fig. 10.1c). The abdominal wall lift is made by pulling up the horizontal arm.

There are two holes in the retractor's handles, placed at different heights, for fixing to the adapter hooks. Usually, the retractors are fixed by means of the inferior hole; the upper one is employed in patients with thick subcutaneous fat. For the

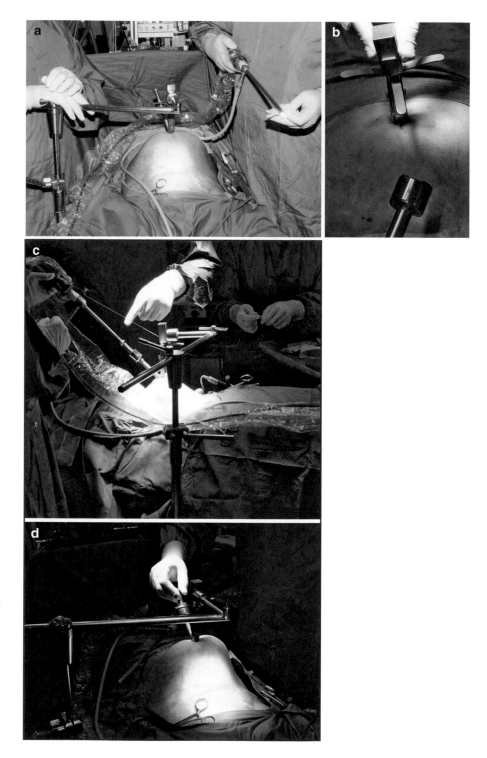

same purpose, two sets of retractors of different sizes are available: The standard set, which consists of retractors 60×13 mm in size, and the other one composed of retractors 85×13 mm in size for use in obese patients. All the parts of the instrument are reusable (Fig. 10.1d).

Since 1999, we have carried out 3,011 gas-less laparoscopy surgical interventions by the GasLup device. We have never had to convert to pneumoperitoneum because of poor visibility, as our device ensures as good pelvic exposition as that with pneumoperitoneum. The only concerns are those of accurate preoperative bowel preparation and a steeper Trendelenburg position.

The Gas-Less Laparoscopic Inspection and Single Hole Surgery Concept

The concept on which our technique is founded is different from that of other laparoscopic combined techniques, such as the laparoscopically assisted vaginal hysterectomy or the laparoscopically assisted minilaparotomic myomectomy. These approaches include conventional laparoscopic steps to support a vaginal or minilaparotomic technique that is often poor by itself. As a result, they add invasiveness to an intervention that a skilled surgeon would have better and quickly performed by the vaginal or minilaparotomic approach alone. Our approach is different.

The idea came to us in March 2000, when a 19-year-old patient presented to our department for evaluation of an ovarian cystic mass that was entirely occupying the abdomen (Fig. 10.2a).

On preoperative work-up the cyst appeared to be unilocular without papillations or solid areas, and the serum markers were in the normal range. The mass was presumed to be a benign serous cystadenoma and the patient consented to undergo transumbilical aspiration and removal of the cyst. At first, we performed a small, vertical incision, 1.5 cm in length, at the umbilicus to enter the abdominal cavity, thus exposing the anterior cystic wall that was perforated in an avascular zone with a Caldwell paracentesis needle connected by a three-way stopcock to a 60-mL syringe (Fig. 10.2b).

In this way enough fluid was aspirated to collapse the cyst and grasp the wall at the needle insertion with ring forceps. The cyst wall was then progressively exteriorized through the umbilicus (Fig. 10.2c) and evacuation of the fluid was completed with the conventional suction device.

At this point, we could extracorporeally clamp and cut the infundibulopelvic ligament. The whole cystic wall was removed and sent for frozen section, while the ovary was sutured (Fig. 10.2d).

Fig. 10.1 (**a**) The Gas-Lup as it is applied. (**b**) The intraumbilical insertion of a part of Gas-Lup retractor-device. (**c**) The Gas-Lup in lateral vision. (**d**) The completing Gas-Lup setting to begin the operation

Fig. 10.2 (**a**) Expanded abdomen caused by a giant ovarian cystadenoma. (**b**) The surgeon visualizes a dermoid ovarian cyst on the monitor and perforates it with an 18-gauge needle connected to a 60-cc syringe and the fluid cyst is aspirated. (**c**) The cyst wall is exteriorized trough umbilical access. (**d**) After removal of whole cystic wall the ovary is sutured by surgeons

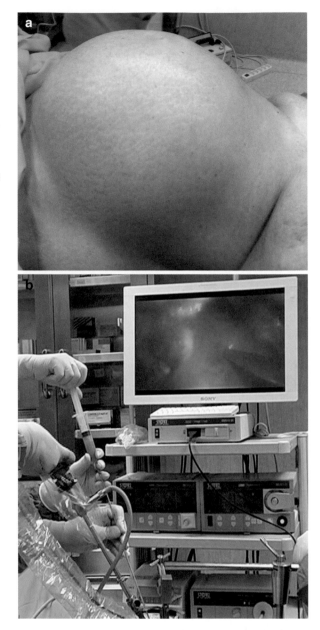

In the meantime, we suspended the abdominal wall with the Gas-Lup and endoscopically explored the upper abdomen and the pelvis to verify the contralateral ovary and the hemostasis. After the pathologist confirmed the lesion to be a serous cystadenoma, we closed the umbilical incision. The recovery of the patient was uneventful; she was discharged the second postoperative day.

Fig. 10.2 (continued)

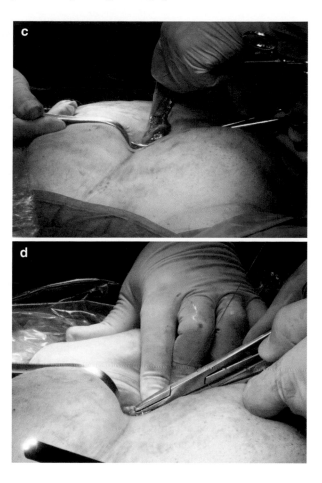

Since then we have performed many oophorectomies, salpingo-oophorectomies, and cystectomies by the transumbilical extracorporeal approach, experimenting with the advantages of this technique.

First, the operating steps and operating technique are the same as the open surgery and are therefore easier. Accordingly, the learning phase is considerably shorter. Second, the invasiveness of the procedure is inferior not only when compared with conventional laparoscopy, but also in regard to the more recent single port laparoscopy, which needs a larger incision. [80] This enhances the cosmetic benefits while minimizing the potential morbidity associated with multiple incisions. Third, the procedure is more cost-effective, because the instruments employed are conventional, which are cheaper and also offer a significantly longer life than laparoscopic instruments, resulting in less frequent repair and replacement. [81]

From these early experiences we developed a new minimally invasive surgical approach named Gas-Less Laparoscopic Inspection and Single Hole Surgery (GLISHS), whose basic steps consist of the preliminary endoscopic inspection of the abdominal cavity to visualize the organ that has to be operated on and to confirm the preoperative diagnosis, the exteriorization of the organ that is operated on by the conventional open technique, and finally, organ repositioning with final laparoscopic control.

Except in the case of a giant ovarian cystadenoma, we choose to enter the abdominal cavity via the suprapubic route through a small transverse incision, 1.5 cm in length, performed according to the open technique (see following text). In this way we operate on benign ovarian tumors, tubal pregnancies, and uterine myomas. In the same manner, we perform tubal sterilization and appendectomies, and we are preparing for cholecystectomies through the incision at the cystic point. Since January 2009, we have performed 530 operations. In none of operated cases was a CO_2 pneumoperitoneum or laparotomic conversion needed and there have been no intraoperative complications.

General Approach

An organized operating room is essential for a successful surgery, and positioning the patient appropriately can facilitate the operation. We prefer that the patient is positioned on the operating table with the legs wide apart at around 30° and with both arms placed at the side. The operator stands between the patient's legs; the assistant stands on the patient's left side, while the Gas-Lup is fixed on the right (Fig. 10.3); the instrument nurse stands on the patient's right side. The video monitor is positioned in front of the operator, to the right of the head of the patient. Because we perform almost all laparoscopic procedures under regional anesthesia, to improve the patient's comfort, we offer them the use of video glasses by which they can see films or relaxing documentaries.

Once the patient is positioned, her abdomen, perineum, and vagina are cleansed with a bactericidal solution and a Foley catheter is inserted. She is draped to expose the abdomen and the perineum, and a Spackman cannula is inserted into the cervical os to manipulate the uterus and for chromoperturbation.

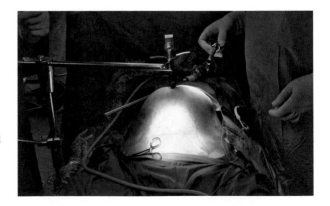

Fig. 10.3 Gas-Less Laparoscopic Inspection and Single Hole Surgery (GLISHS). The Gas-Lup is fixed on the right of the patient's head

The Open Laparoscopy Technique Modified

In 1971, Hasson introduced the open laparoscopy technique to eliminate the risks associated with the insertion of a Veress needle. [82, 83] However, in 1985, Penfield, in reviewing the data from 10,840 open laparoscopies, reported six bowel lacerations: four were recognized and repaired, and two were not suspected until several days postoperatively. [84] To eliminate the risk of such complications, we modified Hasson's technique as follows. A vertical incision, about 1.5 cm in length, is made at the umbilicus or, alternatively, a transverse incision of the same length is made at the suprapubic area with a No. 11 scalpel blade. As the incision is made, two Farabeuf retractors and scissors are used to expose the fascia that is transversely incised with the scalpel. Once the fascia is cut, the intact peritoneum is exposed by blunt dissection with scissors and then perforated by the forefinger. Be aware that in young women the posterior leaf of the rectus sheath is usually strong at the infraumbilical site, and it is very difficult to perforate it by digitoclasia. In these patients, the fibers of the fascia need to be divaricated by opening the scissors' blades up to expose the dome of the peritoneum. Instead, at the suprapubic region, only the attenuated fascia transversalis and peritoneum lie adjacent to the posterior surface of the muscle so resistance is less here. This technique carefully avoids grasping the tissues; it is totally safe and we have performed it in more than 3,011 open abdominal accesses without procured lesions.

At the end of the procedure, the abdominal wall is closed with a vicryl suture attached to a 5/8 curved needle. The needle is loaded in the needle holder as a fish-hook so that the tissues (peritoneum and fascia) can be directly hooked, thus avoiding anti-ergonomic maneuvering and rotating of the needle holder into deep and narrow spaces. To expose the tissues, two small vaginal retractors 1.5 cm large are used and maneuvered with a light rotation in a transverse direction. Finally, the skin is closed with a subcuticular suture. Adopting this technique, we never encountered such complications as bowel injuries or incisional hernias.

Selected Operations

Ovarian Cystectomy

Evolving technique has made it possible to treat most persistent ovarian cysts laparoscopically. However, a serious concern is that an ovarian cyst assumed to be benign subsequently may prove to be an ovarian cancer or a borderline tumor. If the cyst content spills during its aspiration or during the ovarian cystectomy, the risk of abdominal spreading cannot be ruled out. [85- 87, 88, 89, 90, 91] The GLISHS approach avoids this risk. The procedure is as follows for an endopelvic ovarian cyst.

Once the abdominal cavity is entered as previously described through a suprapubic incision 1.5 cm in length, the abdominal wall is suspended with the Gas-Lup and

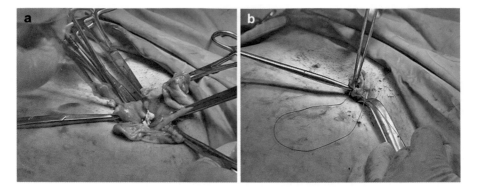

Fig. 10.4 (**a**) The ovarian cyst inner surface was macroscopically explored, (**a**) dermoid cyst is showed in the Fig, through a suprapubic ancillary hole then the surgeon extracorporeally clamped and cut the infundibulopelvic ligament. (**b**) The edges of the ovary are approximated by an extracorporeal suture

the laparoscope is inserted. The cyst wall and the pelvis are inspected for the presence of free fluid, excrescences, or irregular areas that should raise the suspicion of malignancy and prompt a frozen section biopsy.

If this is not the case, the cyst should be gently mobilized with a probe to check for any adhesion that needs to be removed in advance: The gas-less technique works well in this case, as conventional scissors can be inserted through the abdominal incision and a sharp dissection can be accomplished. Then, under endoscopic view, the cyst wall is perforated in an avascular zone with an 18- or 20-gauge needle connected to a 60-cc syringe and enough fluid is aspirated to collapse the cyst and grasp the wall at the needle insertion with ring forceps. At this point, the laparoscope and the Gas-Lup can be removed and the cyst is progressively and gently exteriorized (Fig. 10.4a).

If needed, evacuation of the fluid is accomplished extracorporeally with the suction device: in this way any intraabdominal leakage of fluid is avoided. At this point, it is easy and quick to strip the cyst wall from the ovarian stroma simply using the hands. It is easy to control bleeding from the blood vessels at the base of the capsule as well as the approximation of the edges of the ovarian cortex (Fig. 10.4b).

All such procedures are very time consuming and tedious when performed laparoscopically. The ovary is then repositioned in the pelvis and a final laparoscopic control ensures that hemostasis is appropriate. Closure of the abdominal incision completes the procedure. When the cyst occupies the abdomen, the technique is as previously described through an infraumbilical or suprapubic incision.

Treatment of Tubal Pregnancy

The abdominal cavity is entered as previously described through a suprapubic incision 1.5 cm in length and, with the Gas-Lup in place, the pelvis is inspected. In the presence of hemoperitoneum, a conventional suction device works well for a quick

Fig. 10.5 The tube is gently grasped with a Babcock clamp, the Gas-Lup is removed, and the tube with extrauterine pregnancy inside is then exteriorized

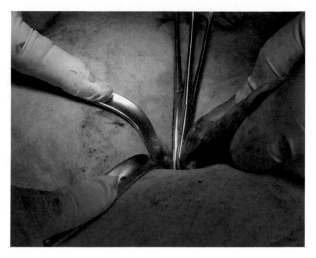

evacuation of intraperitoneal blood and clots. At this point, a slight anti-Trendelenburg position can facilitate the blood flowing toward the cul-de-sac, where it is easily aspirated. The patient is then placed in a reversed Trendelenburg position and the fallopian tubes are inspected to precisely locate the pregnancy.

Because pelvic inflammatory disease is a major risk factor for ectopic pregnancy, it is often necessary to dissect some tubal adhesions to gain a good exposition. Long conventional surgical instruments are suitable for this purpose and can be inserted through the same suprapubic incision. At this point, the tube can be gently grasped with a Babcock clamp, the Gas-Lup is removed, and the tube is exteriorized (Fig. 10.5). Infundibular pregnancies that are about to be extruded can be simply managed by grasping the tissue and completing the process. For unruptured ampullary pregnancies, a salpingotomy is appropriate: A linear incision is made on the antimesenteric surface extending 1–2 cm over the portion of the tube containing the pregnancy. The pregnancy usually protrudes through the incision and can be easily grasped and removed. The tubal incision is not approximated and hemostasis is achieved by coagulation.

Isthmic pregnancies and ruptured tubes are best treated with tubal resection or salpingectomy. Segmental resection is achieved by grasping the proximal and distal boundaries of the tubal segment containing the pregnancy with a Kelly clamp and cutting them from the antimesenteric border to the mesosalpinx. The mesosalpinx under the pregnancy is coagulated, with particular attention given to the anastomosing branches of the ovarian and uterine vessels. After coagulation, the mesosalpinx is cut and the pregnancy removed.

Guidelines for choosing salpingectomy include complete tubal destruction by the pregnancy and a recurrent pregnancy in the same tube. The operation is done by progressively clamping and cutting the mesosalpinx, beginning from the fimbriated end of the tube and progressing to the isthmic portion.

Cornual resection is the traditional management for interstitial pregnancies. This type of ectopic pregnancy is very difficult to manage by conventional laparoscopy, as the uterine cornu is vascular and profuse bleeding may quickly occur. The GLISHS approach follows the steps of the safer open access and avoids this risk. Once the tube and the uterine cornu are exteriorized, a pursestring suture is placed around the interstitial bulge and left untied. An incision is made in the thin part of the cornual region and the conceptus is removed. When the conceptus is completely evacuated, tying of the pursestring is completed, which results in effective cornual closure. If the interstitial pregnancy is advanced and the size of the cornual mass is large, another pursestring suture is placed in a more distal part after the first encircling suture tie is cut.

Finally, whichever procedure has been performed, the Gas-Lup is repositioned and the laparoscopic inspection confirms that the pelvis has been cleansed from clot and trophoblast. A chromopertubation should be performed at this time.

Tubal Sterilization

Although new hysteroscopic sterilization techniques offer effective permanent contraception, they are very expensive for the patient, as our Health Service does not provide patient reimbursement. On the other hand, tubal sterilization by conventional laparoscopy carries the discomfort and the risks of a laparoscopic procedure with general anesthesia. Tubal sterilization by the GLISHS procedure overcomes the disadvantages of both approaches. Indeed, by our technique the operation can be performed under spinal anesthesia, through a single suprapubic incision, and without cost for the patient.

The first steps are the same described in the treatment of tubal pregnancy. Once the tube is exteriorized, a Kelly clamp or scissors are used to create a window in an avascular area of the mesosalpinx just beneath the hystmic portion of the tube, about 3 cm from the uterine cornu. This window is stretched to about 3.0 cm in length by opening the Kelly clamp. Two No. 0 silk ligatures are passed through the window, and the tube is ligated proximally and distally. The intervening segment of tube between the ties is then resected and the hemostasis verified. Care should be taken to avoid undue tractions on the tube, because this could result in tearing of the mesosalpinx and excessive bleeding. At this point, the tube can be repositioned in the abdominal cavity, the Gas-Lup is applied, and the procedure is repeated on the other side.

Myomectomy

The management of leiomyomas endoscopically is one of the more challenging procedures. The ability to enucleate the myoma and repair the defect with a

Fig. 10.6 Myoma extraction trough incision above the pubis by the GLISHS technique

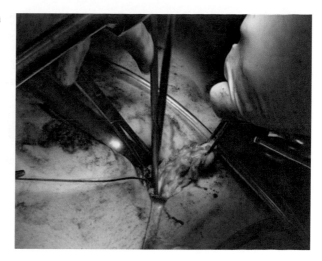

multilayer closure is critical to the success of a laparoscopic myomectomy. This ability to adequately repair the uterus laparoscopically continues to be a subject of debate and possibly plays a role in cases of uterine rupture in subsequent pregnancies. [92, 93]

Our technique overcomes many of the concerns inherent in a laparoscopic myomectomy while retaining its benefits. The abdominal cavity is entered as previously described and the Gas-Lup is positioned: the number, size, and location of myomas should be noted. Special attention should be made of their proximity to the uterine vessels and fallopian tubes. The surgeon must decide if myomectomy is still feasible and desirable, how the myomas will be removed, and in what sequence. If there is any doubt about the safe performance of this procedure via the GLISHS technique (Fig. 10.6), such as the presence of inaccessible posterior or broad ligament myomas, a conventional open access should be performed. Conversion to laparotomy when the myoma is partially dissected will result in increased blood loss owing to the delay, so this decision should be made early. Pedunculated myomas are the least difficult to manage. After one or two ties are placed around the pedicle, the myoma is grasped under laparoscopic vision, over the umbilicus with a tenaculum (Fig. 10.7).

The Gas-Lup is then removed, the top of the myoma is brought to the suprapubic incision, and it is progressively morcellated with a scalpel (Fig. 10.8) until the tied pedicle is reached. It is then carefully dissected from the pedicle. Finally, a horizontal mattress suture is placed in the myometrium incorporating the base of the pedicle and tied tightly. Subserous and deep intramural myomas require more expertise.

The grasped myoma is brought to the suprapubic hole. The surface of the myoma is exposed by means of two small valves and an incision is made on the serosa. The incision is extended until it reaches the pseudo-capsule. You will see that the myometrium retracts as the incision is made and that the myoma bulges outward. A myoma screw can be inserted into the tumor to apply traction while a finger is used

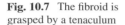

Fig. 10.7 The fibroid is
grasped by a tenaculum

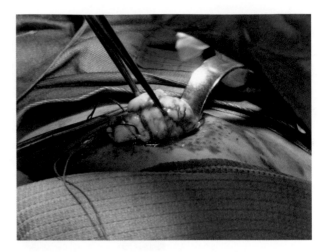

Fig. 10.8 Surgeons show a
fibroid morcellation over on
incision above the pubis

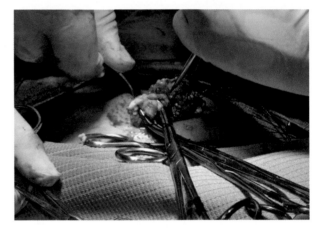

as a blunt dissector. The myoma is shelled and morcellated sequentially using a
No. 11 scalpel blade.

It is most important to re-grasp the remaining edge of the myoma before the
morcellated core of tissue is removed so upward traction is maintained. After complete removal of the tumor, the uterine wall defect shows through the hole and the
repair begins.

The gold standard of myometrial closure after myomectomy is a three-layered
closure beginning at the base of the defect to obliterate the dead space with figure-eight sutures. A second layer of continuous suture is then placed to further approximate the myometrium and finally a continuous 3-0 imbricating suture is placed on
the serosa. After hemostasis is assured, the uterus is dropped back into the pelvis
and the Gas-Lup repositioned for final inspection. The pelvis is irrigated with copious amounts of normal saline and an adhesion prevention barrier is placed over the
uterine incision. The abdominal incision is then repaired in layers as previously
described.

Fig. 10.9 The appendix and
the base of the cecum are
exteriorized

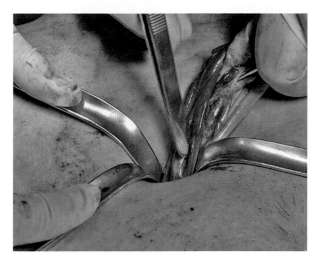

Appendectomy

Acute and chronic right lower abdominal pain frequently represents a diagnostic
challenge for the gynecologist. Hence, it is not infrequent that a woman suspected
to have an adnexal pathology is found to harbor an appendicular disease instead.
Furthermore, acute appendicitis is the most common nonobstetrical pathology
requiring an abdominal operation during pregnancy, occurring in approximately 1
in 1,500 deliveries. Thus, the gynecologist should be trained to properly perform an
appendectomy. This is usually a simple matter, but in some instances a retrocecal
position of the appendix or the presence of adhesions can make it difficult. The
GLISHS technique offers many advantages over the open and conventional laparoscopic approach, as it provides an accurate diagnosis, is safe in the pregnant patient,
and follows standard surgical steps. The procedure is performed through the usual
suprapubic incision.

With the Gas-Lup in place, the appendix is individuated and the mesoappendix is
grasped with a long Kelly clamp near the tip (Fig. 10.9). A Babcock clamp is placed
near the base of the appendix, to further support it, and the Gas-Lup is removed. The
appendix and the base of the cecum are then delivered through the abdominal incision. At this point, the mesoappendix can be ligated en masse. If ligation of the
mesoappendix is not feasible, it is clamped in a succession of small bites and each
segment of the clamped mesoappendix is individually ligated. A pursestring suture is
prepared around the base of the appendix and left untied. The appendix is crushed at
its base with a Kelly clamp and ligated with delayed absorbable suture. A second
Kelly clamp is placed across the appendix a short distance distal to the former, and
the appendix is amputated between the ligature and the clamp. The appendix stump
is finally grasped and inverted, and the pursestring is drawn tight.

We are aware that there are criticisms of an appendectomy technique that includes
burying the appendiceal stump. However, we still prefer to bury the appendiceal

stump rather than run the risk of infection and adhesion formation to an exposed stump. On the other hand, we agree that in case of a gangrenous or perforated appendix the stump should not be buried. The operation ends with closure of the suprapubic access.

Conclusions

Developed as an extension of gas-less laparoscopy, the goal of GLISHS is to improve patient outcomes by minimizing postoperative discomfort, decreasing convalescent time, and optimizing cosmetic results through a tiny hidden incision.

The technique is simple and can be learned easily, allowing more gynecologists—who so far have not performed endoscopic operations because of the inherent difficulty—to now use this approach. As a result, more patients will benefit from the minimally invasive surgery.

In addition, the GLISHS approach offers a cheaper alternative to conventional laparoscopy that can also be adopted in developing countries where hospitals cannot afford expensive instruments. Minimally invasive operations are urgently required in these countries so that patients can be quickly released from the hospital after the operation with further cost savings.

Our experience demonstrates that GLISHS is a safe and feasible technique that can be offered for the most common gynecological operations such as ovarian cystectomy, salpingo-oophorectomy, and myomectomy. Obesity and previous abdominal surgeries do not preclude the performance of GLISHS. Obese patients can maximally benefit from this minimally invasive surgery, because of their greater postoperative morbidity. GLISHS appears to be a promising surgical innovation, and we encourage gynecologists to practice it, because only with larger studies will it be possible to determine the practicality and reproducibility of our technique and definitively validate it.

References

1. Barnett RB, Gordon S, Drizin GS. Pulmonary changes after laparoscopic cholecystectomy. Surg Laparosc Endosc. 1992;2:125–7.
2. Beebe DS, McNevin MP, Crain JM, Letourneau JC, Belani KG, Abrahms JA, et al. Evidence of venous stasis after abdominal insufflation for laparoscopic cholecystectomy. Surgery. 1993;176:443–7.
3. Brown DR, Fishburne JI, Roberson VO, Hulka JF. Ventilatory and blood gas changes during laparoscopy with local anesthesia. Am J Obstet Gynecol. 1976;124:741–5.
4. Fitzgerald SD, Andrus CH, Baudendistel LJ, Dahms TE, Kaminski DL. Hypercarbia during carbon dioxide pneumoperitoneum. Am J Surg. 1992;163:186–90.
5. Ho HS, Gunther RA, Wolfe BN. Intraperitoneal carbon dioxide insufflation and cardiopulmonary function. Arch Surg. 1992;127:928–33.
6. Ivankovic AD, Miletich DJ, Albrecht RF, Heyman HJ, Bonnet RF. Cardiovascular effects of intraperitoneal insufflation with carbon dioxide and nitrous oxide in the dog. Anesthesiology. 1975;42:281–7.

7. Khan RM, Maroof M, Bhatti TH, Hamalawy H, Abbas JS. Correlation of end tidal CO_2 and haemodynamic variation following CO_2 insufflation during laparoscopic cholecystectomy. Anesthesiology. 1992;77:464–7.

8. Lenz RJ, Thomas TA, Wilkins DG. Cardiovascular changes during laparoscopy. Anaesthesia. 1976;31:4–12.

9. Volz J, Koster S, Weis M, Schmidt R, Urbaschek R, Melchert T, et al. Pathophysiologic features of a pneumoperitoneum at laparoscopy: a swine model. Am J Obstet Gynecol. 1996;174:132–40.

10. Kelman GR, Swapp GH, Benzie RJ, Gordon NLM. Cardiac output and arterial blood gas tension during laparoscopy. Br J Anaesth. 1972;44:1155–62.

11. Motew M, Ivankovic A, Bieniarz J, Albrecht RF, Zahed B, Scommegna A. Cardiovascular effects and acid-base and blood gas changes during laparoscopy. Am J Obstet Gynecol. 1973;115:1002–12.

12. Seed RF, Shakespeare TF, Muldoon MJ. Carbon dioxide homeostasis during anaesthesia for laparoscopy. Anaesthesia. 1970;25:223–31.

13. Neuhaus SJ, Watson DI, Ellis T, Rofe AM, Mathew G, Jamieson GG. Influence of gases on intraperitoneal immunity during laparoscopy in tumor-bearing rats. World J Surg. 2000;24:1227–31.

14. Trokel MJ, Bessler M, Treat MR, Whelan RL, Nowygrod R. Preservation of immune response after laparoscopy. Surg Endosc. 1994;8:1385–8.

15. Watson RWG, Redmond HP, McCarthy J. Exposure of the peritoneal cavity to air regulates early inflammatory responses to surgery in a murine model. Br J Surg. 1995;82:1060–5.

16. Akira S, Yamanaka A, Ishihara T, Takeshita T, Araki T. Gasless laparoscopic ovarian cystectomy during pregnancy: comparison with laparotomy. Am J Obstet Gynecol. 1999; 180:554–7.

17. Amos JD, Schorr SJ, Norman PF, Poole GV, Thomae KR, Mancino AT, et al. Laparoscopic surgery during pregnancy. Am J Surg. 1996;171:435–7.

18. Cruz AM, Southerland LC, Duke T, Townsend HG, Ferguson JG, Crone LA. Intraabdominal carbon dioxide insufflation in the pregnant ewe. Uterine blood flow, intraamniotic pressure, and cardiopulmonary effects. Anesthesiology. 1996;85:1395–402.

19. Hess LW, Peaceman A, O'Brien WF, Winkel CA, Cruikshank DP, Morrison JC. Adnexal mass occurring with intrauterine pregnancy: report of fifty-four patients requiring laparotomy for definitive management. Am J Obstet Gynecol. 1988;158:1029–34.

20. Hunter JG, Swanstorm L, Thomburg K. Carbon dioxide pneumoperitoneum induces fetal acidosis in a pregnant ewe model. Surg Endosc. 1995;9:272–9.

21. Carroll BJ, Chandra M, Phillips EH, Harold JG. Laparoscopic cholecystectomy in the heart transplant candidate with acute cholecystitis. J Heart Lung Transplant. 1992;11:831–3.

22. Chamberlain G, Brown JC. Gynaecological laparoscopy: report on the confidential inquiry into gynaecological laparoscopy. London: Royal College of Obstetricians and Gynaecologists; 1978.

23. De Sousa H, Tyler IL. Can absorption of the insufflation gas during laparoscopy be hazardous? Anesthesiology. 1987;67:476–80.

24. Holzman M, Sharp K, Richards W. Hypercarbia during CO2 gas insufflation for therapeutic laparoscopy: a note of caution. Surg Laparosc Endosc. 1992;2:11–4.

25. Johannsen G, Juhl B. The effect of general anaesthesia on the haemodynamic events during laparoscopy with CO_2 insufflation. Acta Anaesthesiol Scand. 1989;33:132–6.

26. Kent RB. Subcutaneous emphysema and hypercarbia following laparoscopic cholecystectomy. Arch Surg. 1991;126:1154–6.

27. Taura P, Lopez A, Lacy AM, Anglada T, Beltran J, Fernandez-Cruz L, et al. Prolonged pneumoperitoneum at 15 mm Hg causes lactic acidosis. Surg Endosc. 1998;12:198–201.

28. Ott DE. Contamination via gynaecologic endoscopy insufflation. J Gynecol Surg. 1989;5:205–85.

29. Canis M, Botchorishvili R, Wattiez A, Mage G, Pouly JL, Bruhat MA. Tumor growth and dissemination after laparotomy and CO2 pneumoperitoneum: a rat ovarian cancer model. Obstet Gynecol. 1998;92:104–8.

30. Canis M, Botchorishvili R, Wattiez A, Pouly JL, Mage G, Manhes H, et al. Cancer and laparoscopy, experimental studies: a review. Eur J Obstet Gynecol Reprod Biol. 2000;91:1–9.
31. Dorrance HR, Oien K, O'Dwyer PJ. Effects of laparoscopy on intraperitoneal tumor growth and distant metastases in an animal model. Surgery. 1999;126:35–40.
32. Gutt CN, Kim ZG, Schmandra T, Paolucci V, Lorenz M. Carbon dioxide pneumoperitoneum is associated with increased liver metastases in a rat model. Surgery. 2000;127:566–70.
33. Hopkins MP, Dulai RM, Occhino A, Holda S. The effects of carbon dioxide pneumoperitoneum on seeding of tumor in port sites in a rat model. Am J Obstet Gynecol. 1999;181:1329–34.
34. Hopkins MP, von Gruenigen V, Haller NA, Holda S. The effect of various insufflation gases on tumor implantation in an animal model. Am J Obstet Gynecol. 2002;187:994–6.
35. Jacobi CA, Sabat R, Bohm B, Zieren HU, Volk HD, Muller JM. Pneumoperitoneum with carbon dioxide stimulates growth of malignant colonic cells. Surgery. 1997;121:72–8.
36. Jones DB, Guo LW, Reinhard MK, Soper NJ, Philpott GW, Connett J. Impact of pneumoperitoneum on trocar site implantation of colon cancer in hamster model. Dis Colon Rectum. 1995;38:1182–8.
37. Smidt VJ, Singh DM, Hurteau JA, Hurd WW. Effect of carbon dioxide on human ovarian carcinoma cell growth. Am J Obstet Gynecol. 2001;185:1314–7.
38. Bacha EA, Barber W, Ratchford W. Port-site metastases of adenocarcinoma of the fallopian tube after laparoscopically assisted vaginal hysterectomy and salpingo-oophorectomy. Surg Endosc. 1996;10:1102–3.
39. Bouvy ND, Marquet RL, Jeekel H, Bonjer J. Impact of gas(less) laparoscopy and laparotomy on peritoneal tumor growth and abdominal wall metastases. Ann Surg. 1996;224(6):694–701.
40. Cavina E, Goletti O, Molea N, Buccianti P, Chiarugi M, Boni G, et al. Trocar site tumor recurrences. May pneumoperitoneum be responsible? Surg Endosc. 1998;12:1294–6.
41. Childers JM, Aqua KA, Surwit EA, Hallum AV, Hatch KD. Abdominal-wall tumor implantation after laparoscopy for malignant conditions. Obstet Gynecol. 1994;84:765–9.
42. Cirocco WC, Schwartzman A, Golub RW. Abdominal wall recurrence after laparoscopic colectomy for colon cancer. Surgery. 1994;116:842–6.
43. Dobronte Z, Wittmann T, Karacsony G. Rapid development of malignant metastases in the abdominal wall after laparoscopy. Endoscopy. 1978;10:127–30.
44. Faught W, Fung M. Port site recurrences following laparoscopically managed early stage endometrial cancer. Int J Gynecol Cancer. 1999;9:256–8.
45. Fusco MA, Paluzzi MW. Abdominal wall recurrence after laparoscopic-assisted colectomy for adenocarcinoma of the colon. Dis Colon Rectum. 1993;36:858–61.
46. Gleeson NC, Nicosia SV, Mark JE, Hofman MS, Cavanagh D. Abdominal wall metastases from ovarian cancer after laparoscopy. Am J Obstet Gynecol. 1993;169:522–3.
47. Hopkins MP, von Gruenigen V, Gaich S. Laparoscopic port site implantation with ovarian cancer. Am J Obstet Gynecol. 2000;182:735–6.
48. Jacquet P, Averbach A, Jacquet N. Abdominal wall metastasis and peritoneal carcinomatosis after laparoscopic assisted colectomy for colon cancer. Eur J Surg Oncol. 1995;21:568–70.
49. Lane G, Tay J. Port site metastasis following laparoscopic lymphadenectomy for adenosquamous carcinoma of the cervix. Gynecol Oncol. 1999;74:130–3.
50. Lehner R, Wenzl R, Heinzl H, Husslein P, Sevelda P. Influence of delayed staging laparotomy after laparoscopic removal of ovarian masses later found to be malignant. Obstet Gynecol. 1998;92:967–71.
51. Leminem A, Lehtovirta P. Spread of ovarian cancer after laparoscopic surgery: report of eight cases. Gynecol Oncol. 1999;75:387–90.
52. Muntz HG, Goff BA, Madsen BL, Yon JL. Port site recurrence after laparoscopic surgery for endometrial carcinoma. Obstet Gynecol. 1999;93:807–9.
53. Naumann RW, Spencer S. An umbilical metastasis after laparoscopy for squamous cell carcinoma of the cervix. Gynecol Oncol. 1997;64:507–9.
54. Nduka C, Monson J, Menzies-Gow N, Darzi A. Abdominal wall metastases following laparoscopy. Br J Surg. 1994;81:648–52.
55. Paolucci V, Schaeff B, Schneider M, Gutt C. Tumor seeding following laparoscopy: international survey. World J Surg. 1999;23:989–95.

56. Tjalma WA, Winter-Roach BA, Rowlands P, De Barros Lopes A. Port-site recurrence following laparoscopic surgery in cervical cancer. Int J Gynecol Cancer. 2001;11:409–12.
57. Volz J, Köster S, Schaeff B, Paolucci V. Laparoscopic surgery: the effects of insufflation gas on tumor-induced lethality in nude mice. Am J Obstet Gynecol. 1998;178:793–5.
58. Wang PH, Yen MS, Yuan CC, Chao KC, Ng HT. Port site metastasis after laparoscopic-assisted vaginal hysterectomy for endometrial cancer: possible mechanisms and prevention. Gynecol Oncol. 1997;66:151–5.
59. Alexander RJT, Jaques BC, Mitchell KG. Laparoscopically assisted colectomy and wound recurrence. Lancet. 1993;341:250–6.
60. Mathew G, Watson DI, Ellis TS, Jamieson GG, Rofe AM. The role of peritoneal immunity and the tumour-bearing state on the development of wound and peritoneal metastases after laparoscopy. Aust N Z J Surg. 1999;69:14–8.
61. Slater NJ, Ratterv AT, Cope GH. The ultrastructure of human abdominal mesothelium. J Anat. 1989;167:47–56.
62. Wang PH, Yuan CC, Chao KC, Yen MS, Ng HT, Chao HT. Squamous cell carcinoma of the cervix after laparoscopic surgery. J Reprod Med. 1997;42:801–4.
63. Koivusalo AM, Kellokumpu I, Ristkari S, Lindgren L. Splanchnic and renal deterioration during and after laparoscopic cholecystectomy: a comparison of the carbon dioxide pneumoperitoneum and the abdominal wall lift method. Anesth Analg. 1997;85:886–91.
64. Koivusalo AM, Kellokumpu I, Scheinin M, Tikkanen I, Makisalo H, Lindgren L. A comparison of gasless mechanical and conventional carbon dioxide pneumoperitoneum methods for laparoscopic cholecystectomy. Anesth Analg. 1998;86:153–8.
65. Lukban JC, Jaeger J, Hammond KC, LoBraico DA, Gordon AM, Graebe RA. Gasless versus conventional laparoscopy. N J Med. 2000;97:29–34.
66. Schulze S, Lyng KM, Bugge K, Perner A, Bendtsen A, Thorup J, et al. Cardiovascular and respiratory changes and convalescence in laparoscopic colonic surgery: comparison between carbon dioxide pneumoperitoneum and gasless laparoscopy. Arch Surg. 1999;134:1112–8.
67. Cravello L, D'Ercole C, Roger V, Samson D, Blanc B. Laparoscopic surgery in gynecology: randomized prospective study comparing pneumoperitoneum and abdominal wall suspension. Eur J Obstet Gynecol Reprod Biol. 1999;83:9–14.
68. D'Ercole C, Cravello L, Guyon F, DeMontgolfier R, Boubli L, Blanc B. Gasless laparoscopic gynecologic surgery. Eur J Obstet Gynecol Reprod Biol. 1996;66:137–44.
69. Johnson PL, Sibert KS. Laparoscopy: gasless vs CO_2 pneumoperitoneum. J Reprod Med. 1997;42:255–9.
70. Kruczynski D, Scaffer U, Knapstein PG. Gasless laparoscopy with conventional surgical instruments. Gynecol Endosc. 1996;5:277–81.
71. Smith RS, Fry WR, Tsoi EK, Henderson VJ, Hirvela ER, Koehler RH. Gasless laparoscopy and conventional instruments: the next phase of minimally invasive surgery. Arch Surg. 1993;128:1102–7.
72. Hill DJ, Maher PJ, Wood HF. Gasless laparoscopy. Aust N Z J Obstet Gynecol. 1994;6:185–92.
73. Paolucci V, Schaeff B, editors. Gasless laparoscopy in general surgery and gynecology. New York: Thieme; 1996.
74. Tanaka H, Futamura N, Takubo S, Toyoda N. Gasless laparoscopy under epidural anesthesia for adnexal cysts during pregnancy. J Reprod Med. 1999;44:929–32.
75. Goldberg JM, Maurer WG. A randomized comparison of gasless laparoscopy and CO2 pneumoperitoneum. Obstet Gynecol. 1997;90:416–20.
76. Guido RS, Brooks K, McKenzie R, Gruss J, Krohn MA. A randomized, prospective comparison of pain after gasless laparoscopy and traditional laparoscopy. J Am Assoc Gynecol Laparosc. 1998;5:149–53.
77. Hashimoto D, Nayeem SA, Kajiwara S, Hoshino T. Laparoscopic cholecystectomy: a new approach without pneumoperitoneum. Surg Endosc. 1993;7:54–6.
78. Nagai H, Kondo Y, Yasuda T. An abdominal wall-lift method of laparoscopic cholecystectomy without peritoneal insufflation. Surg Laparosc Endosc. 1993;3:175–9.
79. Gasbarro N, Lupo P, Brusati M, Leanza V. Chirurgia ginecologica meno invasiva e riparazione lesioni iatrogene. Ed. Abiabè 2006.

80. Fader AN, Rojas-Espaillat L, Ibeanu O, Grumbine FC, Escobar PF. Laparoendoscopic single-site surgery (LESS) in gynecology: a multi-institutional evaluation. Am J Obstet Gynecol. 2010;203:501.e1-6.
81. MacFadyen BV, Lenz S. The economic consideration in laparoscopic surgery. Surg Endosc. 1994;8:748–52.
82. Hasson HM. A modified instrument and method for laparoscopy. Am J Obstet Gynecol. 1971;110:886–7.
83. Hasson HM. Open laparoscopy: a report of 150 cases. J Reprod Med. 1974;12:234–8.
84. Penfield AJ. How to prevent complications of open laparoscopy. J Reprod Med. 1985;30:660–4.
85. Canis M, Mage G, Pouly JL, Wattiez A, Manhes H, Bruhat MA. Laparoscopic diagnosis of adnexal cystic masses: a 12 year experience with long term follow-up. Obstet Gynecol. 1994;83:707–12.
86. Canis M, Pouly JL, Wattiez A, Mage G, Manhes H, Bruhat MA. Laparoscopic management of adnexal tumours suspicious at ultrasound. Obstet Gynecol. 1997;89:679–83.
87. Canis M, Rabischong B, Batchorishvili R, Tamburo S, Wattiez A, Mage G, et al. Risk of spread of ovarian cancer after laparoscopic surgery. Curr Opin Obstet Gynecol. 2001;13:9–14.
88. Ogihara Y, Isshiki A, Kindscher JD, Goto H. Abdominal wall lift versus carbon dioxide insufflation for laparoscopic resection of ovarian tumors. J Clin Anesth. 1999;11:406–12.
89. Querleu D, Childers JM, Dargent D. Laparoscopic surgery in gynaecological oncology. Malden: Blackwell Science; 1999.
90. Shepherd JH, Carter PG, Lowe DG. Wound recurrence by implantation of a borderline ovarian tumour following laparoscopic removal. Br J Obstet Gynaecol. 1994;101:265–6.
91. van Dam PA, DeCloedt J, Tjalma WAA, Buytaert P, Becquart D, Vergote I. Trocar implantation metastasis after laparoscopy in patients with advanced ovarian cancer: can the risk be reduced? Am J Obstet Gynecol. 1999;181:536–41.
92. Leidi L, Brusati M, Vespa MG. A treacherous scar. Am J Obstet Gynecol. 2007;197:553. e1-553. e2.
93. Pelosi 3rd MA, Pelosi MA. Spontaneous uterine rupture at thirty-three weeks subsequent to previous superficial laparoscopic myomectomy. Am J Obstet Gynecol. 1997;177:1547–9.

Chapter 11
First Abdominal Access in Gynecological Laparoscopy: Comparison of Techniques

Antonio Malvasi and Andrea Tinelli

Introduction

The choice of a technique to enter the peritoneal cavity during a laparoscopy depends on diverse variables that do not foster any standardized method. It appears impossible to accurately define which is the best method for the first abdominal access in gynecological laparoscopy.

The preference for one or another technique depends on the surgeon's experience, school and specialty, laparoscopic upgrading and the working environment. Many surgical techniques are not used because of constraints or concerns of some surgeons to change the first access approach, or due to the lack of flexibility of one technique or another. A review of the scientific literature points out that there are two major problems during the first laparoscopic abdominal access, namely, vascular and intestinal complications, and that the percentages may vary.

This study describes a wide range of methods, as well as the most common complications, for open and closed laparoscopies, and direct access, which enable a first abdominal laparoscopic access.

The accurate knowledge of the anatomy in pelvic and abdominal endoscopic surgery is of major importance in order to begin any laparoscopic procedure. It is just as important to have a precise knowledge of the anatomy of the abdominal pelvic viscera and identify the connective structures within which vessels and nerves are located.

A. Malvasi
Department of Obstetrics and Gynecology, Santa Maria Hospital, Bari, Italy

A. Tinelli (✉)
Department of Obstetrics and Gynecology, Division of Experimental Endoscopic Surgery, Imaging, Technology and Minimally Invasive Therapy, Vito Fazzi Hospital, Lecce, Italy
e-mail: andreatinelli@gmail.com

A. Tinelli (ed.), *Laparoscopic Entry*,
DOI 10.1007/978-0-85729-980-2_11, © Springer-Verlag London Limited, 2012

The knowledge of the anatomy of the loose connective tissue that fills the virtual spaces between the pelvic organs (pre-visceral gaps), as well as of the vascular-connective landmark points, will enable access to districts and anatomical structures usually unknown to laparotomic surgery.

For the above reasons, in order to perform a safe laparoscopy, the location of organs, the pelvic structures supporting the muscle and ligaments, and the vessels and nerves has to be clearly illustrated, and should serve as a pattern at the beginning of any surgery [1].

General Principles of Laparoscopic Access

The choice of the site for trocar entry depends mainly on patients' history, suspected adhesions, and any previous laparotomies performed.

The first advice for surgeons approaching laparoscopy is the preoperative positioning of the patient on the surgical operating table for laparoscopic entry (Fig. 11.1).

The inspection of the hepatic dome, gall bladder, diaphragm, stomach, intestinal loops and spleen demands an adequately prepared visual field, making sure not to disregard areas or details that could jeopardize diagnosis and treatment. For several reasons it is of fundamental importance to record and file all endoscopies performed by the surgical team; before introducing any secondary trocar, a transillumination of the wall should be performed in order to detect possible aponeuroses where the instruments have to be introduced [2].

The entry point of the 10-mm diameter central trocar and the entry for the camera is the umbilical region. The entry may be performed in various ways, with different types of trocars, by incision of the skin with a lancet for at least 5 cm in depth, through which the instrument will be introduced. In spite of the diverse theories on

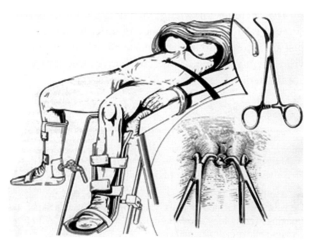

Fig. 11.1 Preoperative positioning of patient on the surgical operating table for laparoscopic entry. In the *right box*, the two Backhaus forceps positioned on the umbilical margins before to entry in abdominal cavity

the introduction of trocars in the abdomen, there still is not one unique and safe method of introduction of the central trocar [3].

The umbilicus is the ideal site of introduction of the lens, because of its thin, non-vascularized skin and because it provides access to all the areas of the pelvis and abdomen. The inner face of the umbilicus, in fact, is adjacent to the middle line; upwards it is adjacent to the falciform ligament, downwards to the urachus cord, downwards and obliquely at 45° to the two fibrous cords of the left and right umbilical arteries [2].

As to closed techniques, it is possible to puncture the anteroposterior intestine without immediate problems and realize it later, or not realize at all. Cases have been described whereby the trocar totally perforated the intestine throughout the entire procedure, without the surgeons realizing the damage caused until the end of the surgery.

For a safe introduction of the central trocars in "open laparoscopy" techniques, by means of a minilaparotomic opening and introduction of a direct-vision Hasson's trocar, the U.S. Food and Drug Administration has recently published a letter reporting that there are no data available stating that trocars thus introduced are safe. Actually it is possible to harm the intestine with any technique, and the only advantage of "open" techniques is that they provide visual access when the intestine is perforated frontally.

The Veress needle has been designed so that, when introduced in the tissues, its mobile central portion detracts against the fibrous or fixed tissue, and passes through loose tissues, with open valves to let air or fluids in. Hence, when the needle is introduced, it is necessary to lift the abdomen so that—in case of a negative pressure in the abdomen—when air is insufflated into the closed cavity, the intestine moves away, spontaneously, from the wall.

The introduction of Veress needle into abdominal wall, requires an incision by surgeon along the bottom rim of the umbilicus or abdominal skin in arched or longitudinal direction. Then surgeon lift up the abdominal skin by his left hand, to separate the abdominal wall from the retroperitoneum. The Veress needle is thus introduced; it will produce a double snap, which corresponds to the passage from the aponeurotic to the peritoneal plane. Subsequently, gas is insufflated into the abdomen.

If the patient is thin, it may be convenient to introduce the needle according to an angle looking towards the uterine fundus or the anterior peritoneum. Conversely, in obese patients, the opposite is suggested, i.e., the needle should be oriented perpendicularly towards the bottom.

In case a pneumoperitoneum is to be produced, it is always desirable to insufflate at least 2–2.5 L of CO_2 into the abdomen at a variable flow speed (up to 30 L/min), with a standard intraabdominal reference pressure of 15 mmHg. The Veress needle is usually introduced into the paraumbilical area, but may also be introduced in the vagina, in the posterior fornix, or in Palmer's point, in the left subcostal area [4].

The Anatomy of the Abdominal Wall

A cross-section of the anterolateral wall of the abdomen is made up of the following overlapping layers: epidermis, dermis, muscles coated by aponeurosis and peritoneum (see Table 11.1).

Table 11.1 Layers of the abdominal wall

Cutis	Subcutaneous layers
	Camper' fascia
	Scarpa's fascia
Aponeurotic muscle layer	Straight band (formed by the merger of the external oblique muscle aponeurosis)
Muscles	Internal oblique muscles (fused in the midline)
	Transverse abdominal muscle
	Fascia transversalis
	Peritoneus

The subcutaneous tissue varies according to the individual's features. It is made up of an upper and a deeper layer, separated by fascia, known as Camper's fascia; if this fascia is thick, abdominal access may be difficult. The abdominal subcutaneous tissue is, in most cases, made up of a single layer a few millimeters thick, including a variable amount of fat; in the lower part of the abdomen, especially in obese females, the subcutaneous tissue is usually divided into two layers—an upper and a deeper one—and, between the two layers there are vessels and superficial nerves. Above the superficial layer there is the external or superficial abdominal fascia (Fig. 11.2).

Between the superficial and the deep layer there is the intermediate fascia—also known as Camper's fascia; and under the deep layer there is the internal or deep abdominal fascia. Camper's fascia plays a major role when the subcutaneous tissue has to be sutured, in so far as reducing dehiscences of trocar scars. Some studies have, in fact, shown that it is sufficient to suture Camper's fascia to reduce complications in laparotomic sutures (Fig. 11.3).

Besides these areas, fascias and muscles also play an important role within the abdominal wall. The fascia of the external oblique muscle, also known as Lauth's fascia, is the common abdominal fascia lining the entire external oblique muscle and its aponeurosis. At the bottom, next to the fold of the groin, it adheres to the inguinal ligament and continues in the fascia of the thigh, medially and, at the bottom on the subcutaneous orifice of the inguinal canal, it forms a lining over the organs contained. The fascia of the internal oblique muscle is very thin and is located on its anterior portion. The fascia of the transverse muscle, also very thin, descends along its front portion.

The fascia transversalis is a connective layer located between the transverse muscle and the parietal peritoneum adhering to the upper rim of the pubis and to the inguinal ligament, and moves down into the endopelvic fascia forming the femoral septum, which closes the femoral ring.

The fascia transversalis is a particularly thick tissue in the ileum-pubic region, extending from the interfoveal ligament to the ligament of Menle. Frontally and medially, this fascia adheres to the conjoint tendon and merges with it. Between the front of the fascia transversalis and the parietal peritoneum, moving downwards, there is a preperitoneal space where the vascular tree passes.

Below the umbilicus, between the fascia transversalis and the peritoneum, lies the prevescical fascia formed by two layers, hosting the median umbilical-vesical

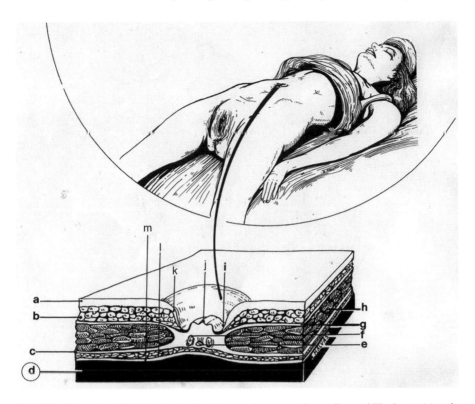

Fig. 11.2 Normal umbilical anatomical region, passing across the median umbilical part: (*a*) cutis (*b*) subcutis (the subcutaneous tissue is absent in umbilical region and the fascia is attached to cutis) (*c*) posterior fascia of right rectus muscle (*d*) right peritoneal cavity (*e*) uracus (*f*) right umbilical artery (*g*) anterior fascia of left rectus muscle (*h*) left rectus muscle (*i*) umbilical line (*j*) umbilical prominence (*k*) umbilical rib (*l*) pre-peritoneal tissue (this tissue is reduced in umbilical area) (*m*) parietal peritoneum

ligament—stemming from the urachus, and the lateral umbilical-vesical ligaments—stemming from the fetus' umbilical arteries.

The abdominal rectal muscle is contained in a fibrous sheath, called aponeurosis of the abdominal rectal muscle, and is made up of two laminae: the anterior or pre-rectal lamina and the posterior or retrorectal lamina, both made up by the aponeurosis of the large muscles of the abdomen.

Above the umbilicus, the anterior or prerectal lamina is made up by the aponeurosis of the internal oblique muscle; whereas, the posterior or retrorectal lamina is made up by the posterior layer of the aponeurosis of the internal oblique muscle and by the aponeurosis of the transverse abdominal muscle. Below the umbilicus, the anterior lamina is made up by the three aponeuroses, as the posterior or retrorectal lamina is missing.

The umbilical structure is the main site for laparoscopic entry. This closed orifice is an excellent entry for the laparoscopic surgeon, as the umbilicus is a scar resulting from the detachment of the umbilical cord and the obliteration of umbilical vessels,

Fig. 11.3 Intraoperative isolation of Camper' fascia during laparotomy. Frontal section of female abdominal wall, with highlighted fascia of large muscles of abdomen raised by two clamps

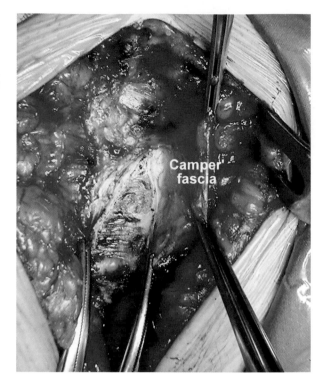

situated in the middle of the anterior wall of the abdomen. The superficial umbilical layers are the cutaneous and the subcutaneous connective tissues. The latter is characterized by a good amount of fat tissue supplied with vessels and nerves. Below this tissue there is a thick and resistant aponeurotic layer corresponding to the linea Alba; below it, there is a loose connective tissue and the peritoneum. The preperitoneal loose connective tissue is thin and has little fat; it is covered by obliterated umbilical vessels (residual fibrous cords) ranging from the umbilicus downwards to the walls of the pelvic cavity (the urachus runs from the umbilicus to the bladder). Superiorly, it forms the hepatic round ligament, which runs upward and back to the anterior portion of the liver. At times, the loose connective tissue adheres to an umbilical fascia—known as Richet's fascia—which is a falciform fibrous structure, depending on the fascia transversalis, which not all individuals have but, when it is found, is a thick structure. It adheres, on the upper rim, to the sheath of the rectal muscles it is enveloped by. On the bottom rim, instead, it takes on the shape of a protruding fold that supports the peritoneum and reinforces the abdominal wall in its weakest point—the umbilical ring—thus enabling the area to bear the endoabdominal pressure [5].

The arcuate line, located 2–3 cm below the umbilicus, is made up by the umbilicus and the inferior rim of the posterior lamina of the rectal muscle's sheath, corresponding medially to the linea Alba. Laterally, instead, it follows along the interfoveal ligament; underneath, the posterior portion of the rectal muscle is lined only by the fascia transversalis. The arcuate line is crossed by the lower epigastric vessels which, subsequently penetrate into the rectal muscle.

The abdominal linea alba is a median, fibrous structure, extending from the xiphoid process of the sternum to the pubis, between the two rectal muscles of the abdomen, and is made up by the crossing fibres of the aponeurosis of abdominal muscles, medial to the aponeurosis of the rectal muscle, and borders bordering with the upper skin and behind the fascia transversalis and the peritoneum.

The abdomen walls are mainly made up of muscles, divided into anterior abdominal muscles (12: i.e., 6 on the right and 6 on the left); the back portion is made up by only one muscle on the right and one on the left. The muscles of the abdominal wall include the following structures: quadratus lumborum, abdominal rectal muscle, external oblique muscle, internal oblique muscle and transverse abdominal muscle. The quadratus lumborum muscle is the posterior muscle of the abdominal wall; it originates in the medial portion of the iliac crest and in the ileolumbar ligament, and connects to the last rib through the fourth lumbar vertebra.

The abdominal rectal muscle is the anterior muscle of the abdominal wall; it stems from the median ribs, approaches the abdomen, and connects to the pubis. It is lined with a fibrous sheath, the rectal muscles' fascia, which partially lines also the external oblique muscle, anterolaterally.

The external oblique muscle originates in the inferior portion of the eighth rib; it connects to the iliac crest superiorly, and to the upper iliac spine, frontally. The internal oblique muscle runs deeply unto the internal oblique muscle; it stems from the iliac crest and the inferior lumbar spine and runs superiorly to its insertions unto the last four ribs. The abdominal transverse muscle is the deepest one and runs from the last six ribs to the iliac crest.

The anterolateral wall of the abdomen is vascularized by the six intercostal arteries, four lumbar arteries and by the upper and lower epigastric arteries. The innervation of the large muscles of the cutaneous and subcutaneous tissues is vascularized by T7-L1 branches; the inguinal and genital region, instead, is innervated by T1-L1branches[5].

General Remarks on the First Laparoscopic Access in the Abdomen

Reviewing literature, most complications during access into the abdomen involve intestinal and vascular lesions. In the former case, literature reports 0.4/1,000 procedures; in the latter, the risk is about 0.2/1,000 cases [6].

A metaanalysis of several studies on gastrointestinal lesions during gynecological laparoscopies pointed out that out of 56 patients with 62 gastrointestinal lesions, in 32% of the cases lesions occurred during the first phase of the procedure (entry into the abdomen). Some patients had electrosurgery lesions (mainly due to the monopolar current); 4–5 days were needed to diagnose lesions [7].

Another study conducted on 5,901 laparoscopic gynecological procedures has shown 2.4 intestinal lesions every 1,000 surgeries [8]. An Australian meta-analysis, instead, conducted in 2002 on the correlations between peritoneal entry techniques and subsequent vascular and intestinal lesions, showed that the latter were found in 0.7/1,000 women, vascular lesions in 0.4/1,000 patients, with an overall prevalence of 1.1/1,000 procedures [2].

The direct access technique is associated with a significant drop in lesion incidence (0.5/1,000 cases), if compared with the open access or to the introduction of the Veress needle (1.1 and 0.9 over 1,000), whereas intestinal lesions at entry are greater in general surgery laparoscopies.

The open access technique is statistically associated with intestinal lesions more than with the direct access or Veress, although vascular lesions seem to be fewer with the open access entry into the abdomen [9].

Despite frequent use of laparoscopy, the optimal technique for the safest access to the abdominal cavity still is debated. Even the European Society for Endoscopic Surgeons (EAES) could not give any strong recommendation in their guidelines of 2002 favoring one technique [10].

Access into the abdomen is the one challenge of laparoscopy that is particular to the insertion of surgical instruments through small incisions. To minimize entry-related complications, several techniques and technologies have been introduced during the last 50 years. This complication rate has remained the same during the last 25 years. The majority of injuries are owing to the insertion of the primary umbilical trocar. Increased morbidity and mortality result when laparoscopists or patients do not recognize injuries early or do not address them quickly.

Currently, four different access methods are the most accepted: the Veress Needle, direct trocar insertion, the direct optical trocar as a closed procedure, and the Hasson technique as open access. Other methods include the use of shielded disposable trocars, optical Veress needle, optical trocars, radially expanding trocars, and a trocarless reusable, visual access cannula (EndoTIP).

At present, there is no evidence that the closed laparoscopic entry is more or less dangerous than the other existing methods of entry. The open (Hasson) entry is an alternative to closed entry. However, it has not prevented visceral and vascular injury. Each of these methods of entry enjoys a certain degree of popularity according to the surgeon's training, experience, and bias, and according to regional and interdisciplinary variability. Anyway, there is evidence that most gynecologists worldwide use the "classic" or closed laparoscopic entry technique [11].

Traditional Access into the Abdomen with Blind Entry

The closed techniques have one thing in common: what is behind the peritoneum cannot be seen.

After the introduction of laparoscopy, carbon dioxide (CO_2) pneumoperitoneum has been accepted as the method of choice compared with gasless lifting techniques.

Therefore, peritoneal access can be achieved with the Veress needle and direct trocar access using the optical trocar or open Hasson technique, even if the closed approach seems to be more popular.

Janos Veress of Hungary (Fig. 11.4) developed a specially designed spring-loaded needle; interestingly, Veress did not promote the use of his Veress needle for laparoscopy purposes. In fact, he used this needle for the induction of pneumothorax in the treatment of pulmonary tuberculosis in 1936.

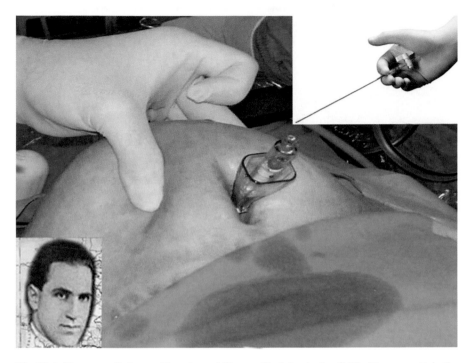

Fig. 11.4 Veress needle inserted into the umbilicus, with abdominal wall lifted by surgeons; in the lower left inset is depicted Janos Veress, the inventor of needle

Currently, the Veress needle is the most important instrument today to create pneumoperitoneum. This needle consists of an outer cannula with a beveled needle point for cutting through tissues. Inside the cannula of the Veress needle is an inner stylet. The stylet is loaded with a spring that springs forward in response to the sudden decrease in pressure encountered upon crossing the abdominal wall and entering the peritoneal cavity (Fig. 11.5).

Under usual circumstances, the Veress needle is inserted in the umbilical area, in the midsagittal plane, with or without stabilizing or lifting the anterior abdominal wall. Literature recommendations call for lifting of the abdominal wall for insertion of the Veress needle to prevent intraabdominal injuries. To determine correct placement of the Veress needle, several techniques or safety tests (Fig. 11.6) have been suggested [12], including the following:

1. The double-click sound of the Veress needle
2. The aspiration test
3. The saline solution hanging drop test
4. The "his" test
5. The syringe test

Although lifting of the abdominal wall results in better protection of retroperitoneal structures, the intestine also may be lifted because the abdominal cavity is a closed physical space (Fig. 11.7).

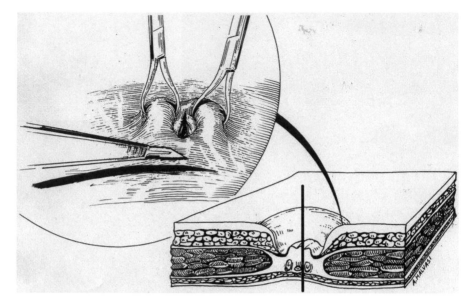

Fig. 11.5 After umbilical incision by scalpel, surgeons lift the abdominal wall facing the umbilical area, by two Backhaus forceps, to remove the underlying viscera. The *black line* represents the correct direction on laparoscopic entries

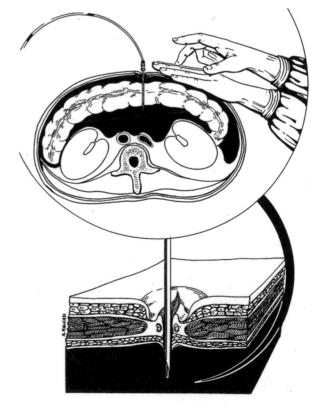

Fig. 11.6 After Veress entry and peritoneal cavity insufflating, the surgeon reproduces a percussion manoeuvre to verify the correct pneumoperitoneum

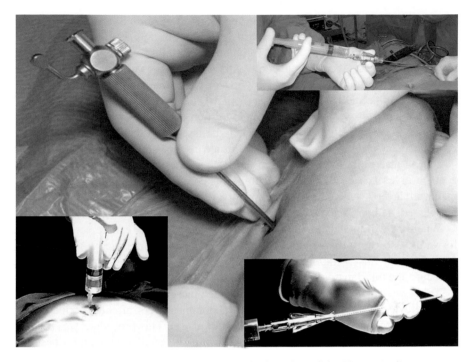

Fig. 11.7 The surgeon lifts the abdominal wall for insertion of the Veress needle to prevent intraabdominal injuries; the inset images show some safety tests

Studies have reported placing the Veress needle into the peritoneal cavity on the first attempt at frequencies of 85.5–86.9%; two attempts were required in 8.5–11.6% of procedures, three attempts in 2.6–3.0%, and more than three attempts in 0.3–1.6%. Complication rates were as follows: at one attempt, 0.8–16.3%; at two attempts, 16.31–37.5%; at three attempts, 44.4–64%; and at more than three attempts, 84.6–100%. Complications were extraperitoneal insufflation, omental and bowel injuries, and failed laparoscopy [12].

Extraperitoneal insufflation is one of the most common complications of laparoscopy, frequently leading to abandonment of the procedure because further attempts to achieve pneumoperitoneum are usually unsuccessful. In one study, preperitoneal insufflation occurred in 2.7%, 15%, 44.4%, and 100% of cases at one, two, three, and more than three attempts, respectively [13].

A prospective study conducted over 1,033 patients, submitted to surgery between 1992 and 1998, compared Veress needle with intraumbilical trocar blind access in two groups of patients: one with no prior abdominal surgery (group 1: 842 patients) and the other group who had undergone prior laparotomies (group 2: 39 patients). Most patients in group 2 showed a difficult access into the peritoneal cavity (4/39) compared to group 1 patients (1/843). Patients who had undergone prior surgery had more adverse events and incidents compared to group 1. No difference was found, in terms of complications, with the introduction of the Veress needle and the intraumbilical trocar in patients with prior laparotomies [14].

As the blind Veress needle entry and the intraumbilical trocar can cause viscero-vascular complications, as well as gas embolisms, some authors developed alternative abdominal access techniques. Nonblind access procedures can reduce lesion risks. According to some authors, techniques used should enable the entry of both instruments and camera, with a direct vision into the peritoneal cavity.

The Veress needle has been further modified to a 2.1 mm diameter and cannula 10.5 cm long to allow insertion of a thin ($\leq$1.2 mm diameter), zero degree, semirigid fiberoptic minilaparoscope. This system may be inserted in the umbilicus or the left upper quadrant, and subsequent ancillary ports are inserted under direct vision [15, 16].

During insertion of the assembled unit (Veress cannula and telescope) the surgeon observes a cascade of monitor color sequences that represent different abdominal wall layers: subcutaneous fat appears yellow, fascia white, anterior rectus muscle red, and peritoneum translucent or shiny bright.

When the Veress needle enters the peritoneum, CO_2 gas can be seen bubbling forwards, and the intraabdominal structures soon come into view. Alternatively, some surgeons insert the optical Veress needle first, secure insufflation, and then introduce the minilaparoscope [17, 18].

This is why, in Germany, a 2.5–2 mm diameter lens has been designed, to be introduced with a specific cannula, across all the abdominal layers, after the periumbilical incision and the insufflation of a small amount of gas. This procedure was used in 184 laparoscopies and has enabled recognition of all layers, thus avoiding adhesions, possible vascular damage, and perforations of the small intestine [19]. The possibility of reducing vascular-enteric lesions is also related to some anatomical and pathological details with which to compare, after introducing the Veress needle.

These features have led to the development, successively, of the optical access devices.

Another example of a blind access involves creating a high pressure pneumoperitoneum. The pressure technique has been adopted by many surgeons worldwide, but the appropriate volume to establish an appropriate intraabdominal pressure remains controversial. It ranges from 10 to 30 mmHg, depending on the surgeons. The rationale for the higher pressure entry technique is that it produces greater splinting of the anterior abdominal wall and a deeper intraabdominal CO_2 bubble than the traditional volume-limited pneumoperitoneum of 2–4 L.

Some authors have used this technique in 3,041 surgical procedures, by raising intraabdominal pressure to 25–30 mmHg and introducing the central trocar without lifting the abdominal wall. This method highlighted two intestinal lesions, but did not produce any vascular lesions or problems caused by the higher intraabdominal pressure [20].

Shamiyeh et al. evaluated the intraabdominal changes during lifting of the fascia with regard to the distance from the fascia to the retroperitoneal vessels and the intestine for access in laparoscopy by Veress needle. They evaluated ten patients scheduled to undergo laparoscopic cholecystectomy. The operation started with the computed tomography (CT) scan, after orotracheal intubation: a CT scan of the umbilical region was performed. After a supraumbilical incision, the fascia was freed and elevated with stay sutures. During maximal elevation, a second CT scan was performed. Distances to the intestinal (small bowel) and retroperitoneal structures (iliac artery, vena cava) were measured. Intraabdominal pressure was measured with a transcystic balloon manometer before and after elevation of the fascia, after insertion of the Veress needle, and after completion of the insufflations.

The authors noted that fascial lifting increased the distance between the fascia and the intestinal structures in the patients with no prior abdominal surgery (mean distance, 1.92 cm; range, 0.87–2.67 cm) and the distance between the fascia and the retroperitoneal vessels (mean distance, 7.83 cm; range, 3–11 cm). The median intraabdominal pressures in terms of cm H_2O were 5.4 for a, 1.1 for b, 1.1 for c, and 12. 5 for d. Authors concluded the elevation of the fascia before the first entrance to the abdominal cavity for laparoscopy may increase safety due to a significant enlargement of distance between the fascia and the retroperitoneal structures [21].

Palmer's Point Entry in Left Upper Quadrant (LUQ)

In patients known or suspected to have periumbilical adhesions, or after failure to establish pneumoperitoneum after three attempts, alternative sites for Veress needle insertion may be sought.

Raoul Palmer, a French surgeon of Paris performed gynecological examinations using laparoscopy in 1944, placing the patients in the Trendelenburg position so air could fill the pelvis. He also stressed the importance of continuous intraabdominal pressure monitoring during a laparoscopic procedure. In patients with previous laparotomy, Palmer advocated insertion of the Veress needle 3 cm below the left sub costal border in the midclavicular line (Fig. 11.8).

This technique should be considered in the obese as well as the very thin patient. In very thin patients, especially those with a prominent sacral promontory and android pelvis, the great vessels lie 1–2 cm underneath the umbilicus. And in obese women, the umbilicus is shifted caudally to the aortic bifurcation.

LUQ insufflation requires emptying of the stomach by nasogastric suction and introduction of the Veress needle perpendicular to the skin. Patients with previous splenic or gastric surgery, significant hepatosplenomegaly, portal hypertension, or gastropancreatic masses should be excluded.

There is significantly more subcutaneous fat at the umbilical area than at the LUQ insertion site [12]. In case of the parietal peritoneum adhered to the undersurface of the ribs at the costal margin, or when it is not easy to enter into the umbilicus, some gynecologists insert the Veress needle through the ninth or tenth intercostal space. The inclusion and exclusion criteria are the same as per LUQ insertion. The Veress needle is inserted directly through the intercostal space at the anterior axillary line along the superior surface of the lower rib to avoid injury to the underlying neurovascular bundle.

Following pneumoperitoneum, established at 20–25 mmHg pressure, 5-mm laparoscopes are introduced at Palmer's point for inspection, followed by additional trocars, inserted under direct vision, to facilitate the required surgery and/or perform adhesiolysis when indicated [22, 23]. A retrospective review of 918 insufflations through the ninth intercostal space found one entry into the stomach and one into the pleural space (causing a pneumothorax) by the Veress needle [24].

Fig. 11.8 A female body
with depicted red area of
Palmer point entry, on the
right side

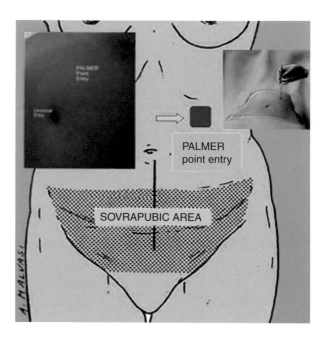

Access into the Abdomen with Direct Access Trocars

The umbilicus, a port with fewer blood vessels in the abdominal wall where muscles and fascias converge, is a preferred site for laparoscopic entry. The maximum resistance of the umbilicus port comes from the incrassate skin and tenacious fascia. Cutting open the umbilicus directly may diminish or even avoid resistance, which can help students get rid of fears for first puncture. It is not CO_2 pneumoperitoneum or the trocars but skills and experience of the surgeon that determine whether a successful laparoscopic access could be achieved [25].

Many surgeons are convinced the open method is safe, but it is time-consuming and associated with difficulty in maintaining the pneumoperitoneum. It is more appropriate for patients who have undergone previous abdominal surgery, are pregnant, or very thin. Especially, previous lower abdominal surgery can leave the bowel adherent to the abdominal wall and a fixed bowel may be damaged during entry into the abdomen. The open method decreases the risk of viscera or vascular injury and allows for surgeons to identify and repair any injury, thus decreasing morbidity and mortality rates.

The direct type of entry is a good alternative whenever the Veress needle is not used for the blind intraabdominal entry to perform a laparoscopy during surgery. When the Direct Access entry is taken, less operative and anesthesia time and less equipment and carbon dioxide are necessary.

Because of the justification that direct trocar insertion, by Direct Access, would cause more hazardous complications, the Veress needle is used widely. Although the Veress needle technique is widely used, it is associated with slow insufflation rates and potentially life-threatening complications. In the vast majority of cases, it is necessary to convert to a laparotomy immediately. Some surgeons use the Veress needle and propose that this is the safest method for the pneumoperitoneum, and some believe that the Direct Access entry is safer than the Veress needle.

Direct trocar insertion without previous pneumoperitoneum has been shown before to be a safe and effective method associated with fewer complications [26–28].

Because meticulous attention to a few key surgical points is critical, Direct Access procedure is thus described in detail.

1. Relaxation: Adequate general anesthesia is essential to assure lower abdominal wall relaxation for proper elevation, especially for obese women because elevation of a heavy abdominal wall can require painful pulling on the skin by two surgeons to achieve the proper anatomical relationships.
2. Sharp Trocar: Sharpness of the trocar should be checked before every entry by this technique, because the force necessary to insert a dull trocar will bring the abdominal wall back down onto the bowel and vessels at the time of entry.
3. Adequate Incision: A horizontal or vertical infraumbilical incision is appropriately made wide enough (1.5–2.0 cm) for the trocar to be inserted without undue resistance from the skin, so that the trocar passes through the fascia and the peritoneum more easily.
4. Technique of elevation of the abdomen: Because most surgeons stand on the patient's left side, the surgeons left hand should grasp the patients lower abdomen at a point midway between the umbilicus and the pubic symphysis. Elevation of the abdominal wall at this point will elevate the umbilicus slightly and stretch it, so that trocar entry can be directed simultaneously: (1) toward the true pelvis (or the uterus), (2) away from the bowels and the large vessels, and (3) at right angles to the skin.

These three simultaneous objectives should be thought of at the time of all entries (Fig. 11.9). The left hand also provides counter traction for the trocar entry by tenting the lower abdomen in a 45° angle.

Altun et al. designed a prospective, nonrandomized study for the comparison of Veress needle and Direct Access insertion techniques. A pneumoperitoneum was created using the Veress needle in 135 patients and using Direct Access insertion technique in 148 patients during a 3-year period. Although no major complication was seen in the Direct Access group, three major complications were seen in the Veress needle group, but there was no statistically significant difference between both groups. More frequent minor complications were seen in the Veress needle group, but it was statistically insignificant. Surgical skill and experience of the surgeon with the entry technique used is an important factor for the selection of the abdominal insufflation technique. Although minor complication rates were higher in the Veress needle group than the trocar group in these studies, major complication rates in both groups were comparable to other studies and there was no significant difference [25].

A North American group of gynecological surgeons has reviewed 1,385 laparoscopies by means of a retrospective study performed between 1993 and 2000, assessed according to entry techniques, demographic characteristics, and complications. This research pointed out that 1223 patients underwent a direct access procedure, 133 a Veress needle procedure, and only 22 an open entry technique. Among the three major complications in 1378 procedures—1 enterotomy, 1 omental herniation, and 1 intestinal herniation—the first occurred during the positioning of the open access

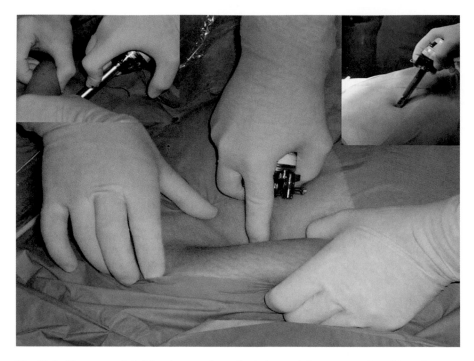

Fig. 11.9 The surgeon's left hand grasps the patient's lower abdomen at a point midway between the umbilicus and the pubic symphysis to introduce, directly, the trocar into the abdomen (direct access technique)

(0.072%); the intestine was sutured laparoscopically. In 1,223 patients submitted to direct access, no lesions related to the trocar entry were found, but 1 patient showed a subsequent omental herniation that required a new laparoscopy after 2 days of hospitalization; another patient showed an intestinal herniation on day 12, which also required a new laparoscopy. The studies concluded and underlined the advantages and safety of the direct access into the abdomen during laparoscopic surgery [29].

An Australian study on 6,173 gynecological laparoscopies, performed by entering into the abdomen with a direct access umbilical trocar technique, and insufflation of CO_2 under vision has shown four intestinal perforations (0.06%) that required a laparotomy, and no lesions of the large vessels or gas embolism. Three of these four intestinal lesions occurred in patients who underwent a prior procedure and had a median subumbilical-pubic scar.

By comparing these data with scientific literature, the review highlighted that the average of visceral or vascular lesions (that required a laparotomy or resuscitation maneuvers) was around 1/1,000 laparoscopies performed with the Veress needle and blind insufflations with the open technique (Hasson's trocar) and with a peri-umbilical direct access. The literature reports also that direct access can reduce the risk of gas embolism by insufflating CO_2 only after confirming the position of the trocar in the abdomen (with a direct intraperitoneal vision); it could even enable an immediate recognition and prompt treatment of major vascular lesions, thus reducing mortality during a laparoscopic procedure.

The author concludes by asserting that data found in literature do not confirm that one technique is better than another in terms of intraabdominal access, and every technique has its pros and cons and a similar morbidity, if performed by expert hands and with the relevant indications. Hence, every technique should be used accordingly by surgeons, depending on the patient and the circumstances [30].

A recently published study compares the most frequently used techniques (Veress needle, direct access, open technique and optical trocar). The study reports that in 578 laparoscopies the use of the direct access, lifting the sheath of the rectal muscle, is a useful, safe, and effective technique with a low rate of surgical complications [31].

A retrospective study performed on 1,500 laparoscopies for cholecystectomies, highlighted six minor lesions (four enterotomies and two omental herniations). Out of the total of the access procedures, 1,375 were performed with the direct access, which produced only three enterotomies with immediate repair of the lesion. The open technique, instead, had caused the others. The study ended by underlining that the direct access technique enabled a safe and effective entry into the abdomen [32].

Prieto-Díaz-Chávez et al. compared the safety and complications of direct trocar insertion without pneumoperitoneum (by Direct Access) with Veress needle in laparoscopic cholecystectomy. They studied 84 patients admitted to our hospital for laparoscopic cholecystectomy, in a random simple blind design, 42 patients were assigned to Direct Access and 42 to Veress needle. The analyzed variables were: procedure complications, laparoscope insertion time, and duration of surgery. In the results, complication percentages between the groups were significantly different (Direct Access 2.3% versus Veress needle 23.8%, $p=0.009$). The duration of surgery between the two groups was also significantly different (Direct Access 56 ± 31 versus Veress needle 71 ± 28 min, $p<0.02$). Finally, laparoscope insertion time between the two techniques was significantly different (Direct Access 1.5 ± 0.5 versus Veress needle 3.0 ± 0.4 min $p<0.001$). Authors concluded that Direct Access to be a safe, efficient, rapid and easily-learned alternative technique, reducing the number of procedure-related complications [33].

Operation time is generally lower in the Direct Access group, compared to the Veress needle group, so as the failed pneumoperitoneum rate is lower with the Direct Access insertion, and with Veress needle use, extraperitoneal insufflation may occur more frequently and this may result in a failed laparoscopy. Due to its fewer complications, direct trocar insertion has been shown to be a safe and efficient alternative method to the VN technique for pneumoperitoneum production [34, 35]. Randomized, prospective trials comparing the Direct Access entry with the Veress needle have failed to demonstrate any difference in major complication rates [36–40].

Access into the Abdomen with the Open Laparoscopy Technique

The type of entry by a small incision and open dissection down through the various layers of the abdominal wall into the abdominal cavity is a good alternative whenever the Veress needle is not used for the blind intraabdominal entry to perform a laparoscopy. Thus, the most important alternative is the "open" laparoscopy described by Harrith Hasson, who first described the open entry technique in 1971 [41]. The suggested benefits are prevention of: gas embolism, preperitoneal insufflation, and possibly visceral and major vascular injury.

The technique involves using a cannula fitted with a cone-shaped sleeve, a blunt obturator, and possibly a second sleeve to which stay sutures can be attached. The entry is essentially a minilaparotomy. A small incision is made transversely or longitudinally at the umbilicus. This incision is long enough to be able to dissect down to the fascia, incise it, and enter the peritoneal cavity under direct vision. The cannula is inserted into the peritoneal cavity with the blunt obturator in place. Sutures are placed on either side of the cannula in the fascia and attached to the cannula or purse-stringed around the cannula to seal the abdominal wall incision to the cone-shaped sleeve (Fig. 11.10).

The laparoscope is then introduced and insufflation is commenced. At the end of the procedure the fascial defect is closed and the skin is reapproximated. The open technique is favored by general surgeons and considered by some to be indicated in patients with previous abdominal surgery, especially those with longitudinal abdominal wall incisions [12]. As mentioned, this technique enables the surgeon to introduce the periumbilical trocar by making a small laparotomy.

Some French gynecologists have compared the risks of major complications during setup procedures for laparoscopy by making two retrospective assessments, i.e., one with the traditional blind entry (creating a pneumoperitoneum and introducing the optical trocar), and the second one with an open laparoscopy performed on two groups of patients. Group A was made up of 8,324 patients submitted to a traditional entry; Group B was made up by 1,562 patients who underwent the open entry technique.

Results of the study pinpointed a higher, statistically significant, risk of failures for the open entry, leading to a laparotomy (three cases versus 0, i.e., 0.19% vs 0%). No differences in the complications between the two groups (four cases versus three cases, i.e., 0.05% for Group A versus 0.19% for Group B). Lesions reported in the group submitted to the traditional entry were the following: one aortic lesion and three intestinal lesions. Complications in the open entry group, instead, were immediate in two cases (intestinal) and subsequent in one case (postop occlusion). The study's conclusions highlight that the open technique did not reduce the risk of major complications during procedures for the laparoscopic surgery setup compared with the blind pneumoperitoneum [42].

Several studies show that cancer patients having to undergo a laparoscopy have a higher risk of complications. Consequently, a group of French laparoscopists performed a study on the possible advantages in using the open entry technique instead of the blind CO_2 insufflation, followed by the introduction of a blind trocar, on 89 cancer patients, who had previously been submitted to severe laparotomy (65%) and/or to radio therapy (17%) or having a large omental plastron (18%).

The study showed one complication in one of the patients who had been submitted to laparotomy for a minor intestinal perforation. Consequently it was underlined that the open access technique was best on cancer patients, for the advantages in terms of safety and reiterability of this technique compared to the blind one [43].

A group of French surgeons evaluated, retrospectively, 1,562 patients who underwent laparoscopic procedures, from 1994 to 2001, performed by eight different surgeons,

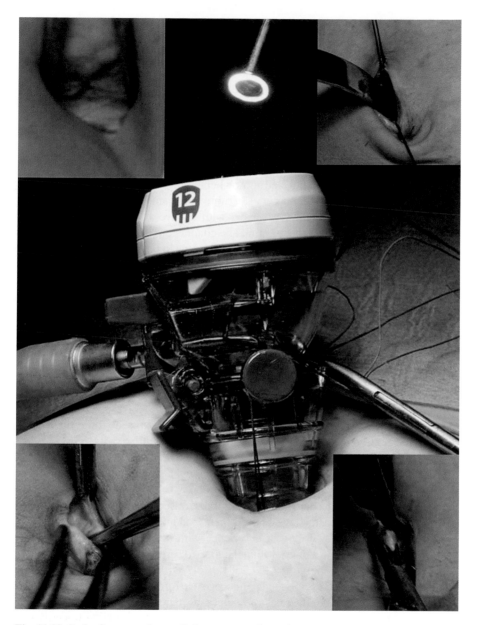

Fig. 11.10 In the figure are shown all the passages of open laparoscopy entry, from the bottom to the top of the figure. After umbilical incision, the incision is long enough to be able to dissect down to the fascia, incise it, and enter the peritoneal cavity under direct vision. Then sutures are placed on either side of the cannula in the fascia and attached to the cannula to seal the abdominal wall incision to the cone-shaped sleeve

who highlighted all intraoperative and postoperative complications. The results of this assessment pinpointed that the major lesions were found in the gastrointestinal tract, with two perforations diagnosed immediately—with no postop occlusion nor death- later treated with a laparotomy (0.19%). In any case there were no vascular or vesical lesions; the group of surgeons therefore reported that the open technique was advisable because of the easy performance and the advantages that reduce the risk of vascular lesions and enables early recognition of the intestinal lesion [44].

A group of US gynecologists performed a retrospective study on 5,284 patients operated with the open access technique between 1970 and 1999. In the study 27 women showed complications related to the primary access (0.5%); 21 suffered a slight infection of the wound, 4 had minor hematomas, 1 developed an umbilical hernia (which required further surgery), 1 more had a small intestine lesion which demanded a major intra-operative repair, with an average access time into the abdominal cavity between 3 and 10 min. The conclusion of the retrospective evaluation showed that such procedure could cause lesions in 0.5% of cases; the authors, therefore, supported this technique instead of the blind access techniques [45].

On the contrary, the literature reports that the percentage of visceral lesions owing to the Veress needle entry technique, or by means of direct introduction, was 0.44 over 1,000 procedures; vascular lesions account for 0.31 over 1,000 procedures [46].

Hasson reviewed 17 publications of open laparoscopy by general surgeons (9 publications, 7,205 laparoscopies) and gynecologists (8 publications, 13,486 laparoscopies) and compared them with closed laparoscopy performed by general surgeons (7 publications, 90,152 patients) and gynecologists (12 publications, 579,510 patients).

Hasson reported that for open laparoscopy the rate of umbilical infection was 0.4%, bowel injury 0.1%, and vascular injury 0%. The corresponding rates for closed laparoscopy were 1%, 0.2%, and 0.2%. Hasson advocated the open technique as the preferred method of access for laparoscopic surgery [47].

Further analysis of Hasson's review suggests that the prospective studies and surveys indicate that general surgeons experience higher complication rates than gynecologists with the closed technique, but experience similar complication rates with the open technique. Using the closed technique, the visceral and vascular complication rates were 0.22% and 0.04% for general surgeons and 0.10% and 0.03% for gynecologists. In a published record of his own 29-year experience with laparoscopy in 5,284 patients, Hasson reports only 1 bowel injury within the first 50 cases [48].

Garry reviewed six reports (n=357,257) of closed laparoscopy and six reports and one survey (n=20,410) of open laparoscopy performed by gynecologists. With the closed entry technique, the rates of bowel and major vessel injury were 0.04% and 0.02%, respectively; with the open entry, they were 0.5% and 0%, respectively. When the survey report (n=8,000) was excluded, the rate of bowel injury with the open technique was 0.06%. Garry concluded that open laparoscopy is an acceptable alternative method that has been shown to avoid the risk of injury almost completely in normally situated intraabdominal structures [49].

After 9 years, Garry, commenting on Journal of Gynecological Surgery the Cochrane review entitled "Laparoscopic entry techniques" of 2008 [50], concluded that this paper provided a very useful review of the relevant literature and trials currently available and proved that serious injuries do rarely complicated various methods of laparoscopic entry. The Cochrane Review gave us no information about the relative safety of each technique; therefore, each surgeon may continue to use their chosen entry technique, for there is no evidence to favor any particular technique [51].

Long et al. performed a retrospective review of 2010 consecutive subjects underwent laparoscopy via open laparoscopic access over an 8-year period from January 1, 1998 to December 31, 2006. Recorded intraoperative complications include enterotomy (0.1%) and failure to enter (0.1%). There were no instances of vascular injury related to entry. Recorded postoperative complications include hernia (0.9%), infection (2.5%), hematoma (0.05%), and noncosmetic healing (0.4%). A statistically significant association existed between obesity and postoperative hernia, and between previous abdominal surgery and postoperative infection. In the conclusion authors affirmed the predominant entry method in gynecologic surgery remains a closed technique. Veress needle has unfortunately been demonstrated in multiple series to have the potential for visceral and vascular injury due to its blind insertion of Veress needles and trocars. The open laparoscopic technique is a safe and effective method of obtaining access to the abdominal cavity with no associated vascular injury [52].

On the contrary, Molloy et al. also reported a statistically significant difference in bowel complication rates: 0.4/1,000 (gynecologists) versus 1.5/1,000 (general surgeons) ($P=0.001$). When all open laparoscopies were excluded from the analysis, the incidence of bowel injuries was 0.3/1,000 in gynecological procedures and 1.3/1,000 in general surgical procedures ($P=0.001$). The authors speculated that the difference may be due to a variety of confounding variables, including heterogeneous data, retrospective data, underreporting of adverse events, differences in clinical practices between centers, and patient selection bias. In addition, they pointed out that gynecologists may have more experience than general surgeons with laparoscopic surgery.

Bowel injuries are reported more frequently with open laparoscopy than with other techniques (0.11%; 0.04% Veress needle entry; 0.05% direct entry). This may be influenced by patient selection bias, as open procedures may be more likely to be chosen for patients who have had previous abdominal surgery. Another potential bias is that the number of practitioners involved in the reports on open entry is likely much smaller than the number reporting on the Veress needle (open: 21,547 patients, Veress: 134,917 patients). Consequently, practitioner experience is not accounted for. The authors conclude that the optimal form of laparoscopic entry in the low-risk patient remains unclear [53].

Authors also proposed modified methods of open laparoscopy, e.g., Liu et al. who reported a modified open trocar first-puncture approach (Yan's open technique) and validated its safety and practicability in a multi-center research. The study was performed in seven gynecological endoscopy centers for 8 successive years from September 1998 to March 2006 involving 17,350 patients who received the modified open trocar first-puncture approach developed by Dr. LIU Yan as the study group (MOT group). This method, called the "Yan's open technique," is based on umbilical incision with a scalpel and then a 10-mm trocar entry into the abdominal cavity through direct trocar puncture or insertion of the cannula sheath via the opened umbilicus under no resistance. As a control group, 4,570 patients received the traditional Veress needle puncture. The first puncture procedures of both groups were performed by 28 experienced gynecologic laparoscopists and 170 students. In

MOT group, the successful achievement rate (AR) of first puncture was 99.99% (17,348/17,350), including smooth manipulation in 17,326 cases and unsmooth manipulation in 22 cases. The remaining two cases failed. First-puncture associated complications occurred in two cases (0.01%). In the control group, the successful AR of first puncture was 99.89% (4,565/4,570), including smooth manipulation in 4,542 cases and unsmooth manipulation in 23 cases. The remaining five cases failed. First-puncture associated complications occurred in four cases (0.09%). There was no significant difference in the successful AR between the experienced gynecologic laparoscopists of the two groups (100% versus 100%, $P>0.05$), but the difference was significant between the learners of the two groups (99.98% versus 99.81%, $P<0.05$). The complication rate of the Veress needle group was significantly higher than that of the MOT group (0.09% versus 0.01%, $P<0.05$) [54].

Access into the Abdomen with Visual Entry Systems

To enter into the abdomen with a scopic vision there are direct vision trocars—single or multiple use—that enable entry into the abdomen with or without a pneumoperitoneum, under optical vision, directly checking the abdominal layers, thus avoiding the blind introduction of the first trocar. Using the optical trocar, vital structures posterior to the peritoneum can be seen, but they may be seen too late to avoid an injury.

This is the current trend followed by most laparoscopists, as the use of such tools enables entry with or without a pneumoperitoneum, with a Veress needle, checking and recording on video acquisition systems the entire procedure, which is also useful for any possible medical-legal instances that may arise.

In the case of single-use trocars, the tools have a transparent sleeve, with a hollow mandrill, equipped with a transparent conical tip, or obturator, where the laparoscopic lens will be placed. The surgeon holds the trocar with the laparoscopic lens connected to the video recording system, in order to see the step-by-step procedure across the abdominal layers, and can stop in case of error or visceral adhesions to the peritoneum [1].

Optical access trocars were introduced in 1994 and two disposable visual entry systems are available that retain the conventional trocar and cannula push-through design: the Endopath optical trocar (Ethicon Endo-Surgery, Inc., Cincinnati, OH) and The Visiport optical trocar, (Covidien, Norwalk, CT).

These single-use visual trocars trade blind sharp trocars for a hollow trocar, in which a zero degree laparoscope is loaded for the distal crystal tip to transmit real-time monitor images while transecting abdominal wall tissue layers. Their application recruits significant axial thrust through the surgeon's dominant upper body muscles to transect abdominal myofascial layers [12].

Real-time visual primary entry enables error archiving and replay capabilities for early mishap detection before irreparable harm is sustained. The single enterotomy was immediately recognized and repaired, resulting in uneventful recovery with no serious health or medico legal consequences. Inadvertent sudden desufflation resulted in loss of abdominal wall and bowel visual cues (situational awareness) contributing to injury.

The Endopath optical trocar comprises a hollowed trocar and a cannula. When insufflation is complete, the Veress needle is withdrawn, and the subcutaneous fatty tissue is dissected off, using peanut sponges, to expose the white anterior rectus fascia. A 5-mm incision is then made with a scalpel to accommodate the visual trocar's lighted pointed tip (Fig. 11.11).

When the Endopath optical trocar is used directly, without preinsufflation, the assistant or first surgeon may grasp the abdominal wall with left hand or towel clips, while the surgeon negotiates the visual trocar [55]. Tilting the tip of the trocar, the handle advances the hydrophobic and winged trocar tip to dissect successive tissue layers on its way towards the abdomen. The cascade of generated entry images displayed on the monitor demonstrates level of penetration and gives safety to surgeons (Fig. 11.12). This technique, called "direct optical entry or direct optical access" was already tested in a large number of women.

Two-hundred two premenopausal women homogeneous in age, parity, and body mass index undergoing laparoscopic surgery for simple ovarian cysts were prospectively randomly assigned to either open laparoscopy or Direct Optical Access or entry. The following parameters were compared: duration of access for entry into the abdomen, occurrence of vascular and/or bowel injury, and blood loss. No statistically significant differences were observed in the occurrence of major vascular and/or bowel injury between the two techniques. However, time for establishment of abdominal

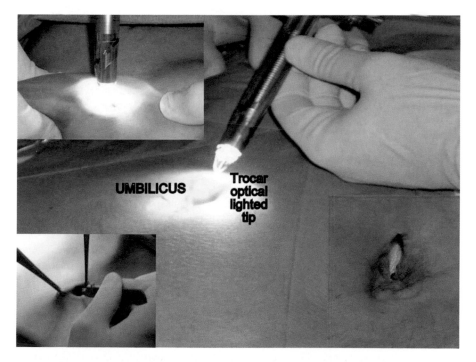

Fig. 11.11 In the figure are shown all the passages of preparation of entry by Endopath optical trocar with lighted tip to introduce into the umbilical incision; this entry is also called "direct optical access or entry"

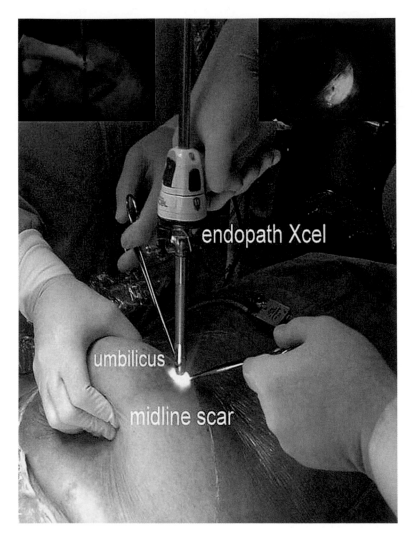

Fig. 11.12 The image shows the "direct optical access or entry" by Endopath optical trocar: the surgeon introduces the lighted optical trocar through the abdominal wall (with the Fascia anchored to two Kocher clamps, as the patient is obese), displaying all the passages into the monitor (on the top left is shown the surgeon's finger through the trocar, on the right top the anterior rectus fascia open through the passage of the trocar)

entry was significantly reduced in the Direct Optical Access group, so as the blood loss ($P<0.05$). The visual entry system with the Direct Optical Access conferred a little statistical advantage over traditional Hasson entry, in term of safety, minimal time saving and in blood loss reducing, allowing a safe and fast visually-guided entry [56].

Then 186 postmenopausal women undergoing laparoscopic surgery for simple ovarian cysts were tested: 89 were assigned to direct optical access (DOA) entry (group 1) and 97 to classical closed Veress needle approach and trocar entry (group 2). The following parameters were compared: time needed for entry into the abdomen, occurrence of vascular and/or bowel injury, and blood loss. In the results no statistically significant differences were observed in the occurrence of major vascular and/or bowel injury, between the two techniques ($P>0.05$), whereas time for abdominal entry was significantly reduced in the DOA group, as well as the occurrence of minor vascular injuries ($P<0.05$). Also in this comparison on the DOA and the Veress methods, the visual entry system offered a statistical advantage over closed Veress needle approach, in terms of time saving and limiting minor vascular injuries, thus enabling a safe and fast visually-guided entry in postmenopausal subjects [57].

Another comparison involved 194 women: 93 assigned to direct optical access (DOA) abdominal entry (group 1), and 101 to classical closed method by Veress needle, pneumoperitoneum, and trocar entry (group 2). All underwent laparoscopic surgery for simple ovarian cysts. No statistically significant differences were observed in the occurrence of blood loss and minor vascular injury between the two techniques; however, time for of abdominal entry, as well as minor bowel injuries, was significantly reduced in the DOA group. The results of this investigation suggested that the visual entry system conferred a statistical advantage over closed entry technique with Veress needle in terms of time saving and because of the minor vascular injuries, thus enabling a safe and expeditious, visually-guided, entry for surgeons [58].

Authors analyzed the safety and efficacy of a modified Direct Optical Entry (DOE) method versus the Hasson method by Open Laparoscopy (OL) in women with previous abdominopelvic surgery in a preliminary prospective case control study. Of 168 women who underwent laparoscopic surgery: 86 were assigned to abdominal DOE (Group A) and 82 to OL (Group B). Statistical differences, in favor of the DOE group ($P<0.01$), were found in duration of entry and blood loss. The vascular and bowel injuries in OL versus DOE were not statistically different.

Because obtaining access to the peritoneal cavity in laparoscopic surgery is a more difficult, time-consuming, and occasionally hazardous procedure in patients with previous abdominopelvic surgery, the authors of the study suggested that DOE was advantageous when compared with OL in terms of saving time and enabling a safe and expeditious visually-guided entry for laparoscopy [59].

Another system of visual entry is the Visiport optical trocar (Fig. 11.13). It is a disposable visual entry instrument that comprises a hollow trocar and a cannula. Every trigger squeeze advances the sharp cutting knife 1 mm to transect tissue in contact with the crystal tip and swiftly retract back into the crystal hemisphere. It is advised that, as with other visual trocars, the Visiport optical trocar is to be applied only after CO_2 insufflation [60]. When insufflation is complete, the Veress needle is withdrawn, and subcutaneous fatty tissue is dissected off the white anterior rectus fascia using peanut sponges.

The Visiport optical trocar is palmed by the surgeon's dominant hand and held perpendicular to the supine patient's CO2 distended abdomen. Once the exact anatomical position of the trocar tip is verified on the monitor, downward axial pressure is applied while activating the trigger. Then downward pressure is relieved, the trigger released, and the trocar tip position verified on the monitor again. This entry sequence is repeated until the peritoneal cavity is entered. The trigger is not fired until the exact anatomical position of the trocar tip is known.

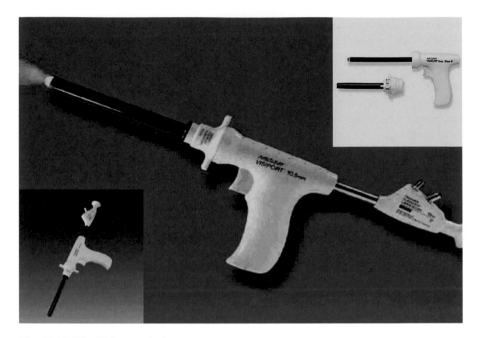

Fig. 11.13 The Visiport optical trocars

The push-through entry design requires significant perpendicular force to drive a trajectory across tissue planes with no means of avoiding trocar overshoot. Sometimes, the anterior abdominal wall may be grasped with the non dominant hand of the surgeon and lifted to offer counter pressure against the advancing trocar. The Visiport optical trocar comes in only one diameter and accommodates only a 10-mm laparoscope [12].

Urologists used the Visiport Optical Trocar as an alternative access technique to facilitate a preperitoneoscopic (extraperitoneal laparoscopic) approach for radical prostatectomy, herniorrhaphy, and other pelvic procedures. A telescope viewing angle of zero degrees telescope was mounted into a Visiport Optical Trocar (Visiport), and via a periumbilical incision was advanced under direct vision at first vertically through different layers of the anterior abdominal wall. Immediately before the posterior rectus sheath, it was redirected caudally and horizontally toward the symphysis pubis. The Visiport was withdrawn and replaced by a dissection balloon that was inflated for developing the working space, and then was substituted with a 12-mm trocar to begin the pneumo-extraperitoneum.

This technique was used in 168 of 179 patients undergoing preperitoneoscopic surgery (97 radical prostatectomies, 80 totally extraperitoneal herniorrhaphies, and 2 urinary bladder diverticulectomies). Operative parameters were compared with 11 preceding patients approached with the open Hasson technique. All of the procedures to create the preperitoneoscopic space were successful, with no complications. For radical prostatectomy, there was a significantly faster access to the preperitoneal space (38 ± 12 versus 540 ± 69 s) and a faster setup of the whole operative space

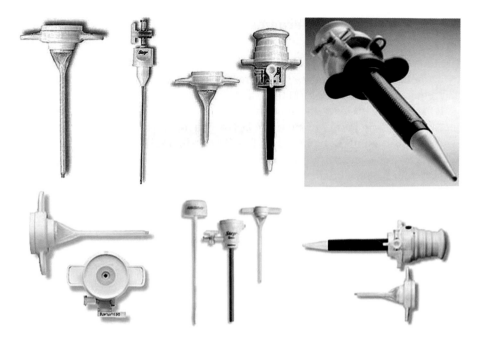

Fig. 11.14 VersaStep consists of a Veress surrounded by an expanding polymeric sleeve; when the needle is removed, the polymeric sleeve can be dilated by inserting a bladeless trocar

(15 ± 5 versus 29 ± 9 min, both $P<.05$) with the new technique. Less pericannular CO_2 leakage was experienced during the preperitoneoscopy with our technique. The Visiport Optical Trocar offered a simple, safe, quick, and effective access for creating a preperitoneoscopic working space [60].

Another visual entry system is the radially expanding access system, the VersaStep, was introduced in 1994. The VersaStep (Covidien, Norwalk, CT) consists of a 1.9-mm Veress surrounded by an expanding polymeric sleeve (Fig. 11.14). The abdomen may first be insufflated using the Veress needle. The needle is removed, and the sleeve acts as a tract through the abdominal wall that can be dilated up to 12 mm by inserting a blunt obturator with a twisting motion [61–63].

The VersaStep bladeless trocars are available in short (70 mm), standard (110 mm) and long (150 mm) working lengths in 5, 11, 12, and 15 mm diameters

The force required to push this trocar through the abdomen in pigs is 14.2 kg compared with forces of 4–6 kg needed for disposable trocars [64].

Several case series and randomized studies have reported no injury to major vessels and no deaths. Abdominal wall bleeding and Veress injury to mesentery have been encountered [61]. In addition, ECTs have demonstrated less postoperative pain and more patient satisfaction with the radially expanding device than with the conventional trocar entry techniques [65–68].

Advantages of this system include elimination of sharp trocars, application of radial force, stabilization of the cannula's position (cannula does not slide in and out), avoidance of injury to abdominal wall vessels, and elimination of the need for suturing of fascial defects.

Visual Entry with the Ternamian Cannula

Dr. Ternamian of Toronto, Canada, introduced in 1997 this method of visual entry. It features a reusable stainless steel–threaded cannula with no sharp components and requires no trocars (ENDOTIP; Karl Storz, Tuttlingen, Germany).

It has a threaded sleeve and, therefore, enables screwing motion of the trocar into the abdomen, both in case of a pneumoperitoneum after using the Veress needle, or when an open minilaparotomy is preferred. The EndoTIP visual cannula system requires no trocar and has no crystal tip compressing and distorting monitor images at the tissue–cannula interface. Interpretations of observed monitor images are identified, layered-entry, and real-time interactive. The EndoTIP consists of a stainless steel cannula with a proximal valve segment and distal hollow threaded cannula section. The conventional valve sector houses a standard CO_2 stopcock, and the cannula's outer surface is wrapped with a single thread, winding diagonally to end in a distal blunt notched tip. The cannula is available in different lengths and diameters for different surgical applications.

A retaining ring keeps the mounted laparoscope from sliding out of focus during insertion.

The technique to utilize is described as follows. After a skin incision and establishment of pneumoperitoneum, the unit (a 0° laparoscope and mounted visual cannula) is inserted in the skin incision and held perpendicularly to the supine patient with the non dominant hand. The cannula is then rotated clockwise with the dominant hand applying minimal downward force. Accumulated subcutaneous fat and debris may be aspirated with the 5-mm suction/irrigation cannula. The cannula's blunt notched tip engages the tissue layers of the abdominal wall and transposes successive tissue layers onto the cannula's outer sheath in accordance with Archimedes' principle (Fig. 11.15).

The yellow fat, white anterior rectus fascia, red rectus muscle, white posterior rectus fascia, yellowish preperitoneal space, and transparent dark-bluish peritoneal membrane are all observed sequentially on the monitor, as in Direct Optical access or entry. It has been observed that the blunt tip of the cannula pushes aside abdominal wall blood vessels, adhesions, and even bowel when adhered to the anterior abdominal wall [69–71].

Conventional primary trocar insertion requires application of considerable axial push-force (2–14 kg) to the trocar and cannula where the anterior abdominal wall dents towards the viscera; entry is blind.

This trocar was used on 143 patients, with both access techniques. During the blind entry procedures, after pneumoperitoneum with Veress needle, intraabdominal adhesions could better be visualized by transillumination. With the open entry technique, after a mini incision of the fascia, visualizing the mass, the omentum, the intestine, and subumbilical adhesions, it was possible, by direct vision, to screw in the Endotip. The main advantage of the equipment consisted in the possibility of getting across the abdominal wall layers, visualizing directly the entry into the cavity. This instrument is a multiple-use tool and enables a more complete vision of the abdominal layers when the central trocar is removed [72, 73].

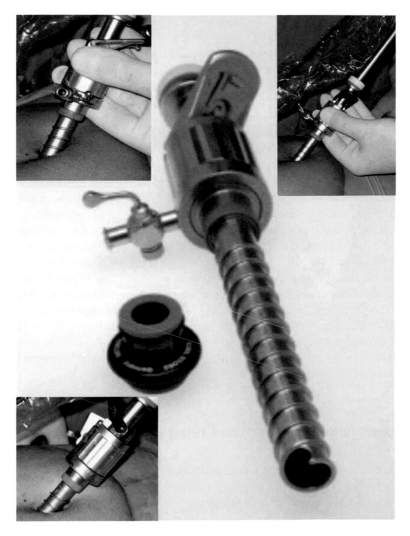

Fig. 11.15 After a skin incision and establishment of pneumoperitoneum, a unit formed by the EndoTIP with a 0° laparoscope mounted inside is inserted into the skin incision and held perpendicularly to the supine patient. The cannula is then rotated clockwise with the dominant hand applying minimal downward force, until entry into the abdominal cavity is achieved

Ternamian et al. estimated the feasibility, reproducibility, and safety of laparoscopic port establishment using a trocarless and externally threaded visual cannula (TVC) by a multicenter, prospective, observational study on 4,724 patients (median age, 34 years; median body mass index, 25) undergoing laparoscopic surgery. After administration of general anesthesia, the Veress needle was inserted at the umbilicus or the left upper quadrant (LUQ) using Veress intraperitoneal pressure of 10 mmHg or less as proxy for correct placement. Transient high intraperitoneal pressure of 20–30 mmHg was attained and primary and ancillary ports were established using the reusable trocarless TVC. Primary umbilical entry was established in 4,598 patients (97.33%), primary LUQ entry in 123 (2.60%), and primary suprapubic entry in 3 (0.06%) patients. Peritoneal preinsufflation was abandoned when 3 consecutive umbilical or LUQ Veress needle insertion attempts failed. Some patients at high risk with known peritoneal adhesions or previous lower abdominal midline scars did not undergo preinsufflation, and the trocarless TVC was applied directly. Surgery was postponed in 3 patients in whom insufflation failed to enable further counseling and appropriate consenting. There were no serious abdominal walls or intraabdominal vascular injuries. One transverse colon, densely adhered to the umbilical region, was injured, which was recognized and repaired intraoperatively. Residents, fellows, or faculty recorded entry-related data on forms postoperatively for study and analysis. Authors concluded that establishing peritoneal ports with the trocarless TVC is feasible, reproducible, and seems to be highly adoptable [74].

No minor or major vascular injuries occurred since adopting the trocarless TVC.

All published visual entry complications involve disposable visual trocars and not the trocarless TVC [49, 75, 76]. Fundamental design and application differences between the two preclude equating safety and complications of one to the other. Knowledge of anatomy, identification of navigational cues, and recognition of monitor images (perceptual awareness) are all important for safe deployment [77, 78].

With consenting high-risk patients (previous abdominal surgery, obesity, or adhesions), the possibility of use of an alternate entry method (visual or open), the probability of a different access site (LUQ), and the likelihood of laparotomy must be discussed [59, 79].

Comparison Between Open and Blind Entry into the Abdomen

All operative methods are prone to risk, and peritoneal entry is no exception. Securing and maintaining ports while averting injury remains a critical first step in laparoscopy.

As the fundamentals of safe surgery are reviewed in general and the mechanisms of inadvertent laparoscopic entry injury are analyzed in particular, five important weaknesses are readily identified: excessive penetration force; sharp, cutting, pointed trocars; nonvisualization of the operative field (blind trocar insertion); sudden loss of surgical instrument or trocar control; and trocar overshoot. Many studies tried to compare the blind and the open entry in abdomen.

A comparison between the techniques (with Veress needle or direct introduction) was proposed by Dutch authors. It referred to complications during a gynecological laparoscopy. The research administered a questionnaire to members of the Dutch Society for Gynecological Endoscopy and Minimally Invasive Surgery; it was also supported by a review of the scientific literature on Medline.

Data included complications reported between 1997 and 2001, listed in a questionnaire, dividing the surgeons into two groups. The first group included surgeons who used the blind technique (with Veress needle or direct introduction); the second group included surgeons promoting the open entry technique. Ninety-eight percent of gynecological surgeons (187) responded and participated in the study, giving the number of laparoscopies performed, the years of experience, and indications for the entry technique. The comparison's outcome is the following: 100 surgeons used only the blind entry technique (57%) with 31 complications over 31,532 procedures (0.1%), also in high-risk patients (for obesity or prior laparotomies). Many gynecologists used an alternative insufflation site (Palmer's point). The remaining surgeons used both techniques, although the open one was used only in specific cases (suspects of adhesions or prior laparotomy in 90% of cases, obesity in 7%, and excessive thinness in 3% of cases) and only in 2% of procedures.

The remaining 81 gynecologists, therefore, referred to 20,027 blind entry procedures and 579 open entry, showing 0.12% and 1.38% complications, respectively, with one statistically significant datum ($P < 0.01$). Furthermore, in the group of treated patients a greater and more significant number of visceral lesions were identified. The conclusions of the study claim that, in spite of the fact that 43% of gynecologists who participated in the survey used this technique; the number of complications is not necessarily lower. Moreover, data reported by general surgeons on complications of the open access technique are in contrast with the ones reported by gynecologists who used the blind method, as the latter refer to a higher number of complications with the open access. There are, therefore, no conclusions leading to the option of an open technique instead of other entry methods. The study, however, delivers one recommendation, i.e., being more accurate and cautious in selecting patients and using one technique or another [80].

A randomized study was conducted in 1999 to compare three different techniques used on 62 patients (compared by age and body mass index) to perform a pneumoperitoneum, i.e., the Veress needle, Hasson's trocar, and a blunt trocar known as TrocDoc. The study's conclusions highlighted that the time needed for the TrocDoc to enter was less than with the other two methods, with a greater effectiveness of the latter method in performing a pneumoperitoneum [81].

A comparison between the direct transperitoneal technique and the Veress needle method—used by some surgeons in cholecystectomies—has shown how 1,030 direct accesses led to 0.9% complications against 14% in 470 Veress needle accesses, which showed two major complications (that being the gastric perforation and the iliac artery lesion). The study underlined that the direct access may be more advantageous than the Veress method in terms of time and lower cost of the equipment [82].

Some surgeons compared the complications rate in a retrospective study when the periumbilical trocar was used with the blind technique and the optic trocar, in 1,546 patients who underwent gynecologic laparoscopies. 1,000 patients were submitted to the blind entry technique with the introduction of a common umbilical trocar (Group 1) and 546 to the introduction of an optical trocar (Group 2). In Group 1 the complications accounted for 0.5%, whereas no complications were found in Group 2. The data highlighted the greater advantage of using an optical vision trocar compared to common sharp trocars (conic or pyramidal) in terms of safety and functionality, especially visualizing periumbilical adhesions, with the aim of avoiding intestinal and vascular lesions [83].

A comparison between the transperitoneal access with the Veress needle and the Otiview trocar pointed out that the latter was more effective at entry. Optiview did not show complications but, when it was not possible to enter into the abdomen with either technique, the open technique using Hasson's trocar was preferred, albeit difficult after the failure of the other two. In using the Veress needle, only four minor complications occurred, namely: one insufflation of the colon, two retroperitoneal hematomas, and one hepatic laceration. These were all solved spontaneously and, for this reason, the authors recommended using the Veress needle instead of the other trocar [77].

The assessment of Optiview was also made by a group of North American doctors in 650 laparoscopic procedures in general surgery. The percentage of complications was of 0.3%, with one intestinal lesion and one gall bladder lesion (immediately detected and solved), with a lower cost and with the first access utilization of this trocar by most colleagues [12].

Some authors, to avoid the double access with Veress needle and blind trocar, published a study on a mini entry into the abdomen by using a small, 2.5–2 mm diameter lens, experimenting with it successfully in 184 laparoscopies. After intraperitoneal insufflation with a specific trocar, this small lens was used to visualize the abdominal cavity and highlight any adhesions, to be detected prior to the entry with the umbilical trocar [11].

Finally, it needs to discuss about closing the fascia: some surgeons have said that it doesn't need to close the fascia if the trocar is 5 mm regardless of site. The evidence shows that ports 10 mm or less do not have to be closed because it is not until the surgeon is above that size that hernias become more likely to occur. It is important to note that significant manipulation of a smaller port, such as with suturing or specimen removal, will increase the size of the fascial defect. Some surgeons always close a 10-mm site regardless of location. Historically, from the beginning of modern-day laparoscopy, only 10-mm laparoscopes were available, and the fascia was never closed. This doesn't mean people didn't get hernias. Some surgeons taught use of the Z technique for insertion to decrease that risk [84].

Although it remains controversial about the need to close a 10-mm umbilical site, most people agree on the need to close lateral trocar sites that are 10 mm or larger. Surgeons close the large lateral ports under direct visualization with one of the various closure needles that are commercially available and observe the site of operation and trocar sites as they decrease the pneumoperitoneum to check for bleeding. Moreover surgeons remove all the trocars under direct vision, including the umbilical. When using an optical trocar, surgeons can withdraw the laparoscope within the trocar sleeve seeing the layers closing behind them. The pressure is dropped before this technique with the camera in place, and someone would be likely to see any significant vascular injury with this method.

Laparoendoscopic Single-Site Surgery Access

Single-incision in laparoscopy (SIL) or laparoscopic single-site-access (LSSA) is gaining interest as a potentially less invasive alternative to standard laparoscopic approaches.

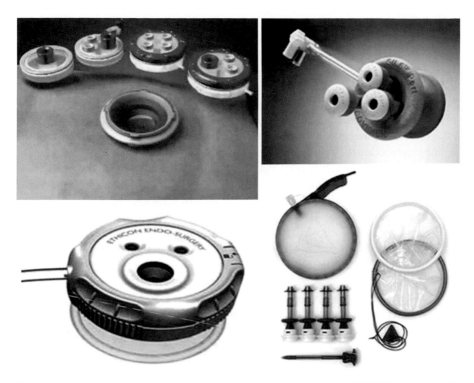

Fig. 11.16 Devices for laparoscopic single-site-access: in the *top left*, the OCTO Port, detachable multichannel port (AFSMEDICAL GmbH, Münich, Germany); in the *top right* is the SILS Port Multiple Instrument Access Port (Covidien, Mansfield, MA); in *bottom left* is the Single-Site Laparoscopy Access System (Ethicon Endosurgery, Cincinnati, OH); and in the *bottom right* is the GelPoint (Applied Medical, Rancho Santa Margarita, CA)

Since Navarra et al. [85] performed the first LSSA laparoscopic cholecystectomy in 1997, the LSSA approach has been applied to most other laparoscopic surgical procedures [86–89].

In contrast to standard laparoscopic surgery, which involves the use of multiple incision sites, LSSA is performed with all ports and instruments placed close together via a single incision access site and a single multiport trocar (Fig. 11.16) at the umbilicus. The principal advantage of the LSSA approach appears to be less visible scarring. However, this approach can be more technically challenging than standard laparoscopy. Some of these challenges include loss of triangulation between the camera and working ports and restricted range of motion due to the close apposition of the ports, instruments, and camera.

So even if LSSA was first developed as a novel approach to laparoscopic cholecystectomy, currently it is being applied to many different laparoscopic procedures in many surgical fields [90–92], although the advantages of this approach over standard laparoscopy through 5-mm (or smaller) incisions is being debated.

Keltz et al., for example, proposed a 5-mm-open laparoscopic technique in a university hospital-based endoscopy practice in 65 consecutive patients undergoing laparoscopy with a single surgeon. They achieved a 71% success rate was achieved using the 5-mm open-entry laparoscopic technique, with complications during any of the laparoscopic procedures, but 29% reverted to a standard 5-mm Veress needle technique. The success of the open-entry technique was independent of prior abdominal surgery, subject age, or body mass index (BMI). In conclusion, the authors affirmed the 5-mm open-entry technique was safe, fast, and cosmetic; moreover it can be easily mastered and may be converted to a standard Veress needle technique if peritoneal entry is not achieved [93].

Piccinni G et al. used in 260 patients a semiopen first umbilical trocar access by a transverse incision above or below the umbilicus of almost 1 cm and, after opening the peritoneum, they preferred to enter the cavity with a Veress needle of 1.9 mm mounted on a radially expandable sleeve, the VersaStep mentioned previously [94]. It is nonetheless gaining momentum among surgeons as a way of performing virtually "scarless" less invasive surgery, with the goal of achieving better cosmetic outcomes for many patients.

In fact, Laparo Endoscopic Single Site (LESS)), you can use all three acronyms, as SIL, LSSA or LESS in the following text improves the cosmetic benefits of minimally invasive surgery by providing only one incision, which also minimizes the potential morbidity associated with multiple incisions. LESS surgery can be performed through a variety of access devices. Conventional, low profile ports of different lengths can help to minimize limitation of movement by the surgeon(s) owing to the extracorporeal interaction of the instruments and camera (known as "sword fighting"). Technological developments have produced multichannel single-port devices as well [95–98].

The prototype access system is the TriPort (Olympus America Inc, Center Valley, PA). This is a Food and Drug Administration-approved device with two components: a retracting component, which consists of an inner and outer ring with a double-barreled plastic sleeve; and a multichannel valve, which has three valves made of a unique elastomeric material. These valves each accommodate one 12-mm and two 5-mm instruments within the same working space (Fig. 11.17). The port comes in various sizes, ranging from 10 to 30 mm, and can be selected according to the size of the fascial incision.

More recently, the Quad-Port, which has four working channels, has been introduced. This port can accommodate one 15-, one 12-, and two 5-mm ports; or four 12-mm ports. While the TriPort can be placed by either an open approach or after insufflation with an introducer, the Quad-Port must be placed by an open-access technique.

Another port that has also been used successfully for LESS procedure is the Uni-X Single-Port Access Laparoscopic system (PNavel systems, Cleveland, OH). This port has three working channels for 5-mm instruments, and it is placed by an open access technique, requiring stitches to secure it to the fascia.

The GelPort or newer generation GelPoint (Applied Medical, Rancho Santa Margarita, CA) devices consist of a combination of the rigid ring of the Alexis wound retractor with a Gelseal cap which maintains pneumoperitoneum during multiple instrument exchanges. Unlike the aforementioned ports, this system allows for the introduction of ports or instruments of varying shapes and sizes directly through the gel.

This device can also be placed into a larger incision, allowing the surgeon to take advantage of the entire fascial incision required during extirpative procedures, and represents an efficient port for tissue removal. The disadvantage of this port, however, is that it may balloon out during insufflation, causing the instruments to be

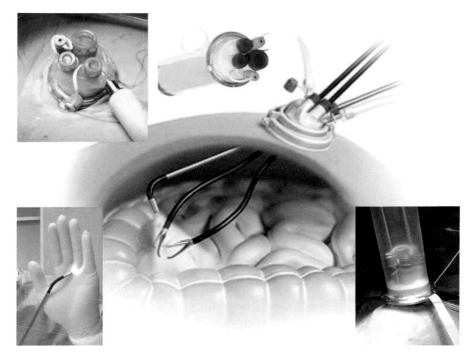

Fig. 11.17 The TriPort system (Olympus America Inc, Center Valley, PA) consists of an inner and outer ring with a double-barreled plastic sleeve and a multichannel valve, which each accommodate one 12-mm and two 5-mm instruments within the same working space, or, possibly, a rotatable 30° Visera EndoEYE laparoscope (Olympus America Inc, Center Valley, PA) at *bottom left*, plus special single-port instrumentation, including flexible and/or articulating instruments

pushed further from the operative field and the fulcrum to be less stable than the other multichannel ports described.

The SILS Port Multiple Instrument Access Port (Covidien, Mansfield, MA) is another multiinstrument access port that allows up to three laparoscopic instruments (three 5-mm cannulas or two 5-mm and one 12-mm cannula) to be used simultaneously through separate flexible channels. This port allows for adjustment of the cannula positions within the flexible port, and there is a separate channel that allows for CO_2 insufflation. The port must be inserted through an open access technique.

Finally, the latest port to be approved is the Single-Site Laparoscopy Access System (Ethicon Endosurgery, Cincinnati, OH), which was introduced on the market in 2010. Two 5-mm seals and one 15-mm seal enable use of a wide range of instrumentation. The advantages of this system include the use of a morcellator through the larger port; the integrated, low-profile system obviates the need for trocars; and the outer seal cap allows for 360° of rotation and reportedly facilitates specimen removal.

Two of the biggest caveats that limit use of the LESS technique are instrument crowding and lack of triangulation. Instrument crowding may occur because of several instruments being passed though a multichannel, single port. Instruments may easily clash with one another or with the laparoscope, all of which are passed through the same surgical fulcrum. Conventional laparoscopes have a large extracorporeal profile with a light cable perpendicular to the telescope. Owing to this latter feature, if the conventional laparoscope is utilized for LESS, instrument clashing may be exacerbated. One method, however, to minimize this problem is by using a lower profile camera system. One system that is currently available is the rotatable 30°Visera EndoEYE laparoscope (Olympus America Inc, Center Valley, PA), which has the unique feature of a video laparoscope integrated with a coaxial light cable in line with the shaft of the telescope. The Olympus EndoEYE is currently the only laparoscope offering this unique feature, and it is available in 5-mm size in 0° and 30° configurations. It is also available with a flexible actively deflectable tip. Other special optics that may facilitate LESS surgery include a 45° telescope (Stryker), which has a coaxial, right-angle light guide adapter to help minimize sword fighting.

Many surgeons are accustomed to the tenet of triangulation, because of the use of conventional laparoscopy, and this practice can be approximated to some degree by utilizing special single-port instrumentation, including flexible and/or articulating instruments. These instruments allow for intracorporeal triangulation, rather than the extracorporeal triangulation utilized in traditional laparoscopy. Those instruments currently available as articulating devices include graspers, shears, endoshears, needle-drivers, and hook electrocautery. Several companies have designed a comprehensive spectrum of these articulating instruments. At this stage in development, bulk and technical challenge pose major obstacles in using articulating instruments.

The routine application of LESS in gynecology not only requires evaluation of safety but also of cost-effectiveness, and these studies must all be performed in larger, prospective studies to definitively answer questions regarding the clinical and economic impact of this novel surgical approach. More detailed data is also needed to further describe the learning curve and the optimal environment for trainees and surgeons to become skilled in LESS procedures [91].

In fact, a recent study compared laparoscopic Single-site-access (LSSA) and multiport (MP) laparoscopy, with predictable results [99]. This study examined the effect of MP versus LSSA skills training on laparoscopic performance using 40 surgically naive medical students, who, at the end of their first year were randomized into two groups. Both groups were trained in four basic laparoscopic drills (peg, rope, bean drop, pattern cutting) using a standard MP setup (group 1) and an LSSA approach (group 2).

The time and number of repetitions required to attain proficiency were recorded. Each group then crossed over to the alternate approach and repeated the sequence. The total times required to attain proficiency for the LSSA and MP approaches were not significantly different between the MP-trained group (234.0 ± 114.9 min) and the LSSA-trained group (216.4 ± 106.5 min) ($P=0.67$). The MP-trained group required less time to reach proficiency on the standard MP setup than the group using the LSSA approach (119.1 ± 69.7 versus. 178.0 ± 93.4 min; $P=0.058$) and significantly fewer repetitions (77.6 ± 42.6 versus. 118.8 ± 54.3; $P=0.027$).

The LSSA-trained group required significantly less time to reach proficiency on the MP setup than the standard MP-trained group (38.4 ± 29.4 versus 119.1 ± 69.7 min; $P=0.0013$) and needed only a mean of 26.9 repetitions. When the standard MP trainees crossed over to the LSSA setup, they required significantly less time to reach proficiency with the LSSA approach than did the LSSA-trained group

(114.8 ± 50.5 versus 178.0 ± 93.4 min; $P = 0.026$) but required more repetitions than with the MP approach (86.2 ± 35.2 versus 77.6 ± 42.6; nonsignificant difference).

In the conclusions, the authors affirmed laparoscopic SSA skills training results in longer times and more repetitions to achieve proficiency than MP training, but the skills acquired transfer well to the MP approach [99].

And the Cochrane Reviews Opinion?

In 2008, a Cochrane review was done to compare the different laparoscopic entry techniques in terms of their influence on intraoperative and postoperative complications.

This review has drawn on the search strategy developed by the Menstrual Disorders and Subfertility Group. In addition, MEDLINE and EMBASE were searched through to July, 2007. Randomized controlled trials were included when one laparoscopic primary-port-entry technique was compared with another. The 17 included randomized controlled trials concerned 3,040 individuals undergoing laparoscopy.

Overall there was no evidence of advantage using any single technique in terms of preventing major complications. On the basis of evidence investigated in this review, there appears to be no evidence of benefit in terms of safety of one technique over another. However, studies were limited to small numbers, excluding many patients with previous abdominal surgery and women with a raised body mass index, who often had unusually high complication rates [50].

Garry lapidary commented [51] this paper highlighting the limitations of Cochrane review: it illustrated either the well-recognized benefits of conducting careful structured reviews of the world literature, or the fallacy of conducting such time-consuming and expensive research on databases that are inherently inadequate for the Cochrane tasks.

The aim of this review was to determine the relative complication rates associated with various methods of laparoscopic entry. With a very comprehensive trawl of the literature, the authors found a total of 3,040 patients in 17 different randomized trials that investigated 10 separate comparisons. The largest number of patients included in any group of studies was 1,909, and the smallest was 62, with most of the other studies being performed on populations of 100–200. Complications related to laparoscopic entry are, however, fortunately very rare, and the number of cases required to demonstrate significant differences in complication rates are correspondingly very large.

Garry previously calculated that to show a difference in bowel injury rate of 50% (i.e., from 0.04% to 0.02%) would require a study population in excess of 800,000.

The inadequacy of the size of the various studies analyzed in this review inevitably led to the conclusion that there was no evidence of benefit in terms of safety of any technique [32].

Varma & Gupta tried in 2008 to establish criteria for safe laparoscopic entry through a systematic literature search and evidence-based medicine appraisal, to determine surgeon preferences for laparoscopic entry in the United Kingdom, and to appraise the medico legal ramifications of complications arising from laparoscopic entry. They performed a systematic literature search of MEDLINE and EMBASE

Table 11.2 Evidence-based criteria for safe laparoscopic entry: ten steps

Step	Intervention	Level of evidence	Levels of evidence	Grades of recommendation
1	Suitability criteria: consider alternative entry (e.g., Palmer's point or open [Hasson] technique) for patients with risk factors such as previous abdominal surgery, obesity, extremely thin physique, or known abdominal adhesions	2++, B	2++ High-quality systematic reviews of case-control or cohort studies High-quality case-control or cohort studies with a very low risk of confounding, bias, or chance and a high probability that the relationship is causal	A At least one metaanalysis, systematic review, or RCT rated as 1++ and directly applicable to the target population, or a systematic review of RCTs or a body of evidence consisting principally of studies rated as 1+, directly applicable to the target population, and demonstrating overall consistency of results
2	Safety criteria: patient should be lying flat with an empty bladder; palpation should be used for the abdominal aorta, any masses; and the Veress needle should be checked for spring action and gas patency	4, GPP	2+ Well-conducted case-control or cohort studies with a low risk of confounding, bias, or chance and a moderate probability that the relationship is causal	B A body of evidence including studies rated as 2++, directly applicable to the target population and demonstrating overall consistency of results; or extrapolated evidence from studies rated as 1++ or 1+
3	Incision: 10-mm vertical intraumbilical incision starting deep inside the umbilicus pit and extending caudally	4, GPP	2− Case-control or cohort studies with a high risk of confounding, bias, or chance and a significant risk that the relationship is not causal	C A body of evidence including studies rated as 2+, directly applicable to the target population and demonstrating overall consistency of results; or extrapolated evidence from studies rated as 2++

			3 Non analytic studies (e.g., case reports, case series)	4 Expert opinion	D Evidence level 3 or 4; or extrapolated evidence from studies rated as 2+
4	Insertion of the Veress needle: at the deep umbilical pit, 90° to the skin, with or without stabilizing or elevating the umbilical sheath/fascia or anterior abdominal wall, and in a controlled manner with insertion of <2 cm of the Veress needle tip	2+, C (indirect evidence from knowledge of abdominal anatomy)			
5	No movement of the Veress needle after insertion to avoid converting a possible needlepoint injury into a large complex tear	4, GPP			
6	Safety abdominal pressure check of Veress placement: most reliably achieved by using a Veress IAP of <10 mmHg	2+, C			
7	Safety abdominal pressure check for primary trocar: the IAP should be 25 mmHg to achieve the maximum safe distance between the anterior abdominal wall and the underlying abdominal contents	2+, C			
8	Vertical primary trocar insertion: inserted in a controlled two-handed screwing manner vertically at 90° to the skin, with only the tip of the trocar inserted through the abdominal wall	2+, C>			
9	Injury check: an initial 360° laparoscopic check for intraperitoneal organ injury is performed	4, GPP			
10	No epigastric for secondary trocar(s) insertion: inserted under direct vision in a controlled two-handed manner at 90° to the skin, avoiding inferior epigastric vessels	2+, C (indirect evidence from knowledge of abdominal anatomy)			

Adapted from Varma and Gupta [100]

GPP Good practice points: recommended best practice based on the clinical experience of the guideline development group, *RCT* randomized clinical trial, *IAP* intraabdominal pressure

The acronyms SCIIN (suitability, criteria, incision, insertion, no movement), SAVE (safety abdominal Veress), SAVING (safety, abdominal pressure Veress), SAVING (safety, abdominal pressure [trocar], vertical trocar, injury check, no epigastrics) are suggested for the ten steps

(1996–2007) as well as by a national surgeon survey by questionnaire (May–December 2006). Laparoscopic entry criteria involving ten steps (see Table 11.2) were established based on the systematic literature search and evidence-based critical appraisal.

The national survey had 226 respondents, with the majority aware of the Middlesbrough consensus or Royal College of Obstetricians and Gynecologists [RCOG]-sourced guidance. There was considerable variation in preferred laparoscopic entry techniques. Currently, there is clear judicial guidance on the medicolegal stance toward laparoscopic entry-related complications.

Despite widespread awareness of laparoscopic entry guidelines, the authors concluded there remains considerable variation in the techniques adopted in clinical practice. Unless practice concurs with recommended guidance, women undergoing laparoscopy will be exposed to increased unnecessary operative risk. Laparoscopic entry-related injury in an uncomplicated woman is considered negligent practice according to UK legal case law [100].

Conclusions

At the moment, it is not yet possible to state which is the best technique for the periumbilical laparoscopic access into the abdomen. There is a wide range of entry techniques, which does not facilitate standardization of a unique access.

Preference for one or another technique depends on the surgeon's experience, his school and specialty, as well as on the laparoscopy school and the working environment. Some techniques cannot yet be selected owing to concerns and constraints of some surgeons in changing the entry approach or the lack of flexibility of one or another technique.

A laparoscopist should be trained by many mentors and should be knowledgeable in many different techniques, with no fears or uncertainties, but rather with expertise and versatility in applying the best method to a specific case.

We believe that the best technique to access the uterine cavity has not yet been found. Nevertheless, technology advances, and the increasingly widespread laparoscopic practice will soon lead to detecting a single, reiterable, safe, practical, and expeditious technique.

References

1. Molloy D, Kaloo PD, Cooper M, Nguyen TV. Laparoscopic entry: a literature review and analysis of techniques and complications of primary port entry. Aust N Z J Obstet Gynaecol. 2002;42:246–54.
2. Kaloo P, Cooper M, Molloy D. A survey of entry techniques and complications of members of the Australian Gynaecological Endoscopy Society. Aust N Z J Obstet Gynaecol. 2002;42:264–6.
3. Munro MG. Laparoscopic access: complications, technologies, and techniques. Curr Opin Obstet Gynecol. 2002;14:365–74.
4. Nazareno J, Ponich T, Gregor J. Long-term follow-up of trigger point injections for abdominal wall pain. Can J Gastroenterol. 2005;19:561–5.

5. Testut L, Jacob O. Trattato di Anatomia Topografica: Le pareti dell'addome. 1977.
6. Vellinga TT, De Alwis S, Suzuki Y, Einarsson JI. Laparoscopic entry: the modified alwis method and more. Rev Obstet Gynecol. 2009;2(3):193–8.
7. Chapron C, Pierre F, Harchaoui Y, Lacroix S, Beguin S, Querleu D, et al. Gastrointestinal injuries during gynaecological laparoscopy. Hum Reprod. 1999;14:333–7.
8. Rongieres C, Gomel V, Garbin O, Fernandez H, Frydman R. C-reactive protein should accelerate the diagnosis of bowel injury after gynecologic surgery. J Am Assoc Gynecol Laparosc. 2002;9:488–92.
9. Stany MP, Winter III WE, Dainty L, Lockrow E, Carlson JW. Laparoscopic exposure in obese high-risk patients with mechanical displacement of the abdominal wall. Obstet Gynecol. 2004;103:383–6.
10. Neudecker J, Sauerland S, Neugebauer E, Bergamaschi R, Bonier HJ, Cuschieri A, et al. The European Association for Endoscopic Surgery clinical practice guideline on the pneumoperitoneum for laparoscopic surgery. Surg Endosc. 2002;16(7):1121–43.
11. Vilos GA. The ABCs of a safer laparoscopic entry. J Minim Invasive Gynecol. 2006;13:249–51.
12. Vilos GA, Ternamian A, Dempster J, Laberge PY, The Society of Obstetricians and Gynaecologists of Canada. Laparoscopic entry: a review of techniques, technologies, and complications. J Obstet Gynaecol Can. 2007;29(5):433–65.
13. Teoh B, Sen R, Abbott J. An evaluation of four tests used to ascertain Veres needle placement at closed laparoscopy. J Minim Invasive Gynecol. 2005;12:153–8.
14. Riek S, Bachmann KH, Gaiselmann T, Hoernstein F, Marzusch K. A new insufflation needle with a special optical system for use in laparoscopic procedures. Obstet Gynecol. 1994;84:476–8.
15. McGurgan P, O'Donovan P. Optical Veress as an entry technique. Gynaecol Endosc. 1999;8:379–92.
16. Noorani M, Noorani K. Pneumoperitoneum under vision—a new dimension in laparoscopy. Endo World. 1997;39-E:1–8.
17. Meltzer A, Weiss U, Roth K, Loeffler M, Buess G. Visually controlled trocar insertion by means of the optical scalpel. Endosc Surg Allied Technol. 1993;1:239–42.
18. Lecuru F, Leonard F, Philippe JJ, Rizk E, Robin F, Taurelle R. Laparoscopy in patients with prior surgery: results of the blind approach. JSLS. 2001;5:13–6.
19. Schaller G, Kuenkel M, Manegold BC. The optical "Veress-needle"–initial puncture with a minioptic. Endosc Surg Allied Technol. 1995;3:55–7.
20. Reich H, Ribeiro SC, Rasmussen C, Rosenberg J, Vidali A. High-pressure trocar insertion technique. JSLS. 1999;3:45–8.
21. Shamiyeh A, Glaser K, Kratochwill H, Hormandinger K, Fellner F, Wayand WU, et al. Lifting of the umbilicus for the installation of pneumoperitoneum with the Veress needle increases the distance to the retroperitoneal and intraperitoneal structures. Surg Endosc. 2009;23:313–7.
22. Lam KW, Pun TL. Left upper quadrant approach in gynecologic laparoscopic surgery with reusable instruments. J Am Assoc Gynecol Laparosc. 2002;9:199–203.
23. Golan A, Sagiv R, Debby A, Glezerman M. The minilaparoscope as a tool for localization and preparation for cannula insertion in patients with multiple previous abdominal incisions or umbilical hernia. J Am Assoc Gynecol Laparosc. 2003;10:14–6.
24. Agarwala N, Liu CY. Safe entry technique during laparoscopy: left upper quadrant entry using the ninth intercostal space: a review of 918 procedures. J Minim Invasive Gynecol. 2005;12:55–61.
25. Altun H, Banli O, Kavlakoglu B, Kücükkayikci B, Kelesoglu C, Erez N. Comparison between direct trocar and Veress needle insertion in laparoscopic cholecystectomy. J Laparoendosc Adv Surg Tech A. 2007;17:709–12.
26. Dingfelder JR. Direct laparoscope trocar insertion without prior pneumoperitoneum. J Reprod Med. 1978;21:45–7.
27. Copeland C, Wing R, Hulka JF. Direct trocar insertion at laparoscopy: an evaluation. Obstet Gynecol. 1983;62:656–9.
28. Byron JW, Fujiyoshi CA, Miyazawa K. Evaluation of the direct trocar insertion technique at laparoscopy. Obstet Gynecol. 1989;74:423–5.
29. Jacobson MT, Osias J, Bizhang R, Tsang M, Lata S, Helmy M, et al. The direct trocar technique: an alternative approach to abdominal entry for laparoscopy. JSLS. 2002;6:169–74.

30. Woolcott R. The safety of laparoscopy performed by direct trocar insertion and carbon dioxide insufflation under vision. Aust N Z J Obstet Gynaecol. 1997;37:216–9.
31. Gunenc MZ, Yesildaglar N, Bingol B, Onalan G, Tabak S, Gokmen B. The safety and efficacy of direct trocar insertion with elevation of the rectus sheath instead of the skin for pneumoperitoneum. Surg Laparosc Endosc Percutan Tech. 2005;15:80–1.
32. Rahman MM, Mamun AA. Direct trocar insertion: alternative abdominal entry technique for laparoscopic surgery. Mymensingh Med J. 2003;12:45–7.
33. Prieto-Díaz-Chávez E, Medina-Chávez JL, González-Ojeda A, Anaya-Prado R, Trujillo-Hernández B, Vásquez C. Direct trocar insertion without pneumoperitoneum and the veress needle in laparoscopic cholecystectomy: a comparative study. Acta Chir Belg. 2006;106:541–4.
34. Biojo RG, Manzi GB. Safe laparoscopic surgery: tubal ligation without prior pneumoperitoneum. Surg Laparosc Endosc. 1995;5:105–10.
35. Lazarus HM. An alternative technique to create the pneumoperitoneum for laparoscopic surgery. Surg Laparosc Endosc. 1995;5:205–8.
36. McMahon AJ, Baxter JN, O'Dwyer PJ. Preventing complications of laparoscopy. Br J Surg. 1993;80:1593–4.
37. Fletcher DR. Abdominal insufflation for laparoscopy: can the risks be reduced? Aust N Z J Surg. 1995;65:462.
38. Hanney RM, Alle KM, Cregan PC. Major vascular injury and laparoscopy. Aust N Z J Surg. 1995;65:533–5.
39. Byron JW, Markenson G, Miyazawa K. A randomized comparison of Veress needle and direct trocar insertion for laparoscopy. Surg Gynecol Obstet. 1993;177:259–62.
40. Agresta F, DeSimone P, Ciardo LF, Bedin N. Direct trocar insertion versus Veress needle in nonobese patients undergoing laparoscopic procedures: a randomized, prospective, single-center study. Surg Endosc. 2004;18:1778–81.
41. Hasson HM. A modified instrument and method for laparoscopy. Am J Obstet Gynecol. 1971;110:886–7.
42. Chapron C, Cravello L, Chopin N, Kreiker G, Blanc B, Dubuisson JB. Complications during set-up procedures for laparoscopy in gynecology: open laparoscopy does not reduce the risk of major complications. Acta Obstet Gynecol Scand. 2003;82:1125–9.
43. Decloedt J, Berteloot P, Vergote I. The feasibility of open laparoscopy in gynecologic-oncologic patients. Gynecol Oncol. 1997;66:138–40.
44. Cravello L, Banet J, Agostini A, Bretelle F, Roger V, Blanc B. Open laparoscopy: analysis of complications due to first trocar insertion. Gynecol Obstet Fertil. 2002;30:286–90.
45. Hasson HM, Rotman C, Rana N, Kumari NA. Open laparoscopy: 29-year experience. Obstet Gynecol. 2000;96:763–6.
46. Jansen FW, Kolkman W, Bakkum EA, de Kroon CD, Trimbos-Kemper TC, Trimbos JB. Complications of laparoscopy: an inquiry about closed- versus open-entry technique. Am J Obstet Gynecol. 2004;190:634–8.
47. Hasson HM. Open laparoscopy as a method of access in laparoscopic surgery. Gynaecol Endosc. 1999;8:353–62.
48. Hasson HM, Rotman C, Rana N, Kumari NA. Open laparoscopy: 29-year experience. Obstet Gynecol. 2000;96:63–6.
49. Garry R. Towards evidence based laparoscopic entry techniques: clinical problems and dilemmas. Gynaecol Endosc. 1999;8:315–26.
50. Ahmad G, Duffy JMN, Phillips K, Watson A. Laparoscopic Entry Techniques. Cochrane Database Syst Rev. 2008;16:CD006583.
51. Garry R. Surgeons may continue to use their chosen entry technique. Gynecol Surg. 2009;6:87–92.
52. Long JB, Giles DL, Cornella JL, Magtibay PM, Kho RMC, Magrina JF. Open laparoscopic access technique: review of 2010 patients. JSLS. 2008;12:372–5.
53. Molloy D, Kalloo PD, Cooper M, Nguyen TV. Laparoscopic entry: a literature review and analysis of techniques and complications of primary port entry. Aust N Z J Obstet Gynaecol. 2002;42:246–54.
54. Liu HF, Chen X, Liu Y. A multi-center study of a modified open trocar first-puncture approach in 17,350 patients for laparoscopic entry. Chin Med J. 2009;122(22):2733–6.

55. McKernan J, Finley C. Experience with optical trocar in performing laparoscopic procedures. Surg Laparosc Endosc. 2002;12:96–9.
56. Tinelli A, Malvasi A, Hudelist G, Istre O, Keckstein J. Abdominal access in gynaecological laparoscopy: a comparison between direct optical and open access. J Laparoendosc Adv Surg Tech A. 2009;19:529–33.
57. Tinelli A, Malvasi A, Guido M, Istre O, Keckstein J, Mettler L. Initial laparoscopic access in postmenopausal women: a preliminary prospective study. Menopause. 2009;16:966–70.
58. Tinelli A, Malvasi A, Istre O, Keckstein J, Stark M, Mettler L. Abdominal access in gynaecological laparoscopy: a comparison between direct optical and blind closed access by Veress needle. Eur J Obstet Gynecol Reprod Biol. 2010;148:191–4.
59. Tinelli A, Malvasi A, Guido M, Tsin DA, Hudelist G, Stark M, Mettler L. Laparoscopic entry in women with previous abdomino-pelvic surgery. Surg Innov. 2011; [Epub ahead of print].
60. Tai HC, Lai MK, Chueh SC, Chen SC, Hsieh MH, Yu HJ. An alternative access technique under direct vision for preperitoneoscopic pelvic surgery: easier for the beginners. Ann Surg Oncol. 2008;15(9):2589–93.
61. Turner DJ. Making the case for the radially expanding access system. Gynaecol Endosc. 1999;8: 391–5.
62. Bhoyrul S, Mori T, Way LW. A safer cannula design for laparoscopic surgery: results of a comparative study. Surg Endosc. 1995;9:227–9.
63. Turner DJ. A new radially expanding access system for laparoscopic procedures versus conventional cannulas. J Am Assoc Gynecol Laparosc. 1996;3:609–15.
64. Tarnay CM, Glass KB, Munro MG. Entry force and intra-abdominal pressure associated with six laparoscopic trocar cannula systems: a randomized comparison. Obstet Gynecol. 1999;94:83–8.
65. Yim SF, Yuen PM. Randomized double-masked comparison of radially expanding access device and conventional cutting tip trocar in laparoscopy. Obstet Gynecol. 2001;97:435–8.
66. Lam TY, Lee SW, So HS, Kwok SP. Radially expanding trocars: a less painful alternative for laparoscopic surgery. J Laparoendosc Adv Surg Tech A. 2000;19(5):269–73.
67. Bhoyrul S, Payne J, Steffes B, Swanstrom L, Way LW. A randomized prospective study of radially expanding trocars in laparoscopic surgery. J Gastrointest Surg. 2000;4:392–7.
68. Feste JR, Bojahr B, Turner DJ. Randomized trial comparing a radially expandable needle system with cutting trocars. JSLS. 2000;4:11–5.
69. Ternamian AM. Laparoscopy without trocars. Surg Endosc. 1997;11:815–88.
70. Ternamian AM. A trocarless, reusable, visual-access cannula for safer laparoscopy; an update. J Am Assoc Gynecol Laparosc. 1998;5:197–201.
71. Ternamian AM. A second-generation laparoscopic port system: EndoTIP. Gynecol Endosc. 1999;8:397–401.
72. Ternamian AM, Deitel M. Endoscopic threaded imaging port (EndoTIP) for laparoscopy: experience with different body weights. Obes Surg. 1999;9:44–7.
73. Ternamian AM. How to improve laparoscopic access safety: ENDOTIP. Minim Invasive Ther Allied Technol. 2001;10:31–9.
74. Ternamian AM, Vilos GA, Vilos AG, Abu-Rafea B, Tyrwhitt J, MacLeod NT. Laparoscopic peritoneal entry with the reusable threaded visual cannula. J Minim Invasive Gynecol. 2010;17:461–7.
75. Fuller J, Ashar BS, Carey-Corrado J. Trocar-associated injuries and fatalities: an analysis of 1399 reports to the FDA. J Minim Invasive Gynecol. 2005;12:302–7.
76. Corson SL, Chandler JG, Way LW. Survey of laparoscopic entry injuries provoking litigation. J Am Assoc Gynecol Laparosc. 2001;8:341–7.
77. String A, Berber E, Foroutani A, Macho JR, Pearl JM, Siperstein AE. Use of the optical access trocar for safe and rapid entry in various laparoscopic procedures. Surg Endosc. 2001;15:570–3.
78. Tinelli A, Malvasi A, Schneider AJ, Keckstein J, Hudelist G, Barbic M, et al. First abdominal access in gynecological laparoscopy: which method to utilize? Minerva Ginecol. 2006;58:429–40.
79. Sharpe HT, Dodson MK, Draper ML, Watts DA, Doucette RC, Hurd WW. Complications associated with optical-access laparoscopic trocars. Obstet Gynecol. 2002;99:553–5.
80. Bemelman WA, Dunker MS, Busch OR, Den Boer KT, de Wit LT, Gouma DJ. Efficacy of establishment of pneumoperitoneum with the Veress needle, Hasson trocar, and modified blunt trocar (TrocDoc): a randomized study. J Laparoendosc Adv Surg Tech A. 2000;10:325–30.

81. Yerdel MA, Karayalcin K, Koyuncu A, Akin B, Koksoy C, Turkcapar AG, et al. Direct trocar insertion versus Veress needle insertion in laparoscopic cholecystectomy. Am J Surg. 1999;177:247–9.
82. Jirecek S, Drager M, Leitich H, Nagele F, Wenzl R. Direct visual or blind insertion of the primary trocar. Surg Endosc. 2002;16:626–9.
83. Marcovich R, Del Terzo MA, Wolf Jr JS. Comparison of transperitoneal laparoscopic access techniques: optiview visualizing trocar and Veress needle. J Endourol. 2000;14:175–9.
84. Soderstrom RM. Basic operative technique. In: Soderstrom RM, editor. Operative laparoscopy: the masters' techniques. New York: Lippincott Raven Press; 1998. p. 27–36.
85. Navarra G, Pozza E, Occhionorelli S, Carcoforo P, Donini I. One-wound laparoscopic cholecystectomy. Br J Surg. 1997;84:695.
86. Vidal O, Valentini M, Ginestà C, Martì J, Espert JJ, Benarroch G, et al. Laparoendoscopic single-site surgery appendectomy. Surg Endosc. 2010;24(3):686–91.
87. Uppal S, Frumovitz M, Escobar P, Ramirez PT. Laparoendoscopic single-site surgery in gynecology: review of literature and available technology. J Minim Invasive Gynecol. 2011;18(1):12–23.
88. Nguyen NT, Slone J, Reavis K. Comparison study of conventional laparoscopic gastric banding versus laparoendoscopic single site gastric banding. Surg Obes Relat Dis. 2010;6(5):503–7.
89. Canes D, Berger A, Aron M, Brandina R, Goldfarb DA, Shoskes D, et al. Laparo endoscopic single site (LESS) versus standard laparoscopic left donor nephrectomy: matched-pair comparison. Eur Urol. 2010;57(1):95–101.
90. Symes A, Rane A. Urological applications of single-site laparoscopic surgery. J Minim Access Surg. 2011;7(1):90–5.
91. Fader AN, Levinson KL, Gunderson CC, Winder AD, Escobar PF. Laparoendoscopic single-site surgery in gynaecology: a new frontier in minimally invasive surgery. J Minim Access Surg. 2011;7(1):71–7.
92. Diana M, Dhumane P, Cahill RA, Mortensen N, Leroy J, Marescaux J. Minimal invasive single-site surgery in colorectal procedures: current state of the art. J Minim Access Surg. 2011;7(1):52–60.
93. Keltz MD, Lang J, Berin I. A 5-mm open-entry technique achieves safe, single-step, cosmetic laparoscopic entry. JSLS. 2007;11:195–7.
94. Piccinni G, Merlicco D, Centonze A, Sciusco A, Petrozza D, Testini M, et al. The semiopen first umbilical trocar access technique in laparoscopic surgery: easy and safe. J Laparoendosc Adv Surg Tech A. 2008;18(6):865–8.
95. Dutta S. Early experience with single-incision laparoscopic surgery: eliminating the scar from abdominal operations. J Pediatr Surg. 2009;44:1741–5.
96. Stein RJ. Robotic Laparoendoscopic single-site surgery using gelport as the access platform. Eur Urol. 2010;57:132–7.
97. Merchant AM. Transumbilical gelport access technique for performing single-incision laparoscopic surgery (SILS). J Gastrointest Surg. 2009;13:159–62.
98. Kommu SS, Rane A. Devices for laparoendoscopic single-site surgery in urology. Expert Rev Med Devices. 2009;6:95–103.
99. Cox DR, Zeng W, Frisella MM, Brunt LM. Analysis of standard multiport versus single-site access for laparoscopic skills training. Surg Endosc. 2011;25(4):1238–44.
100. Varma R, Gupta JK. Laparoscopic entry techniques: clinical guideline, national survey, and medicolegal ramifications. Surg Endosc. 2008;22(12):2686–97.

Chapter 12
Blind Entry at Gynecological Laparoscopy Is Substituted by Entry Under Sight: Complications in Conventional Laparoscopic Entry

Liselotte Mettler, Wael Sammur, and Antonio Malvasi

Introduction

As witnesses to the early gynecological endoscopic surgical years of Kurt Semm in Kiel, Germany, since 1970, we have observed enormous changes in this challenging surgical field for more than 40 years.

Progress in understanding the hazards, advantages, and disadvantages of open versus conventional laparoscopic and robotic surgery together with the immense technical development in access and surgical possibilities in the individual cavities of the human, visualization, and instrumentation, as well as apparatus development should also lead to stabilization of entry technique.

Is this really the case for abdominal entry by laparoscopic surgery today?

Development of Gynecological Endoscopic Surgery

The development of gynecological endoscopic surgery from 1901 to 2012, including the "safety steps" of the Kiel School of Gynecological Endoscopy has been well written in six textbooks and publications:

- 1970–1985 [1–3]
- 1979–2010 [4–7]

L. Mettler (✉)
Department of Obstetrics and Gynecology, Kiel School of Gynaecological Endoscopy, University Hospitals Schleswig-Holstein, Kiel, Germany

W. Sammur
Department of Obstetrics and Gynecology, German Medical Centre, DHCC, Dubai, UAE

A. Malvasi
Department of Obstetrics and Gynecology, Santa Maria Hospital, Bari, Italy

A. Tinelli (ed.), *Laparoscopic Entry*,
DOI 10.1007/978-0-85729-980-2_12, © Springer-Verlag London Limited 2012

This chapter concentrates on laparoscopic entry and does not comment on hysteroscopy. It details a few developments.

Imaging and Gynecological Laparoscopy

Georg Kelling performed the first "laparoscopy," called "coelioscopy" by him, in 1901 on a dog using Nitze's cystoscope and air insufflation mechanism in Hamburg, Germany at an Assembly of German Natural Scientists. This technique was developed further by Raoul Palmer, Hans Frangenheim, and (after 1960) mainly by Kurt Semm. Semm initiated diagnostic and operative laparoscopy for gynecologists and operative endoscopic surgery for many other medical specialities [2].

Work on "imaging" progressed from camera and light source development to the rod-lens invention, from one chip to three chips, to HDTV and Endocameleon cameras as well as from direct view to 2D or 3D view on the TV monitor. Apparatus and instrument development, in continuous cooperation with the medical technical industry, brought new features for coagulation, suturing, and robotics. Instruments went from two to multiple degrees of liberty, from straight to rotating, multifunctional, articulated, and robotic forms. Precision surgery by means of an enlarged visual image and small or even single port entries for an instrument set with multiple degrees of liberty has become a reality. Imaging surgery on the video screen is the technique of the future and is already used for most benign and some malignant diseases in the field of gynecology [6, 7].

It is applied for vaginal natural orifice surgery and can replace laparotomy in approximately 80% of cases. Only Caesarean sections, hysterectomies for very large uteri, and specific cancer surgeries are still performed by laparotomy.

As newer versions of laparoscopic surgery, single port entry with already quite fancy entry systems, and robotic surgery, which uses conventional laparoscopic entries, need special attention.

Robotic Laparoscopic Surgery

The growing popularity of laparoscopic surgery focused new attention on the need for both improved laparoscopic camera control and instrument range in terms of motion and dexterity.

The first robotic camera assistant used in endoscopic surgery was the automated endoscopic system for optimal positioning (AESOP; Computer Motion, Santa Barbara, CA). This hand-, foot-, or voice-controlled arm allows the surgeon to perform complex laparoscopic surgery faster than with an assistant holding the camera [8].

The next surgical robot was a voice-controlled robot, ZEUS (Computer Motion) that consists of an AESOP to hold the camera and two additional AESOP-like units, which have been modified to hold the surgical instruments.

The modern robot generation named the da Vinci Surgical System is based on the technologies of computer motion, which have been developed further by Intuitive Surgical (Sunnyvale, CA). The da Vinci Surgical System was approved by the FDA in May 2005 for clinical use in gynecology and was first used in reproductive gynecology for tubal surgery [9] and later in oncologic surgery [10, 11].

There are four main components of the da Vinci S Surgical System:

- Surgeon's console: The surgeon sits viewing a magnified 3D image of the surgical field.
- Patient side-cart: This system consists of three instrument arms and one endoscope arm;
- Detachable instruments (endowrist instruments and intuitive masters): These detachable instruments allow the robotic arms to maneuver in ways that simulate fine human movements. There are seven degrees of freedom, which offer considerable choice of rotation in full circles. The surgeon is able to control the amount of force applied, which varies from a fraction of a gram to several kilos. Tremor and scale movements are filtered out. The movements of the surgeon's hand can be translated into smaller ones by the robotic device.
- 3D vision system: The camera unit or endoscope arm provides enhanced 3D images with the result that the surgeon knows the exact position of all instruments in relation to the anatomical structures. The patient lies in a horizontal position with both arms tucked alongside the body. Four trocars are placed next to the optic trocar. The surgeon sits at the console and the first surgical assistant is seated, in most cases on the patient's left side. This assistant controls the left accessory ports into which are inserted the instruments that are used for vessel sealing, retraction, suction, irrigation, and suturing. The middle robotic arm is attached to the optical trocar, with two lateral working arms to the right and one to the left. The robotic arms are connected at the beginning of the procedure and disengaged from the trocars at the end of the operation. The incisions are stitched and the incision lines are re-approximated (da Vinci S Surgical System). The core technology of the da Vinci Surgical System has been further refined to now include the da Vinci S Surgical System and the da Vinci Si Surgical System.

The da Vinci Surgical System has captured the imagination of the surgical community worldwide; however, the costs are very high and remain at the same level for each new surgical procedure. On the other hand, smaller innovative robotic systems with instruments with up to seven degrees of liberty are coming on the market. New HDTV systems allow the surgeon to work in what is almost a 3D field.

Safety Steps for Abdominal Entry at Laparoscopy

The following safety measures are advised before insertion of the Veress needle for CO_2 insufflation of the abdomen.

Fig. 12.1 The palpation of aorta test (Mettler [6]. Reprinted with permission)

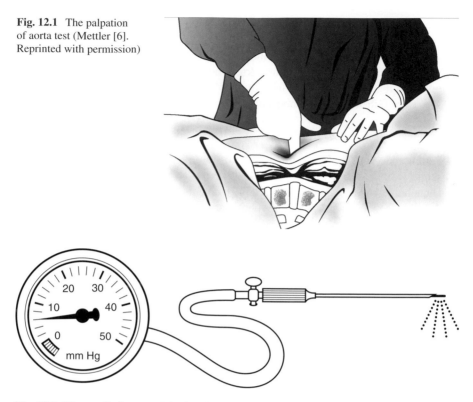

Fig. 12.2 The needle flow test (Mettler [6] . Reprinted with permission)

- *"Palpation of aorta" test:* If the abdominal aorta can be palpated directly below the umbilicus, the bifurcation must be further toward lower pelvis. It cannot be injured by oblique insertion of a Veress needle. If the bifurcation is felt above the umbilicus, perpendicular insertion with the anterior abdominal wall lifted up is suitable (Fig. 12.1).
- *Needle flow test:* To ensure flawless insertion of the Veress needle, the manometer should be set to a resistance of maximum 4–6 mmHg with a gas flow rate of 1 L/min. If the resistance is high, there is some obstruction inside the Veress needle (Fig. 12.2).
- *Insertion of the Veress needle:* Veress needle insertion must be always at a right angle. (An obliquely inserted needle becomes a scalpel!)
- *"Snap" test:* During insertion of the Veress needle through the skin, subcutaneous fat tissue, fascia, musculature, and peritoneum, a snap can be heard because of the CO_2 gushing through the respective layers (Fig. 12.3).
- *Hiss phenomenon:* After successful perforation of the anterior abdominal wall, a soft hissing sound is produced during the insertion of the Veress needle in the elevated abdominal wall as a result of negative pressure in the abdominal cavity.
- *Aspiration test:* Injection of 5–10 mL normal saline solution results in negative aspiration if the Veress needle is correctly placed, but gives blood-tinged aspirate or aspirate with intestinal contents if the needle is placed either in a blood vessel or intestine (Fig. 12.4).

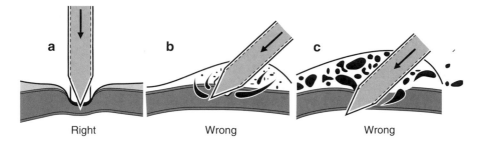

Fig. 12.3 The snap test (Mettler [6]. Reprinted with permission)

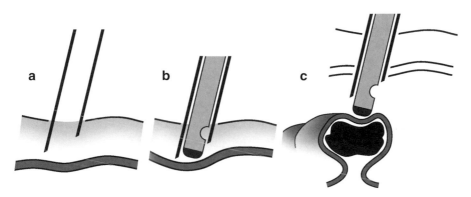

Fig. 12.4 The aspiration test (Mettler [6]. Reprinted with permission.)

- *Quadro test:* The four parameters measured are insufflation pressure, intraabdominal pressure, gas volume per minute, and total volume of instilled gas (Fig. 12.5). When the anterior abdominal wall is lifted up because of the negative pressure created in the abdominal cavity, if the pressure drops to below zero, then only CO_2 should be insufflated to a pressure of 15–20 mmHg.
- *Sounding test:* CO_2 is aspirated in a syringe containing 20 mL of normal saline solution and the result examined. When the tip lies free in the abdominal gas, CO_2 bubbles are visible in the normal saline solution during respiration, indicating the position in the free abdominal cavity (Fig. 12.6). When planning Z-insertion, the aspiration must be carried out horizontally toward the right or left and caudally, depending the planning.
- *Panoramic viewing after Z-insertion:* The panoramic viewing facilitates to uncover any pathological changes in the vicinity of the lower pelvis, e.g., in the intestines, liver, gallbladder, and spleen (Fig. 12.7).

Abdominal Entry Possibilities

Entry possibilities are given for single port, multiple ports, and robotic surgical entries by laparotomy, vaginal access, and laparoscopic open and closed approach, blind entry or laparoscopic entry under sight or vision,.

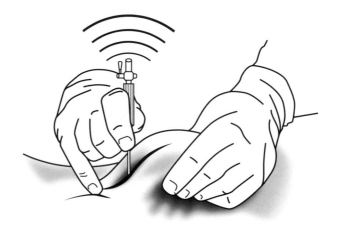

Fig. 12.5 The quadro test (Mettler [6]. Reprinted with permission)

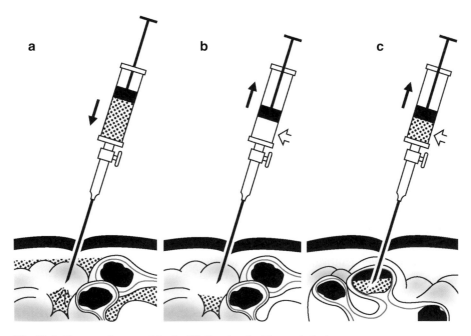

Fig. 12.6 The sounding test (Mettler [6]. Reprinted with permission)

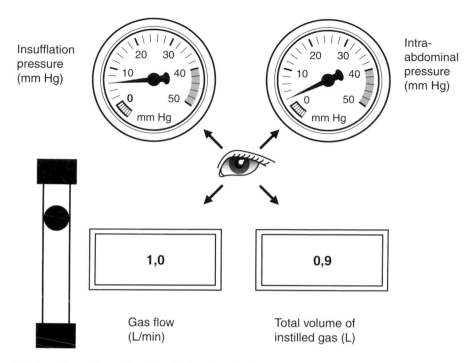

Insufflation pressure (mm Hg)

Intra-abdominal pressure (mm Hg)

1,0

0,9

Gas flow (L/min)

Total volume of instilled gas (L)

Fig. 12.7 Inspection of the abdominal cavity, after insertion of a laparoscope under CO_2 abdomino-pelvic distention (panoramic viewing after Z-insertion) (Mettler [6]. Reprinted with permission)

The anterior abdominal wall has four muscles that are penetrated at all entries:

- Rectus abdominis
- External obliquus abdominis
- Internal obliquus abdominis

The transversus abdominis and four structures lead from the medial to the lateral abdominal wall—urachus, inferior epigastric vessels, umbilical lateral ligament, and the superficial epigastric vessels. At laparotomy the incision possibilities are transversal with the conventional Pfannenstiel incision in the lower abdomen, a little higher the high fascial opening called the Misgav-Ladach Caesarean section incision described by Joel Cohen and Michael Stark and the longitudinal incision to the umbilicus or around it.

The gynecological surgeon and general surgeon have four routes of entry to the abdomen to treat intraabdominal disease surgically or by needle puncture with aspiration or instillation. These entry possibilities can remain the same under imaging techniques such as an MRI or CT scan; however, focused ultrasound destruction for fibroids controlled by magnetic resonance imaging (MRI) is possible today as well; techniques are changing [12].

Fig. 12.8 Veress needle entry. After skin incision the needle penetrates the umbilicus, the subcutaneous fat tissue and the fascia as well as the peritoneum. In position 1, 2 and 3 CO_2 bubbles are aspirated into the syringes from the free abdominal cavity. (Mettler [6]. Reprinted with permission)

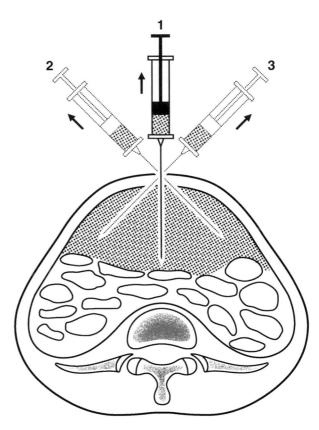

1. *Open abdominal:* Laparotomy in its different forms always dissects all abdominal layers to gain enough access to study and heal the respective disease. It always requires the closure of the wound in different layers by sutures.
2. *Laparoscopic:* Closed and open—multiple ports, single port, robotic.

In the *closed* access technique, the pneumoperitoneum is created by the Veress needle. This is a blind entry and has been the most commonly practiced entry by surgeons and gynecologists worldwide since the invention this spring–needle system by the Hungarian gynecologist Janos Veress (Fig. 12.8).

After pneumoperitoneum, the 5–10-mm conic trocar insertion principles are the following. After making the incision with a scalpel, enter with a 5-mm trocar sleeve and conical mandrin, pushing through the skin, subcutaneous fat tissue, and fascia; advance the trocar with a conical tip toward the right with rotational movements through the musculature till the peritoneum is reached; avoid the umbilical aponeurosis; and insert the conical elliptical trocar through the peritoneum by rotational movements.

It is easy to insert the Veress needle and create the pneumoperitoneum mostly through the umbilicus or at Palmer's point (= left upper abdomen, about 2 cm under the palpable rib in preoperated patients), but lacerations of vessels and more seldom bowel loops do occur.

Direct access or entry by the *open* technique, without creating pneumoperitoneum or using insufflators, has been described by Hasson [13].

It is also called the Scandinavian or Fielding technique. Some surgeons perform blind trocar insertion without pneumoperitoneum. The vascular lesions and bowel lesions appear to be similar.

3. Conventional *vaginal entry*, with colpotomy and single port systems for transvaginal surgery. Vaginal surgery with colpotomy has a long tradition and is the entry of choice for the gynecologist if the individual patient situation does not require a visual check of the abdominal cavity. Even vaginal hysterectomy is performed by pulling out the organs before transecting them and the vision is poor. Single port systems for a small 12–15-mm entry through the posterior cul-de-sac are in development

4. *Natural orifice transluminal endoscopic surgery* (NOTES), which includes the transgastric and transvaginal approach and *natural orifice surgery* (NOS): coming mostly from the field of general surgery, various systems through the entry point of the stomach and umbilicus are available and facilitate surgical interventions with only one incision: Single port entries (SILS, Single Port Laparoscopic System, Covidien), Laparoendoscopic Single Site surgical technique (LESS, Olympus), and X-CONE (Storz, Rochester, NY).

All access possibilities that are done blind through the Veress needle or with the trocar directly (using sharp, edgy, conic, or blunt trocars) carry a certain danger of lacerating structures immediately adherent to the abdominal wall as adhesions or bowel loops, deeper structures such as bowels or vessels, and abdominal organs (stomach, bladder). Entries under sight with the optical Veress needle and with Visiport, Optiview, and Endo-TIP have been described for closed access and give a certain security; however, basically the open and closed access techniques even under sight give a similar numbers of lesions in patients with bowel loops adherent to the anterior abdominal wall.

We think in 2011 that entry under sight has to be required for the primary trocar because this reduces lacerations in all situations in which bowel is not adherent to the abdominal wall.

The Choice of Gas for the Pneumoperitoneum

In the early years air was used for insufflation, but because of the increased risk of air embolism it was quickly replaced by CO_2 or N_2O gas. CO_2 is 200 times more diffusible than O_2. It is rapidly cleared by the lungs and does not support combustion. N_2O is only absorbed in blood up to 68% compared with CO_2, but has the advantage of a mild analgesic effect. Thus it is preferably used in laparoscopic procedures under local anesthesia. Helium gas, being inert in nature, is also applied in some centers but does not have added benefit over CO_2. Of course, gasless laparoscopy, as advised by some studies, carries no danger of any gas insufflation, but

Fig. 12.9 The right direction of trocar insertion at first entry gives a panoramic view of the laparoscope with the opportunity to discover any pathological changes in the minor pelvis and outside (Mettler [6]. Reprinted with permission)

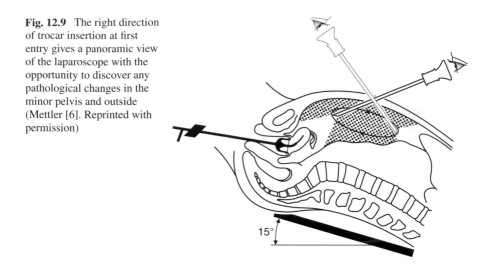

needs abdominal wall retractors etc. However, it does facilitate the use of conventional surgical instruments.

Trocars for Closed Laparoscopic Abdominal Entry

Surgeons can apply conic trocars, beveled trocars, multi-edged sharp trocars, threaded trocars such as the Endo-TIP (entry without force but with feeling, under sight), and visual trocars during first access. After the pneumoperitoneum is reached through the Veress needle, the optical trocar is placed.

Should it be conical with one point of laceration, or multi-edged and more dangerous to make cuts, if adherent bowel is not detected by the security steps, but does not need so much abdominal wall penetration force to enter the abdominal cavity? One of the most important steps for the first trocar insertion is its direction of insertion, because the wrong direction could cause considerable damage (Fig. 12.9).

Beveled trocars need larger incisions. All the trocars for robotic work need larger incisions anyway, because of the 12-cm size of the instruments. Single port entries all need larger incisions and certain tricks to access the abdomen safely. Direct trocars and radially expanding trocars are other trocars that can be used for laparoscopic entry. For a safe entry into the abdominal cavity, blind entry can be replaced by sharp trocars under vision. This is also called entry under sight. After skin incision penetration through skin and subcutaneous fat tissue with the trocar up to the fascia, insert the scope and reduce the CO_2 flow, cutting through the fascia and musculature to the peritoneum. Under vision, guide the tip of the scope on the peritoneum to a place where there are no bowel loops against it. Perform sharp perforation of the peritoneum under visualization. Put off CO_2 and inspection of the abdominal cavity. No specific trocars have shown to be superior in preventing vascular and visceral lacerations.

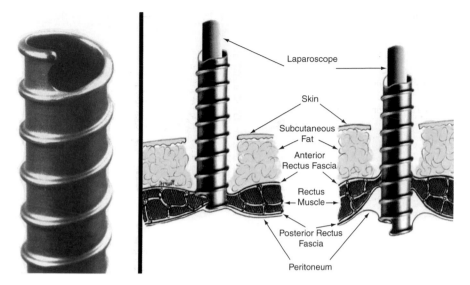

Fig. 12.10 Trocar insertion with Endo-TIP cannula, under vision

Optical Trocars

Optical trocars combine the advantages of a certain kind of vision in all different entry techniques. The Endo-TIP cannula was introduced by Artin Ternamian of Toronto, Canada (4). It features a reusable stainless steel-threaded cannula with no sharp components, and it requires no trocars (Endo-TIP; Karl Storz, Tuttlingen, Germany). After skin incision and establishment of pneumoperitoneum, the unit (a zero-degree laparoscope and mounted visual cannula) is inserted in the skin incision and held perpendicularly to the supine patient with the nondominant hand. The cannula is then rotated clockwise with the dominant hand applying minimal downward force. Accumulated subcutaneous fat and debris may be aspirated with the 5-mm suction/irrigation cannula. The cannula's blunt notched tip engages the tissue layers of the abdominal wall and transposes successive tissue layers onto the cannula's outer sheath in accordance with Archimedes' principle. The yellow fat, white anterior rectus fascia, red rectus muscle, white posterior rectus fascia, yellowish preperitoneal space, and transparent dark-bluish peritoneal membrane are all observed sequentially on the monitor. It has been observed that the blunt tip of the cannula pushes aside abdominal wall blood vessels, adhesions, and even bowel when adjacent to the anterior abdominal wall, but not, however, when really firmly adhered (Figs. 12.10 and 12.11).

Radially Expanding Trocars

Our experience with radially expanding trocars shows that the only advantage in comparison with conventional primary trocar entries is the reduced degree of postoperative pain (Figs. 12.12 and 12.13).

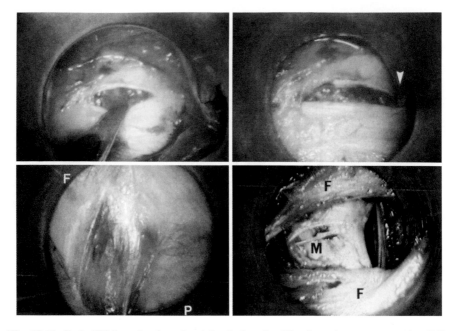

Fig. 12.11 Endo-TIP insertion into the abdominal cavity. The tissue layers are parted radially when the cannula penetrates the peritoneum

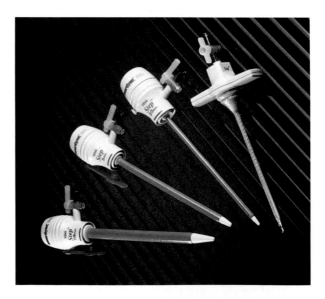

Fig. 12.12 Radially expanding trocars

According to a French retrospective study, the incidence of serious trocar accidents was evaluated from 103,852 laparoscopic operations involving almost 390,000 trocars. Seven perioperative deaths occurred (mortality 0.07/1,000), arising almost exclusively from vascular injuries. The incidence of vascular injuries was 0.4/1,000. There were injuries to almost all the abdominal organs and most of the abdominal vascular tree.

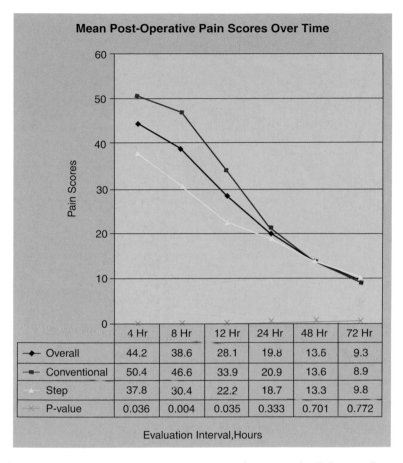

Fig. 12.13 Pain score after gynecological laparoscopy conic trocars and radially expanding trocars

Complications and Laceration Possibilities During First Access

The following series of figures compares correct and incorrect needle and trocar positions as well as cutting procedures (Figs. 12.14–12.25).

Abdominal Access Complications

Abdominal access complications occur at trocar placement with lacerations of the bowel, vessels, or if no abdominal entry is possible. At trocar entry, primary bowel lesions on adherent bowel loops to the anterior abdominal wall occur at both laparoscopy and laparotomy. By placing the Veress needle a vessel can be opened and intravascular insufflation may occur under CO_2 insufflation.

Several mechanisms may lead to gas embolism. Any cut into an abdominal wall or peritoneal vessel can cause CO_2 gas to be forced into the vessel, and if the Veress

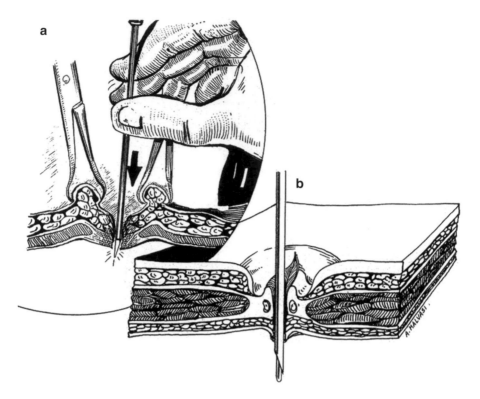

Fig. 12.14 Correct Veress needle introduction trough the umbilical fascia by perpendicular direction. (**a**) Surgeons lift the umbilical area by two Backhaus forceps and introduce the Veress needle. (**b**) The correct intraabdominal positioning of Veress needle

needle is put directly into a vein or parenchyma organ, this may cause gas embolism. Lacerations of the epigastric inferior arteries by placing secondary trocars under vision occur again and again because colleagues are not really using the abdominal translucency technique to see and avoid these vessels. In obese patients the tranluminency test gives poor visualization. The percentage of women requiring more than one attempt at laparoscopic entry is highest in the obese and particularly morbid obese patients. Epigastric arteries and even ureter are more difficult to identify.

The angle of the optical trocar if under vision or blind should not be more than 45°. It is important to palpate the aorta to find out whether the bifurcation is above or below the umbilicus.

Case Report: Persistent Ductus Omphalos Entericus

With the Veress needle at blind entry I once punctured a persistent, still blood-filled, ductus omphalos entericus that gave a heavy arterial bleed. The situation was visualized

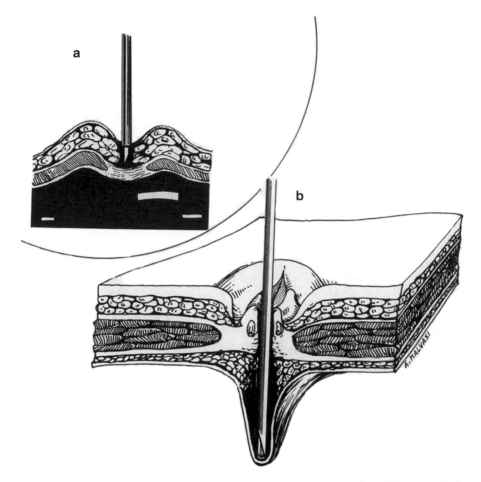

Fig. 12.15 (a) Normal introduction of Veress needle. (b) Wrong introduction of Veress needle in the pre-peritoneal space with the curtain effect

by quickly entering the optical trocar as well as two lower abdominal trocars and the duct grasped and coagulated. The arterial bleeding was immense; the patient had more than 1 L of fresh blood in the abdomen.

Laparoscopic entry lesions are classified as follows:

- *Type 1 Injuries:* Damage by Veress needle or trocar to major blood vessels and normally located bowel (1–4 per 1,000 patients)
- *Type 2 Injuries:* Damage by Veress needle or trocar to bowel adherent to the abdominal wall or vessels in the abdominal wall.

Type 2 lesions may occur whether the mode of access is by laparotomy or laparoscopy. The incidence of primary trocar lesions is 0.4–0.8% and the incidence of secondary trocar lesions is 0.8–0.12%. Bowel lesions occur in 4 per 1,000 cases

Fig. 12.16 Minor vascular
injury. Accidental needle
puncture of intraomental
blood vessel, adherent to
abdominal wall

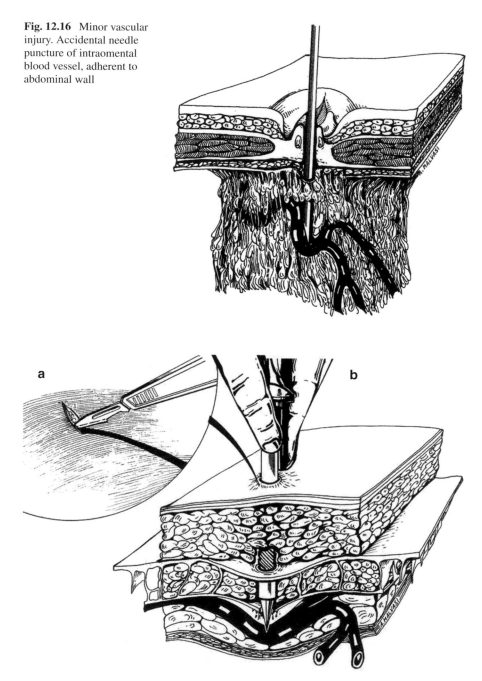

Fig. 12.17 Minor vascular injury during ancillary trocar introduction. (**a**) Abdominal wall lateral
incision to introduce the ancillary trocar. (**b**) Injury of epigastric artery during the ancillary trocar
introduction. This lesion is more frequent in obese women, in whom the Camper fascia switch the
trocar direction

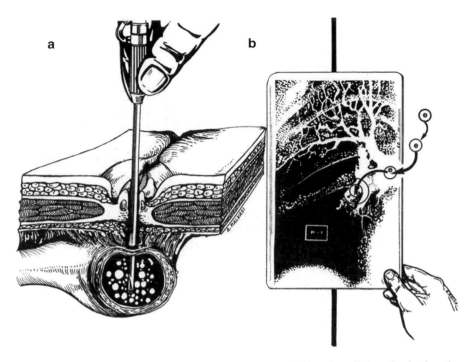

Fig. 12.18 Veress needle entry and possible embolism. (**a**) Accidental needle introduction into the blood vessel adherent to abdominal wall and wrong CO_2 insufflation. (**b**) Radiographic image of left lung infarct (*E* Embolism, *PA* pulmonary infarct)

(obtained from 350,000 laparoscopies in multicenter studies). Even with the most experienced laparoscopic and laparotomic surgeon, bowel lesions are not always avoidable.

The vascular lesions occur in 2 per 1,000 cases. According to the German Laparoscopic registry (Arbeitsgemeinschaft Gynäkologische Endoscopie, AGE) bowel and vascular lesions are found in 2–4 per 1,000 patients. Open laparoscopy offers no advantage in avoiding these lesions. Immediate action upon recognition of complications guarantees the safety of the patient.

In a retroperitoneal vascular laceration with the Veress needle or the tip of the optical trocar without an immediate fast-growing hematoma that requires direct action: All medical actions are immediately to be done by anesthetists, nurses, colleagues and vascular surgeons helps. Such a small retroperitoneal hematoma can also be carefully observed while doing the surgical planned procedure. A small hematoma does not have to be opened and must not necessarily be revised.

As I learned from my teacher, Kurt Semm [1], in every laparoscopic theater special vascular clamps, such as right-angled Kelly clamps, Adson-Schmidt, DeBakey hemostat, or Crawford clamps must be at hand. No attempt should be made to grasp any injured vessel with nonvascular instruments.

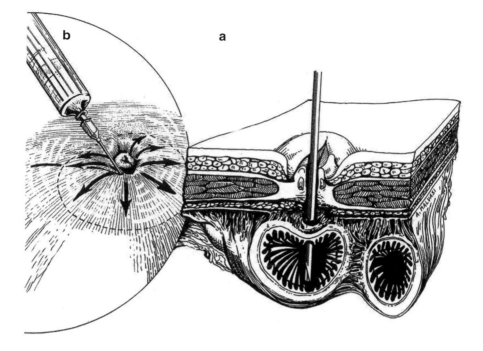

Fig. 12.19 Bowel injury during Veress introduction. (**a**) Accidental Veress introduction into small bowel, adherent to anterior abdominal wall. (**b**) Safety maneuver to check correct needle introduction

Immediate Complications

They occur during surgical interventions such as *bowel, vessel, bladder, and ureter* lesions, as well as anesthesia-related or general complications, such as pulmonary embolism, massive bleedings, consecutive to *major vessel injuries* or *intravascular insufflation* and heart arrest. In our gynecological field we have to be aware that even during the clearest laparoscopic hysterectomy and particularly in cancer situations, veins are opened and gas enters into the venous system and may even reach the right side of the heart [14]. Bowel lesions are not always avoidable, even with the most experienced laparoscopic and laparotomic surgeon. Primary bowel lesions occur by direct cutting, traction at adhesiolysis, or as thermal injuries in about 1% of laparoscopies [5].

Case Report: Bowel Lesion

Here I want to share the reader's opinion on a bowel perforation recognized at the end of the laparoscopy with entry of the primary optical trocar at Palmer's point and positioning of two lower umbilical trocars under sight.

The case report involved a 37-year-old patient with ovarian cancer, in stage III, who underwent radical hysterectomy with bilateral adnexectomy, pelvic systematic lymphadenectomy, and adjuvant chemotherapy.

Fig. 12.20 Wrong
introduction of a poly-use
trocar in the pre-peritoneal
space with the curtain effect

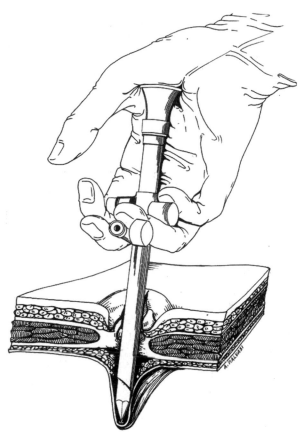

At second-look laparoscopy, surgeons caused a lesion of small bowel during placement of a secondary port under suboptimal vision. The question is, Was it avoidable?

After taking a biopsy doing some adhesiolysis and really diagnosing all the small
cancerous implants, we found that the right secondary trocar had *totally perforated
a small bowel loop*. Surgeons entered a Foley catheter through the port. Together
with a general surgeon we took the bowel loop outside, resected the perforated part,
and performed an end-to-end anastomosis of the bowel loop (Fig. 12.26a–c).

Differentiation of the Different Major Lesions Occurring During a Laparoscopic Procedure

Vascular Lesions

Major vessel injuries can occur during the operative part of the surgery and particularly at retroperitoneal dissection. Normally, the distal abdominal aorta, as well as
the common and external and internal iliac arteries, lie in the retroperitoneal space

Fig. 12.21 Accidental
introduction of a poly-use
trocar in the omentum tissue
adherent to abdominal wall

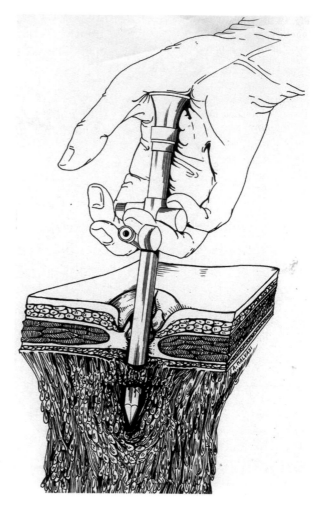

of the retroperitoneum. Luckily, lacerations of these vessels occur rarely [15–17].
Most venous injuries other than to the vena cava are accompanied by injury of the
overlying arteries. The large number of injuries to the aorta and vena cava are sur-
prising, because these vessels are above the umbilicus in most women. In most
aortic or vena cava lacerations, periumbilical trocars were placed at angles >45°
from the plane of the spine.

The first steps in effective management of major vessel injury are early recognition, minimizing the bleeding, performing a laparotomy if the bleeder cannot be
laparoscopically compresses or stilled, calling a vascular surgeon, and being aware
of intravascular insufflation (end-tidal carbon dioxide, decreased oxygen satura-
tion, millwheel murmur, tachyarrhythmia, and right-side heart strain with ST-T

Fig. 12.22 Frontal and sagittal section of uterus (**a**) and lower genitourinary system: left ureter (**b**) and bladder (**c**). Accidental ureteral partial cutting by endoscopic Mayo scissors during laparoscopic total hysterectomy

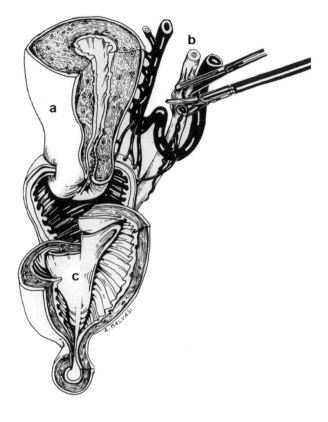

changes). Direct compression of the bleeder is possible with a midline approach at laparotomy until a vascular surgeon arrives. If an additional surgeon with vascular repair experience is not at hand, tight packing of the pelvis with dry laparotomy pads and temporary abdominal closure as well transport of the patient to a larger center are advisable.

Bowel Lesions

Many intraoperative bowel lesions can be sutured. Partial excision and sutures as well as resection of lacerated areas have to be applied, including end-to-end anastomosis. In many cases of endometriosic infiltration of the bowel, a primary resection is planned and the bowel is prepared preoperatively. In cases of unprepared bowel we suggest a careful disinfection of the area and multiple irrigations after the procedure.

Abdominal access and the creation of a pneumoperitoneum carry a significant risk of bowel injuries. Such injuries are more frequent in laparoscopic surgery and

Fig. 12.23 Frontal and sagittal section of uterus (**a**) and lower genitourinary system: left ureter (**b**) and bladder (**c**). Accidental ureteral section by endoscopic Mayo scissors during laparoscopic total hysterectomy

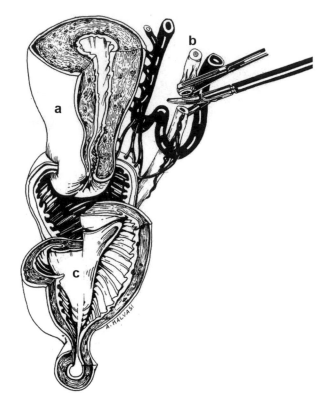

are often avoided in open surgery. Although these catastrophic injuries are uncommon, they represent a major reason for mortality from laparoscopic procedures, and a significant source of the morbidity associated with any laparoscopic procedure. Shea and colleagues examined 78,747 patients in a metaanalysis of 98 laparoscopic cholecystectomy studies. Fourteen percent of 1,400 conversions were from complications such as bleeding and bowel injury [18].

Despite the rapid evolution of laparoscopic surgery in the past decade, the surgical community has failed to adequately report and study this tragic complication. As a result, most case reports and large series reporting these injuries are derived from older gynecological literature. It was largely believed that newer instrumentation and knowledge would reduce the risk of these complications; however, reports from the general surgical literature suggest that this not the case.

In fact, these injuries occur with greater frequency. Most disturbing, surgeons have been oblivious to the risk by failing to associate postoperative complication with the possibility of trocar injury, thus failing to recognize bowel perforation until it is too late. Laparoscopic cases are scheduled in outpatient clinics lacking blood, vascular operative instruments, and expertise.

Bowel injury is the third cause of death from laparoscopic procedures after major vascular injury and anesthesia [19]. Unlike major vascular injuries, in which

Fig. 12.24 Frontal and sagittal section of uterus (**a**) and left uterine artery (**b**). Accidental partial cutting of descending uterine artery branch by endoscopic Mayo scissors during laparoscopic total hysterectomy

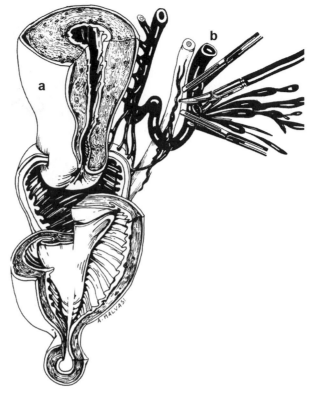

the risk and presentation are immediate, many bowel injuries go unrecognized at the time of the procedure. Consequently, patients present postoperatively, often after discharge, with peritonitis. This delay makes it a significant cause of morbidity and mortality [20].

A large survey of nearly 37,000 gynecological laparoscopies in the United States revealed a 0.16% incidence of bowel injury: 39.8% of vascular and intestinal injuries were caused by the Veress needle, 37.9% by insertion of the primary trocar, and 22% by the secondary trocar. The remaining gastrointestinal injuries resulted during dissection, electrocoagulation, or grasping [21].

Importantly, these investigators noted that the experience of the surgeons was an important factor in the overall complication rate and in the incidence of intestinal injury.

Surgeons operating on the abdomen and pelvis should be familiar with the management of iatrogenic injuries of the gastrointestinal tract. These injuries should be recognized and appropriately managed, to minimize morbidity [22].

Dr. Brosens from Belgium and Dr. Alan Gordon from the United Kingdom organized a multinational survey using the experience of members of the International Society of Gynecological Endoscopy (ISGE), who were requested

Fig. 12.25 Frontal and
sagittal section of uterus (**a**)
and left uterine artery (**b**).
Accidental total section of
descending uterine artery
branch by endoscopic Mayo
scissors during laparoscopic
total hysterectomy

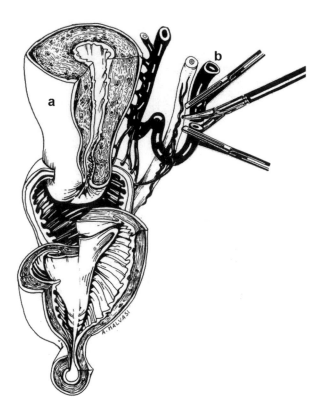

to report the details of bowel trauma over 2 years and thereby learn from each others' experiences [23].

A sound knowledge of laparoscopic anatomy is essential to understand the distorted anatomy often present in disease. Most injuries can be accounted for by failure to keep to tissue planes, blunt dissection, diathermy in close proximity to the intestine, excessive traction, and poor visualization.

Previous surgery, endometriosis, chronic pelvic inflammatory disease (PID), malignancy, or radiotherapy may distort anatomy and obliterate tissue planes [24].

All high-risk patients should be warned about the possible risk of gastrointestinal injury. Bowel preparation is advisable before major pelvic surgery [25].

Injuries may result from mechanical or thermal forces. Damage to the rectum is less common, but carries a higher potential for complications and may occur during pelvic dissection or adhesiolysis [26].

Injuries with healthy edges can be repaired primarily using tension-free, single-layer, interrupted sero-submucosal 3-0 Vicryl [27].

For more extensive injuries, resection and primary anastomosis are required. Persistent pyrexia, tachycardia or ileus in the postoperative period should raise the index of suspicion for bowel injuries. Laparotomy followed by resection and defunctioning with an end stoma may be required [28].

Fig. 12.26 Laparoscopic
bowel lesion and repair.
(**a,b**) Small bowel loops
are totally adherent to the
abdominal wall. (**c**) The
secondary trocar
perforated the adherent
small bowel loop. (**d**)
surgeons entered a Foley
catheter through the port

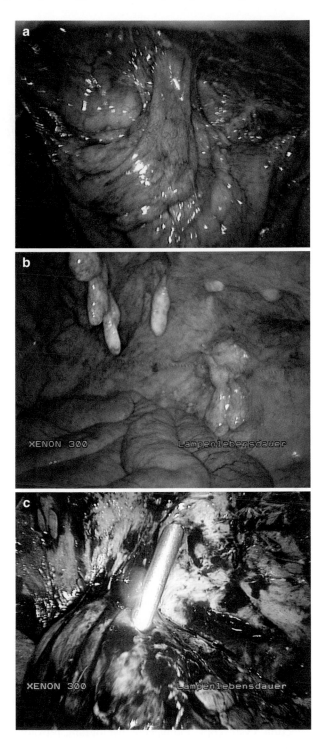

Fig. 12.26 (continued)

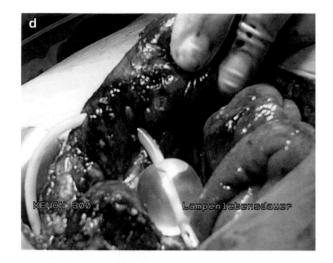

Proctosigmoidoscopy can be performed at the end of the surgery to evaluate intraluminal abnormality or rectosigmoid injury. The pelvis is then filled with isotonic fluid and observed laparoscopically for air leakage [29, 30].

Bladder and Ureter Injuries

Routine intraoperative cystoscopies after many major gynecological operations allow an early recognition to facilitate a repair at the primary surgery with less morbidity for the patient. The intraoperative demonstration and dissection of the ureter is often necessary and required if the surgery is performed in the ureteric area. Of course, an open bladder can also be detected by direct emission of urine. Sometimes the Foley catheter bag fills with CO_2 and indicates a bladder lesion.

Urinary tract injuries associated with laparoscopic surgery differ in substantial manner from laparoscopic major vessel or intestinal iatrogenic injury. The former rarely result in the death of the patient, whereas the latter two are associated with mortality. Urinary complications are seldom the result of needle or trocar trauma (i.e., entry related). By far bladder and ureteral injuries happen as the result of the operative aspect of the laparoscopy [31].

The most cogent factors related to ureteral damage are (1) suboptimal knowledge of pelvic anatomy, (2) failure to open into and dissect retroperitoneally, (3) employment of energy devices with marginal knowledge relating to the physics as well as the tissue interaction of these devices, (4) imprecise application of stapling devices, and (5) pelvic adhesions, particularly dense adhesions located in and around the ovarian fossa [32].

Injury to the ureter sustained is egregiously compounded by late postoperative recognition. Failure to order suitable diagnostic tests (e.g., indigo carmine dye injection, cystoscopy, intravenous pyelogram, retrograde pyelograms) will accrue additional damage.

Bladder injuries may be less serious than ureteral injuries, particularly if lacerations are recognized intraoperatively and are repaired appropriately in a timely manner. As with ureteral injury, the instillation of a dye (e.g., methylene blue) into the bladder will lead to early diagnosis, as will intraoperative cystoscopy.

Injury to the trigone may be avoided by doing a cystoscopy before or during bladder laceration closure. Resecting a significant portion of the bladder during a gynecological surgical procedure reflects a deficit in knowledge of pelvic anatomy.

Similarly, the creation of a vesicovaginal fistula or ureterovaginal fistula is clearly a failure of recognition and is associated with compromise to the blood supply to the bladder or ureter.

A number of recently published reports have quantified the incidence of urologic (bladder and ureter) injuries associated with laparoscopic surgery. These range from 0.3 to 4.0%. The risk of urologic injury was greater with total laparoscopic hysterectomy compared to LAVH: 4.0% versus 0.49% [33–36].

Baggish studied 75 cases of bladder and ureteral injuries over a period of 24 years (1984–2008). Data included single or multientry procedures, primary diagnostic or operative procedures, description of pathology encountered, type of bladder or ureteral injury, instrument or device, symptoms and signs, etiologic factor(s) resulting in injury, time of diagnosis, diagnostic tests ordered, performance of ameliorative procedures, results of repair, subsequent surgery, morbidity, and follow-up. Of the 75 injuries, the bladder accounted for 33 (44%) and the ureter 42 (56%). Clearly the majority of entries (trocar)-related injuries were sustained by the urinary bladder. Of the 12 entry injuries, 10 were inflicted by the primary entry trocar and two by means of secondary entry devices. The single ureteral entry injury was caused by a 5-mm secondary trocar ostensibly placed under direct vision. Adhesions between the bladder and uterus were significant in the etiology of bladder lacerations.

Trocar puncture trauma accounted for more than one-third of the bladder injuries and thermal devices for another one-third of the bladder injuries. Stapling devices, electrosurgical, and ultrasonic devices accounted for 28=42% or 67% of ureteral injuries. Depending on the particular instrument and technique associated with the ureteric injury, the locations of the injury site varied [37].

Parpala-Spurman et al. reported in 2008 ureteric injuries associated with laparoscopic surgery in three 7-year time periods; between 1986 and 1992, only five injuries were observed, whereas 28 were observed between 1993 and 1999, and 39 were reported between 2000 and 2006. Sixty-four percent of the injuries were in association with gynecological operations. Only 11% occurred with urological procedures [38].

Assimos et al. likewise reported a rise of ureteral injuries over a 5-year period in gynecological patients. The rate increased from 13 to 41 per 10,000 admissions [39].

Analysis of factors contributing to urological injuries was a high priority goal of the current study. Failure to secure the ureter by exposing the retroperitoneal space and deficient anatomical knowledge of the bladder and ureter, including their relationships, were critical factors associated with complications. The presence of adhesions and particularly a history of Caesarean section surgery placed the patient in a high-risk category for bladder injury.

A history of major intraabdominal surgery and the presence of adhesions were likewise strong indicators for ureteric injuries. The presence of significant endometriosis and accompanying inflammation as well as scar formation was high-risk factors for ureteric complications [40].

Prevention of injury and recognition of injury are sentinel pillars for high-quality medical practice standards. Varying opinions have been reported relative to ureteral catheter placement for the prevention of injury during major surgery and particularly relating to laparoscopic surgery [41].

The latter is cogent because one drawback of laparoscopic surgery relates to a lack of tactile sensation. Late diagnosis of bladder and ureteral injuries may lead to greater difficulties for the patient who underwent surgery as well as the surgeon who performed it [42].

Although urinary tract injuries are rarely lethal, they can and do lead to significant morbidity, sometimes chronic. The risk of injuries especially to the ureter is increased with the laparoscopic approach and particularly with gynecological laparoscopic operations. The reason for the higher risk with laparoscopy may be explained on the basis of lack of tactile sensation, decreased mobility, reduced vision, especially depth perception and panoramic view, reluctance of the gynecologist to open into the retroperitoneal space, suboptimal knowledge of pelvic anatomy, and reliance on hemostatic devices, which increase the risk for urinary tract injury.

Late Complications

The late complications are secondary bowel lesions associated with peritonitis and massive intraabdominal infection. Often small vascular lesions are not recognized until a haematoma appears and ureter lesions are sometimes only recognized after the development of a urinoma. This may occur many days after the surgery. These lesions occurring in the postoperative period are also called secondary lesions and occur in 0.5% [5]. Patients have to be informed to immediately report adverse feeling or situations, whether or not they are still in the hospital. This is a very important fact to be transmitted to patients before any surgery.

Future Developments and Prevention of Complications

To prevent complications you must have a thorough understanding of anatomy as well as the pathophysiology of the disease you are trying to treat, know your instruments, work gently and with a plan, acquire laparoscopic suture techniques, and do not depend on coagulation alone. A defect can occur even with the most modern instruments. Never work alone, but let your assistant to both help and criticize you, and certainly train your nurses to help you. Every laparoscopic surgeon needs to know his or her apparatuses, coagulation techniques, and settings, and must never completely depend on nurses, technicians, or colleagues.

Prior to trocar entry we advise palpation of aorta, horizontal positioning of the patient, and a quick aspiration test. The intraabdominal pressure can be as high as 25 mmHg at trocar entry, but has to be reduced after the trocar is in the right position to 12–15 mmHg for the continuing surgery. Alternative entry sites for the Veress needle are Palmer's point that is the left upper quadrant and any other area in the abdomen suitable after multiple previous surgeries.

In any type of laparoscopic surgery, the trocar entry points should follow a certain pattern in every team, but the surgeon should be open to schedule different settings for individual cases required by the tumor or the patient's previous surgeries. If the uterus to be taken out laparoscopically by whatever method reaches the umbilicus, the optic trocar has to be placed higher up in the abdomen. In cases of suspected midline adhesions, the 5-mm trocar could be placed at Palmer's point, and if desired, the umbilical trocar placed under sight. This may require extensive adhesiolysis in the umbilical area immediately before placement of a trocar in the umbilical area. After trocar insertion, mostly through the umbilicus, the laparoscope should be rotated through 360°. This circular view affords the possibility of assessing suspected and unsuspected pathology.

Even with all the entry technologies available today, the entry under sight with the Endo-TIP cannula of Artin Ternamian (which follows the principle of Kurt Semm), established in the early 1980s, represents the method of choice for the primary trocar.

It does take a bit of time and a little larger incision; however, with good 5-mm optics the entry can also be performed by using the threaded 5-mm Endo-TIP cannula and a 5-mm optic. For single port entry and robotic laparoscopic surgery the entries are large in any case. An optical entry of the primary trocar in robotic surgery may be helpful as well.

We compared [43] the safety and efficacy of a modified direct optical entry versus Hasson's method by open laparoscopy in women with previous abdominopelvic surgery in a preliminary prospective case-control study. Statistical differences were found in favor of the direct optical entry in both the time span of entry and blood loss. There was no difference in vascular or bowel injuries. The study suggested that direct optical entry is advantageous in comparison with open laparoscopy in terms of saving time in preoperated patients, thus facilitating safe visually guided entry for laparoscopy. Hemostasis by modern instrument development became easier as well; however, no technology is without risk.

All abdominal entry possibilities, even under direct vision, carry inborn risk.

For prevention of complications, we doctors can never be careful enough and all need God's protection.

Acknowledgments The authors thank Nicole Guckelsberger, as office manager, for her continuous support; and Wael Sammur, Department of Gynecology, Obstetrics and Female Infertility, German Medical Center, Dubai Healthcare City, United Arabian Emirates (UAE), for his contribution in chapter editing and formatting.

References

1. Semm K. Pelviskopie und Hysteroskopie. Farbatlas und Lehrbuch. Stuttgart: Schattauer; 1976.
2. Semm K. Operationslehre für Endoskopische Abdominal-Chirurgie. Stuttgart: Schattauer; 1984.
3. Semm K. Operative manual for endoscopic abdominal surgery. Chicago: Year Book Medical Publishers; 1986.
4. Mettler L, Giesel H, Semm K. Treatment of female infertility due to tubal obstruction by operative laparoscopy. Fertil Steril. 1979;32:384–8.
5. Mettler L. Endoskopische Abdominal-Chirurgie in der Gynäkologie. Stuttgart: Schauttauer; 2002.
6. Mettler L. Manual for laparoscopic and hysteroscopic gynecological surgery. New Delhi: Jaypee Brothers; 2006. ISBN 31-8061-632-0.
7. Mettler L. Manual of new hysterectomy techniques. New Delhi: Jaypee Brothers; 2007.
8. Mettler L, Ibrahim M, Jonat W. One year of experience working with the aid of a robotic assistant (the voice-controlled optic holder AESOP) in gynaecological endoscopic surgery. Hum Reprod. 1998;13(10):2748–50.
9. Advincuala AP, Wang K. Evolving role and current state of robotics in minimally invasive gynaecologic surgery. J Minim Invasive Gynecol. 2009;16(3):291–301.
10. Mettler L, Schollmeyer T, Boggess J, Magrina JF, Oleszczuk A. Robotic assistance in gynecological oncology. Curr Opin Oncol. 2008;20(5):581–9.
11. Bandera CA, Magrina JF. Robotic surgery in gynaecologic oncology. Curr Opin Obstet Gynecol. 2009;21(1):25–30.
12. Stewart EA, Gostout B, Rabinovici J, et al. Sustained relief of leiomyoma symptoms by using focused ultrasound surgery. Obstet Gynecol. 2007;110:279–87.
13. Hasson HM. A modified instrument and method for laparoscopy. Am J Obstet Gynecol. 1971;110:886–7.
14. Kim CS, Kim JY, Kwon JY, et al. Venous air embolism during total laparoscopic hysterectomy. Anesthesiology. 2009;111:50–4.
15. Soderstrom RM. Injuries to major blood vessels during endoscopy. J Am Assoc Gynecol Laparosc. 1997;4:395–8.
16. Fuller J, Ashar BS, Carey-Corrado J. Trocar-associated injuries and fatalities: an analysis of 1399 reports to the FDA. J Minim Invasive Gynecol. 2005;12:302–7.
17. Azevedo JL, Azevedo OC, Miyahira SA, et al. Injuries caused by Veress needle insertion for creation of pneumoperitoneum: a systematic literature review. Surg Endosc. 2009;23:1428–32.
18. Shea JA, Healey MJ, Berlin JA, Clarke JR, Malet PF, Staroscik RN, et al. Mortality and complications associated with laparoscopic cholecystectomy. A meta-analysis. Ann Surg. 1996;224(5):609–20.
19. Tian YF, Lin YS, Lu CL, Chia CC, Huang KF, Shih TY, et al. Major complications of operative gynecologic laparoscopy in southern Taiwan: a follow-up study. J Minim Invasive Gynecol. 2007;14(3):284–92.
20. Kyung MS, Choi JS, Lee JH, Jung US, Lee KW. Laparoscopic management of complications in gynecologic laparoscopic surgery: a 5-year experience in a single center. J Minim Invasive Gynecol. 2008;15(6):689–94.
21. Chandler JG, Corson SL, Way LW. Three spectra of laparoscopic entry access Injuries. J Am Coll Surg. 2001;192:478–91.
22. Harkki-Siren P, Kurki T. A nationwide analysis of laparoscopic complications. Obstet Gynecol. 1997;89:108–12.
23. Brosens I, Gordon A. Bowel injuries during gynaecological laparoscopy: a multinational survey. Gynecology. 2001;10(3):141–5.
24. Schäfer M, Lauper M, Krähenbähl L. Trocar and Veress needle injuries during laparoscopy. Surg Endosc. 2001;15(3):275–80.

25. Wu M, Koh L, Chow S. Can bowel injury be prevented during laparoscopic surgery? A case report and literature review. Taiwan J Obstet Gynecol. 2004;43(4):219–21.
26. MacCordick C, Lécuru F, Rizk E, Robin F, Boucaya V, Taurelle R. Morbidity in laparoscopic gynecological surgery: results of a prospective single-center study. Surg Endosc. 1999;13(1):57–61.
27. Leng J, Lang J, Huang R, Liu Z, Sun D. Complications in laparoscopic gynecologic surgery. Chin Med Sci J. 2000;15(4):222–6.
28. Wang PH, Lee WL, Yuan CC, Chao HT, Liu WM, Yu KJ, et al. Major complications of operative and diagnostic laparoscopy for gynecologic disease. J Am Assoc Gynecol Laparosc. 2001;8(1):68–73.
29. Leonard F, Lecuru F, Rizk E, Chasset S, Robin F, Taurelle R. Perioperative morbidity of gynecological laparoscopy. A prospective monocenter observational study. Acta Obstet Gynecol Scand. 2000;79(2):129–34.
30. Tarik A, Fehmi C. Complications of gynaecological laparoscopy—a retrospective analysis of 3572 cases from a single institute. J Obstet Gynaecol. 2004;24(7):813–6.
31. DeCicco C, Schonman R, Craessaerts M, et al. Laparoscopic management of ureteral lesions in gynecology. Fertil Steril. 2009;92:1424.
32. Baggish MS. Analysis of 31 cases of major vessel injury associated with gynecologic laparoscopy operations. J Gynecol Surg. 2003;19:63.
33. Saidi MH, Sadler RK, Vancaillie TG, et al. Diagnosis and management of serious urinary complications after major operative laparoscopy. Obstet Gynecol. 1996;87:272.
34. Tamussino KF, Lang PF, Breinl E. Ureteral complications with operative gynecologic laparoscopy. Am J Obstet Gynecol. 1998;178:967.
35. Aslan P, Brooks A, Drummond M, et al. Incidence and management of gynecological related ureteric injuries. Aust N Z J Obstet Gynecol. 1999;39:178.
36. Wang PH, Lee WL, Yuan CC, et al. Major complications of operative and diagnostic laparoscopy for gynecologic disease. J Am Assoc Gynecol Laparosc. 2001;8:68.
37. Baggish MS. Urinary tract injuries secondary to gynecologic laparoscopic surgery: analysis of 75 cases. J Gynecol Surg. 2010;26(2):79–92.
38. Parpala-Spurman T, Paananen I, Santala M, et al. Increasing numbers of ureteric injuries after the introduction of laparoscopic surgery. Scand J Urol Nephrol. 2008;42:422.
39. Assimos DG, Patterson LC, Taylor CL. Changing incidence and etiology of iatrogenic ureteral injuries. J Urol. 1994;152:2240.
40. Schonman R, DeCicco C, Cornoa R, et al. Accident analysis: factors contributing to a ureteric injury during deep endometriosis surgery. BJOG. 2008;115:1611.
41. DeCicco C, Ret Davalos ML, Van Cleynenbreugal B, et al. Iatrogenic ureteral lesions and repair: a review for gynecologists. J Minim Invasive Gynecol. 2007;14:428.
42. Oh BR, Kwon DD, Park KS, et al. Late presentation of ureteral injury after laparoscopic surgery. Obstet Gynecol. 2000;95:337.
43. Tinelli A, Malvasi A, Guido M, Tsin DA, Hudelist G, Stark M, et al. Laparoscopy entry in patients with previous abdominal and pelvic surgery. Surg Innov 2011; [Epub ahead of print].

Chapter 13
Natural Orifice Surgery: Surgical Procedures Through Natural Body Openings

Michael Stark and Tahar Benhidjeb

Introduction

The art of surgery has a long history in human culture, and it is important to follow its development to understand its current state. Different surgical procedures were practiced in ancient times, as can been shown by archaeological findings in countries with a rich history of high culture, such as China and Egypt.

In Egypt, medical and midwifery schools are known to have existed during the Fourth Dynasty, when different surgical procedures were taught and practiced. We know also that women studied and practiced medicine, and there is evidence that a woman called Peseshet who graduated around 2400 BCE from the medical school (Perianch) in Sais, was not only a practicing physician and surgeon, but also supervised other doctors [1]. The original doctor's title was *wabau*. This title has a long history that repeated for centuries.

Royalty employed their own private physicians. There is evidence of inspectors of doctors, overseers, and chief doctors. The earliest recorded physician in the world, Hesy-Ra, was the official Chief of Dentists and Physicians to King Djoser during the twenty-seventh century BCE. There were many other titles, ranks, and

M. Stark (✉)
The New European Surgical Academy (NESA),
Berlin, Germany

The USP Hospital Palmaplanas of Mallorca, Mallorca, Spain

T. Benhidjeb
Department of General, Visceral and Thoracic Surgery,
University Medical Center Hamburg-Eppendorf,
Hamburg, Germany

The New European Surgical Academy (NESA),
Berlin, Germany

A. Tinelli (ed.), *Laparoscopic Entry*,
DOI 10.1007/978-0-85729-980-2_13, © Springer-Verlag London Limited 2012

sub-specializations in the fields of medicine and surgery, the existence of which demonstrate the large variation in practiced medicine and surgery.

The ancient Egyptian specialties that are known to have existed were ophthalmology, gastroenterology, proctology (the ancient Egyptian term for proctologist, *neru phuyt*, translates literally as the "the anus shepherd"), dentistry, and "doctor who supervises the work of the butchers."

Hospitals, which were called *Houses of Life*, treated inpatient and ambulant patients and are known to have existed in ancient Egypt in the First Dynasty.

Different kinds of surgical procedures are also known to have been performed as early as in the third millennium BCE. Surgical equipment such as scalpels, tooth forceps, scissors, and gynecological specula very similar to the instruments in daily use today were extensively used by the Romans, and can still be seen in different archaeological museums.

Because of the lack of anesthesia as we understand it today, the spectrum and extent of surgery was limited. Opium and alcohol were used as anesthesia, and the surgical procedures had to be done very quickly because of their weak effectiveness. Indeed, even surgical procedures that were described in the eighteenth and nineteenth centuries, such as Chopart's [2] and Lisfranc's amputations [3], respectively, were designed in a way that allowed them to be performed very quickly.

The era of abdominal surgery as it is known and understood today began in 1809, when Ephraim McDowell in Kentucky, Missouri performed the first successful ovarian cystectomy using longitudinal incision [4]. The longitudinal incision has been in use ever since.

This operation was done before the introduction of ether anesthesia. After ether was first introduced by William T. G. Morton in Boston, on October 16, 1846 [5], the development of more sophisticated, prolonged, and complicated surgical procedures, such as the two types of the Billroth stomach operations for peptic ulcers and the Wertheim operation for cervical malignancies, were introduced [6, 7].

Toward the end of the nineteenth century, and during the era of existing general anesthesia, Johannes Pfannenstiel modified the lower abdominal incision by performing it transversely [8]. Despite the longer time required, the transverse incision proved to have advantages over the longitudinal incision regarding postoperative pain, mobility, and cosmetic effects. However, because this modification took place before the era of today's evidence-based surgery, the first comparative study between longitudinal and transverse incisions (in Caesarean sections) was performed 74 years after the Pfannenstiel incision was first introduced [9]. Longitudinal incisions in the lower and upper abdomen and variations such as the Kocher incision [10] as well as transverse low abdominal incisions are still in use. In some procedures, such as Caesarean sections, they continue to be used owing to lack of an alternative.

Laparotomy is associated with postoperative discomfort as well as complications such as febrile morbidity or eventration. Therefore, to optimize laparotomy, in 1972 Joel Joel-Cohen introduced an alternative transverse incision in which the opening of the fascia was above the *linea arcuata* [11].

At this anatomical level, cranial to the Mm. Pyramidalis, the fascia does not adhere to the muscles, and contrary to the need to separate it from the muscles, can

Fig. 13.1 The returning of the blood vessels to the anatomic site at the end of the operation

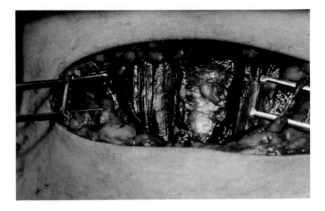

be separated in a relatively nontraumatic way. This method has been integrated into the Misgav Ladach Caesarean section with some modifications. In this method the longitudinal muscles and blood vessels are stretched laterally manually, similar to the strings on a musical instrument, to create access to the abdominal cavity. At the end of the operation, the muscles and blood vessels return back to their original anatomical position (Fig. 13.1).

The nineteenth century was the era of open surgery, in which great surgical traditions were developed, and various physiological and pathological processes were studied with the help of—and parallel to—the development of Roentgen imaging and laboratory and pathological skills and knowledge.

The Era of Laparoscopy

New ideas emerged at the beginning of the twentieth century when, in 1904, Georg Kelling in Germany performed the first known experimental endoscopic procedure on a dog [12].

During the twentieth century, new developments such as the introduction of endotracheal intubation [13], light sources and insufflators that control intraabdominal pressure [14], and the introduction of monitors enabled the continuation of this pioneering approach to endoscopy.

In the 1970s, when laparoscopy gradually became accepted, it was used mainly for diagnostic purposes, such as detection of unexplained and acute abdominal pain [15], detection of the source of unexplained bleeding, and confirmation or ruling out of pathological situations such as extrauterine pregnancies. However, gradually parallel to the development of modified and optimized surgical instruments, endoscopy was developed into a new surgical discipline, and various procedures such as tubal sterilization became part of the daily gynecological arsenal [16].

In the beginning laparoscopy was used mainly by gynecologists [17]. However, soon it was accepted in other disciplines, and today all the surgical disciplines are using endoscopic procedures as an alternative to most of the time-honored established open abdominal operations [18].

The most common endoscopic procedures today are the cholecystectomy [19], laparoscopically assisted vaginal hysterectomy [20], total abdominal hysterectomy [21], colectomy [22], nephrectomy [23], appendicectomy [24], and splenectomy [25].

It was shown that patients undergoing endoscopic operations use less postoperative analgesics and present decreased morbidity with shorter hospital stay [22]. However, endoscopic operations require sophisticated surgical know-how and advanced training, which includes the use of simulators before clinical application. At the same time these procedures require sophisticated equipment such as cameras and disposable instruments. Therefore, they are not yet in general use, definitely not in countries with limited resources.

At the end of the twentieth century most of the abdominal surgical, urological, endocrinological, and gynecological procedures had endoscopic solutions. The only abdominal operation that remains without alternative is the Caesarean section, and this in a time in which its use is increasing yearly [26]. Therefore it is of utmost importance to re-analyze and optimize this procedure, as was done when the Misgav Ladach Vaesarean section was introduced [27, 28].

Most of the discomfort associated with surgery is caused by the abdominal incision. When abdominal and vaginal hysterectomies are compared, it is shown that the vaginal hysterectomy is associated with a significantly lower need for analgesics, shorter hospital stay, as well as a quicker return to mobility and work.

Endoscopy can be optimized as well, either by introducing sophisticated instruments, such as modified morcellators [29] which enable one to remove the specimen through the trocar in use without needing an extra incision, or the development of different methods to improve the cosmetic effect, such as the small laparoscopic incision placement (SLIP) method, [30] or the single port system, which enables the performance of various operations through one incision, such as hernias [31], urological operations [32], endocrinological operations like adrenalectomies [33] or gynecological procedures [34].

Hybrid operations are still currently in use because certain operative methodologies using the single port approach are not yet established in various operations, such as cystectomies [35].

It is probable that during the twenty-first century many pathological conditions will be prevented or treated by nonsurgical means, such as chemical or genetic measures. It seems that certain developing techniques, such as identifying and applying targeted treatment to cancer stem cells, will open new horizons toward early identification and treatment of malignancies [36].

Other nonsurgical methods, such as the emission of ultrasound waves, are already in use for treatment of uterine fibroids using an MRI-guided punctual focal heating of small areas of tissues, which causes local degeneration within the fibroid and results in shrinkage of the fibroid within a couple of weeks [37].

At the moment, however, as the mentioned methods are still at an early stage of development, we have to continue to look for optimal future surgical methods that will make operations safe and efficient, solve the pathological condition, and at the same time result in as little discomfort to the patient as possible, with an as short as possible hospital stay, and will enable the patient to return as soon as possible to her or his family and work.

Natural Orifice Surgery

The question at the beginning of the twenty-first century is, therefore, whether the peak level of today's development of surgical solutions has already been achieved or the development and/or optimization of new surgical approaches and methods can still be sought.

It seems that when the development of sophisticated imaging methods and surgical tools is taken into consideration, the next logical step is the search for novel methods that will perform the necessary procedures for pathological conditions but entirely without or with minimal discomfort while taking into account the cosmetic outcomes associated with abdominal scars.

The only way to perform sophisticated surgical procedures without cutting the surface of the body is the use of natural body openings for entry to the abdomen or other parts of the body. We believe that if this approach will be extensively studied and become feasible and optimal, the twenty-first century will become the era of natural orifice surgery (NOS).

The idea to perform operations through natural openings is not new. Tonsillectomies were performed transorally for more than 2,000 years [38]. Celsus (ca 25 BCE to 50 CE) described a method of digital removal of the tonsils. Tonsillectomy is still in use for various indications such the treatment of obstructive sleep apnea [39].

Another time-honored use of the natural opening is the vaginal hysterectomy. This method is has been in use for more than 100 years. Over the years some variations in the operative method have been introduced, although not always founded on evidence-based facts. Recently the vaginal hysterectomy became subject of reanalyzing. Six different methods were examined for their different steps and sequences, and only those common to all the operative descriptions (and therefore probably the most essential) were used in a prospective randomized study. It was shown that using the so-called Ten-Step Vaginal Hysterectomy results in reduced operation time and a lower need for analgesics [40].

When vaginal hysterectomy is compared with abdominal hysterectomy, the vaginal route results in less discomfort and fewer complications, such as postoperative infections [41].

For many years gastroenterologists used the natural openings of the body for various diagnostic and operative procedures such as gastroscopy, duodenoscopy, rectoscopy, and colonoscopy. Polyps are routinely removed currently during colonoscopies after a relative short colon preparation. Colonoscopy is also used as a routine periodical examination in elderly people, especially in those with a family history of colon cancer and those who are genetically affected.

Transrectal endoscopic microsurgery (TEM) was introduced in the 1980s [42, 43].

With this method, rectal adenomas and malignancies were successfully operated transanally, thus avoiding abdominal incisions. Pituitary adenomas have been operated trans-sphenoidally, which provides a relatively easy access to the sella turcica [44].

The Transgastric Approach

Anthony Kalloo from the Division of Gastroenterology at the Johns Hopkins Hospital was the first to report an experimental transgastric intraabdominal peritoneoscopy [45].

This approach was followed by other gastroenterologists. When the gastroenterologists reached the intraperitoneal cavity through the wall of the stomach, the term Natural Orifice Transluminal Endoscopic Surgery (NOTES) was introduced to describe procedures performed through natural body openings. As soon as other body openings became the target, this term was found irrelevant as the vagina, for example, cannot be described as a lumen. The term NOS (Natural Orifice Surgery) is therefore more appropriate because it is descriptive and includes the transgastric approach [46].

Gastroenterologists penetrated the wall of the stomach using a gastroscope when using the transgastric approach for diagnostic and therapeutic procedures [47]. Many research groups followed [48, 49].

Most of the known works are preclinical studies in which the topics of research are the development of designed surgical instruments for the gastric incision, intraperitoneal manipulation, suturing and/or coagulation, the removal of specimens, and the secure suturing of the gastric wall. However, there are questions to be answered and problems to be solved before extensive clinical application.

1. How to prevent bacteriological contamination, as the gastroscope is introduced after passing through contaminated areas that can be cleaned but practically cannot be sterilized.
2. The diameter of the esophagus limits the size of the instrument in use.
3. Today's existing multichannel endoscopes have to be improved and adapted to the special requirements prescribed by the anatomy.
4. The diameter of the esophagus and the lack of adapted morcellator do not allow the retrieval of specimens with a diameter wider than the esophagus. Therefore, a second entry to the abdomen is necessary.
5. The acidity of the stomach is an important factor to be considered when the transgastric approach is planned. It should be neutralized medically or by repeated washing before, during, and probably also after the procedure, because the healing of the entry might take some days.
6. Ergonomic aspects. Performing the so-called NOTES operation requires a much higher muscular workload when compared with traditional laparoscopy. When compared, these operations take much longer. Lee and co-workers concluded that

performing transluminal operations was a much more significant challenge for surgeons than traditional laparoscopy, combined with higher ergonomic risks [50].

The transgastric approach is feasible. However, the question is, What does it improve? We have to calculate whether the benefit of avoiding small abdominal incisions justifies such a complex and challenging approach. To prevent damage to the intestines or blood vessels by creating a security space between them and the abdominal wall, each endoscopic procedure starts with insufflation of CO_2, sometimes up to 20 mmHg and more [51].

The introduction of the Veress needle is then relatively safe, and is performed manually with the opportunity to ensure that the peritoneal cavity has been reached before introduction of the trocar, which might cause severe complications, such as injury to the major blood vessels [52].

Transgastric insufflation is associated with risks, not just because of the lack of hand-guided feedback, but also because of the different anatomical considerations. When the abdominal wall is insufflated during laparoscopy, it is elevated, usually creating space between the posterior wall and the abdominal wall, but when an incision is created through the stomach, there is no direct way to make sure that there is a secured free space beyond and no way to control the presence of intestinal loops just next to the incision, although of course hybrid maneuvers are possible [53].

A Veress needle can be introduced before stomach penetration, but without an optical device inserted into the peritoneal cavity before the penetration, safety remains uncertain.

The transgastric approach is still in a very early stage of evolution, although its potential use is already being suggested. To make it acceptable, effective, and safe, the challenges have to be solved; for example, instruments have to be designed and constructed, and surgical methods that allow for safety and efficacy have to be studied and developed. Other challenges also exist, such as the prevention of leaks from anastomosis. Meanwhile, methods are being examined for the safe closure of the stomach, such as the double layer Queen method [54] or clips [55].

Should these challenges be solved, training programs will have to be developed, preferably using designed simulators, when they become mainstream therapy.

The Trans-Douglas Approach

The pouch of Douglas offers relatively easy and safe access to the peritoneal cavity in women. The opening of the pouch of Douglas is one of the first steps in every vaginal hysterectomy, with or without descensus. It is carried out easily by cutting the vaginal wall transversally about 1–2 cm above the external os and then lifting the posterior aspect of the cervix with a tooth tennaculum, identifying the pelvic peritoneum between the sacrouterine ligament, pulling it with surgical forceps, cutting it with round scissors, inserting the scissors into the peritoneal cavity, and pulling the scissors out while holding them open with both hands [40]. This method has proved to be safe, does not require insufflation before the maneuver, and can be done under epidural and/or spinal anesthesia. In recent years the pouch of Douglas has been used as an entry for infertility evaluation and treatment using the so-called fertiloscope [56].

We believe that because of the relative ease of the entry into the abdominal cavity and its and safety, the use of the pouch of Douglas will become more prevalent during the twenty-first century provided that adapted instruments will be designed. Various abdominal operations have already been performed transvaginally. In 2001, Tsin published a preliminary report on culdo-laparoscopy [57], and in 2003 he reported on a procedure of a combined transvaginal hysterectomy and hybrid cholecystectomy in an 81-year-old woman [58].

A transvaginal cholecystectomy has been reported by Zorrón in Brazil [59]. Bessler in the United States reported in 2007 about a hybrid endoscopic cholecystectomy [60]. These approaches were followed by Marescaux in France [61].

The transvaginal approach for urological, gynecological, and surgical indications is establishing itself gradually, not just because of its relatively easy access through the pouch of Douglas, but also because of the relatively wide diameter of the entry, which enables an uncomplicated retrieval of specimens.

In a study conducted to estimate the physiological diameter of the pouch of Douglas, the mean diameter was found to be 2.6 cm with a range of 2.0–3.4 cm [62]. This was an anatomical study, and it seems that in living patients the elasticity of the pouch of Douglas is even higher. These results are important when instruments are designed that could be used without causing damage to the pelvic floor owing to overstreching.

The theoretical advantages of the trans-Douglas approach are as follows:

1. Easy and relatively nontraumatic entry into the abdominal cavity.
2. Possible wide diameter of the inserted instruments.
3. When performing vaginal hysterectomy, the pouch of Douglas can be opened under vision, and the traditional 15 mmHg pressure is not needed. For some procedures much lower intraabdominal pressure in needed; therefore, these can be performed with epidural anaesthesia.
4. The vaginal wall repairs without scars.
5. Specimens with large diameters can be retrieved.

A questionnaire showed that women primarily chose to be operated on via the vaginal approach because of their conclusion that the vagina's sensitivity did not change and they were encouraged by knowing that the operation did not leave any scarring [63].

Recently, with accumulating experience, more sophisticated trans-Douglas procedures are being performed, such as hybrid hemicolectomy [64] or transvaginal nephrectomy [65, 66]. The feasibility of hybrid trans-Douglas nephrectomy combined with mini-laparotomy was evaluated in five patients by Porpiglia et al. [67]. Although the average operation time was relatively long (120 min), the blood loss was minimal and all reported operations were performed without complications.

The feasibility of a combined abdominal and transvaginal sleeve gastrectomy in morbidly obese women was reported by Choillard et al. [68]. Although in six

Fig. 13.2 The TED in S-shape for procedures in the upper abdomen (schematic representation)

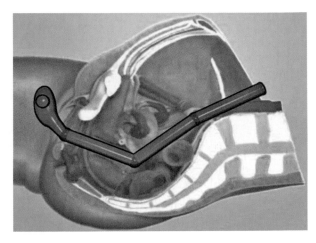

patients a conversion (to laparoscopy) became necessary, no complications were reported. The mean hospital stay was 72 h, with a range of 24–144 h. The average operation time, however, was long (116 min, with a range of 54–231 min).

Therefore it seems that in women the trans-Douglas surgery is more suitable and involves fewer risks than the transgastric approach. Unlike the transgastric approach, which must be done endoscopically, the access through the pouch of Douglas is direct and can be performed manually. Closure is done manually and directly compared with the challenging and indirect way used in the transgastric approach. The contamination risk is minimal and the ergonomics are optimal. The trans-Douglas approach does not leave scars, whereas the effect of the transgastric approach still has to be assessed [61].

In 2006, the New European Surgical Academy (NESA) established in Berlin the first Europe-based working group on natural orifice surgery (NOS). The members of the NOS working group are scientists, physiologists, surgeons, gynecologists, urologists, and pharmacologists from Germany, United Kingdom, the Netherlands, Denmark, Austria, Italy, France, Switzerland, Israel, the United States, and Canada, as well as representatives from the industry. In the working group's meetings, the concept of natural orifice surgery and the published research data are presented and discussed, and the idea for a novel instrument, a single port endoscope, the so-called Transdouglas Endoscopic Device (TED) has been introduced.

This device should enable performing complex and complete surgical procedures through transvaginal entry so as to avoid hybrid procedures [69]. There will be no need for any additional abdominal wall incisions. Any trans-Douglas endoscopic instruments have to take pelvic anatomy into account, and the TED can assume an S-shape for procedures in the upper abdomen and a U-shape for those in the lower abdomen (Figs. 13.2 and 13.3). The TED should contain a light source, camera as well as two triangulated working arms containing the surgical instruments as well as instruments for flushing and sucking (Figs. 13.4 and 13.5). The theoretical advantages of single-port trans-Douglas procedures are as follows:

Fig. 13.3 The TED in U-shape for procedures in the lower abdomen (schematic representation)

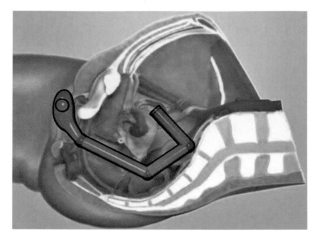

Fig. 13.4 The TED in closed mode

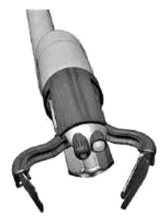

Fig. 13.5 The TED in open mode

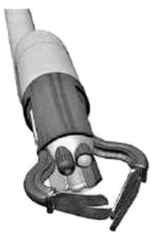

Fig. 13.6 (**a**) Opening the pouch of Douglas by insertion and traction of curved scissors with prolapsus. (**b**) Opening the pouch of Douglas by insertion and traction of curved scissors without prolapsus

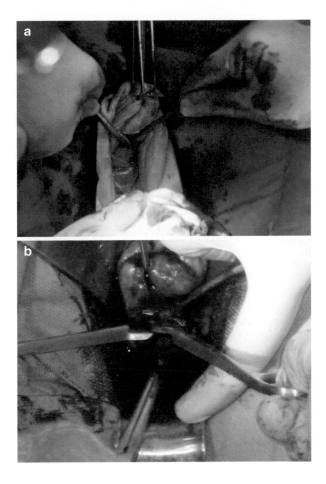

1. The vagina, unlike the mouth and stomach, can be cleaned completely, thus minimizing the risk of infection.
2. The opening and suturing of the vaginal wall is safe as it is known from more than 100 years of experience with vaginal hysterectomy (Fig. 13.6a, b).
3. The vaginal wall lining repairs without leaving scars and without any long-term discomfort or dysfunction [63].
4. In the conventional laparoscopy the Veress needle is inserted vertical to the major blood vessels. Therefore, alternative ways of entry were suggested, such as open access [70]. Life-threatening conditions happen because of the vertical insertion of the Veress needle and the trocars [71]. In the trans-Douglas approach the instruments are inserted under vision, and more important, parallel to the major blood vessels, hence the safety.
5. The reason for the use of the traditional 15 mmHg pressure is to produce space between the abdominal wall and the intraabdominal organs and blood vessels. Such high pressure cannot be achieved without the use of intratracheal intubation and positive pressure respiration resulting from the high CO_2 pressure on the dia-

phragm. Such a high pressure in not necessary when the trans-Douglas approach is used; therefore, just minimal pressure is needed. Some procedures could be done using peridural anaesthesia.

6. The large diameter of the pouch of Douglas enables the insertion of relatively wide instruments and the retrieval of specimens without a need to use a morcellator [72].
7. Contrary to abdominal incisions, the pouch of Douglas cannot cause herniation or eventration.
8. Ergonomic aspects. The trans-Douglas approach can be performed while the surgeon is seated comfortably.

The vaginal route has been used to remove appendices [71, 73], and also, following endoscopic cholecystectomy, a large gall bladder with stones [74]. Different gynecological procedures, such as the removal of uterine fibroids, are routinely performed transvaginally [75, 76].

Trans-Douglas hybrid procedures are routine. Federlein et al. reported 115 cases and found that transvaginal cholecystectomy is safe and easy-to-learn with minimal trauma to the abdominal wall, whereas postoperative pain scores were similar to those of laparoscopy. Most of the patients were satisfied with the procedure [77]. The trans-Douglas route was also recently used for a hybrid hemicolectomy [64].

Transoral Thyroidectomy

Total or partial thyroidectomy is traditionally done through a transverse incision in the neck. The resulting scars are aesthetically disturbing. As a result, methods have been developed to reduce the size of the scar. The technique of minimally invasive video-assisted thyroidectomy (MIVAT) developed by Miccoli [78] is the method that has become most widespread so far. The limiting factors of this method include the bothersome 20-mm cervical incision and consequent specimen size to remove.

Other methods were introduced to completely avoid these scars. Such approaches are via the chest, axillary, a combined axillary bilateral breast or a bilateral axillary breast approach [79–82]. Several papers have been published that describe access outside the front neck region. Recently, a paper describing a transaxillary approach in 338 patients using the da Vinci system was reported. In this series, three cases of damage to the recurrent nerve and one of Horner's syndrome were recorded [83]. The other approach in use is the transmammillar pathway [84].

The development of cervical scarless thyroid surgery is indeed a great step toward better cosmetic outcomes. However, these techniques just moved the scars from the front neck region to the axilla or the chest where they are still visible. Indeed, the mentioned minimally invasive accesses as well as conventional approaches to the thyroid gland do not respect the anatomical surgical planes. This may result in patient complaints, e.g., scar development and swallowing disorders. Furthermore, the extracervical approaches do not comply with the use of the term *minimally invasive* because they are associated with an extensive dissection of the chest and neck region, thus being rather maximally invasive for the patients. The main aim should be the introduction of a technique of thyroid resection that fulfils the following criteria:

1. Respecting anatomical planes and minimizing surgical trauma in thyroidectomy
2. Achieving an optimal cosmetic result by performing a scarless operation
3. Achieving these optimal cosmetic results with scarless surgery in combination with minimal trauma
4. Achieving a minimally invasive procedure by the access itself being close to the thyroid gland
5. Not compromising patient safety by use of a minimally invasive approach with an optimal cosmetic result

The technique that meets all these criteria is the transoral access because the distance between the sublingual place and the thyroid gland is short, thus avoiding extensive dissection maneuvers. Furthermore, the mouth mucosa can be sutured without difficulty, and repairs itself without leaving any visible scars. Feasibility of the transoral access has been recently demonstrated in a porcine model by using a modified axilloscope [85].

However, the described technique is a hybrid because an additional medial access (3.5-mm incision) 15 mm below the larynx was necessary for the insertion of a fixation forceps through a trocar. The main aim of our project was the investigation and introduction of a technique of totally endoscopic thyroid resection that is minimally invasive and safe for the patient and at the same time cosmetically optimal (scarless). For this purpose a total of five human cadavers were used. In three cadavers, safety and reproducibility to reach and resect the thyroid gland was assessed according to a defined road map. At the end of the procedure the cadavers were dissected to evaluate all defined anatomical key structures regarding possible injuries, and also to allow an evaluation of the surgery performed.

The totally TransOral Video-Assisted Thyroidectomy (TOVAT) was performed on two further human cadavers with the help of one 5- and two 3-mm trocars that were introduced through the mouth floor and the vestibulum of the mouth subplatysmal. A working space was created by insufflating CO_2 at a pressure of 4–6 mmHg ("air dissection"). Surgical dissection of the further working space was realized with 3-mm bipolar scissors.

The TOVAT procedure consists of the following steps [86]:

- 5-mm small incision between the carunculae sublinguales
- Insertion of a 5-mm trocar
- Blunt dissection subplatysmally by CO_2 insufflation ("air dissection")
- CO_2 insufflation (4–6 mmHg) and creation of a working space
- Insertion of two 3-mm trocars in the vestibulum oris on the right and left side
- Division of the linea alba coli and exposure of the strap muscles
- Separation of the strap muscles from the thyroid gland
- Isthmus transection and blunt dissection of the thyroid gland from the trachea
- Dissection and division of the upper pole arteries and medial thyroid vein closely to the gland
- Division of branches of the inferior thyroid artery closely to the gland

- If necessary, preparation of the retro-thyroidal area, including visualization of the recurrent laryngeal nerve
- Thyroid resection from cranially to caudally and transoral removal of the specimen through the 5-mm midline incision

The TOVAT technique is still experimental, but is a promising approach that needs further refinements of access and instruments before its widespread use can be recommended. The patient's safety, ethical principles, reliability, and seriousness of scientific conduct are mandatory [87]. Paradigms, unlike religions, depend on current knowledge and development of the human spirit. Innovative ideas, which at the beginning seem unfeasible, might make their way into the mainstream.

The Future of Natural Orifice Surgery

Today, when reports concerning surgical procedures are emerging from all over the world, it is clear that to avoid hybrid operations it is necessary to introduce designed instruments that will provide safety and surgical perfection. These instruments should contain optics, irrigation and suction, coagulation, triangulation, stability, and stiffness.

To perform a single port trans-Douglas cholecystectomy safely (as often the anatomical relations are complex), it is necessary to have instrument stability, as well as the ability to tie or coagulate safely, and optimally the potential to be performed by a single surgeon.

Today's challenge is to secure optimal vision, stability, and accuracy, which are difficult and require high specialization. Any optimal operation should be structured in such a way that every surgeon will use the same surgical steps that proved to be the most optimized by comparative studies matched for age groups [88], simplicity [89], or methodology [90].

The time for surgical champions is over. The outcome of operations performed according to evidence-based methods, with the same steps and sequence should not defer significantly. The essential secure standardized performance of single port or hybrid procedures will be brought about by adapted optimized tools.

During the last 20 years some so-called "robotic" systems were introduced, with the purpose of value-added accuracy and precision. The description of these systems as "robotics" is misleading. No artificial intelligence is behind them, as they follow the instructions of the surgeon. These systems (da Vinci, ZEUS) improve surgery through better ergonomics and manipulation as well as nontremor and articulated instrumentation; however, the most important problem is still unanswered, namely, the haptic sensation.

Musicians use their fingertips to play the piano or manipulate strings. The feedback they get is the key to sensitivity and excellence. Surgeons traditionally used their fingertips when holding scalpels or forceps, and more important, when palpating the anatomical and pathological findings. When endoscopy was introduced, palpation and sight became indirect.

Fig. 13.7 The TELELAP
ALF-X in action

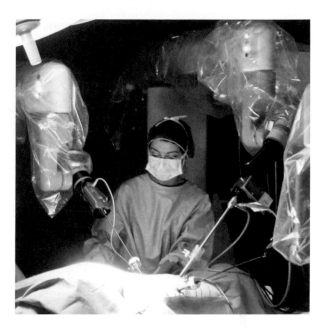

Despite the proved advantages in endoscopic operations as well as in some of the robotic systems concerning postoperative pain and cosmetic outcome, the sensitivity of the fingertips seems to have been lost. Most of the endoscopic instrumentation is manipulated by the fists or the proximal part of the fingers, in which the most sensitive parts, namely the fingertips, are not in use anymore. The optimal future surgical tools should follow the concept of "back to the fingertips" [90].

When performing endoscopy, the eyes are looking to the monitor, and the surgeon is unable to watch his or her own hands, which is of utmost importance concerning the coordination of movements. To solve these problems, a new concept has evolved, followed by construction of a novel system, the TELELAP ALF-X (Figs. 13.7 and 13.8).

The TELELAP ALF-X in not a robot, but rather an advanced surgical tool enabling the surgeon not just to see the operative site, but at the same time, use his or her own hands and the tips of the instruments. The surgeon also can feel the consistency of the tissues, to detect hidden structures such as lymph nodes and feel the force exerted while stitching and tying knots.

This system proved to be efficient, reliable, and useful with optimal ergonomics. This system, which includes a 3D vision and eye tracking system, makes surgery as similar as possible to traditional laparotomy with all the advantages of endoscopy concerning postoperative pain and hospital stay. It becomes the "prodromos" (forerunner) of a new era, the Renaissance of abdominal surgery. This system can be easily adapted for use in natural orifice surgery with all the advantages involved.

This system will enable the surgeon to execute complicated procedures far away from the instrument's entry point and secures stability, nontremor, and good site

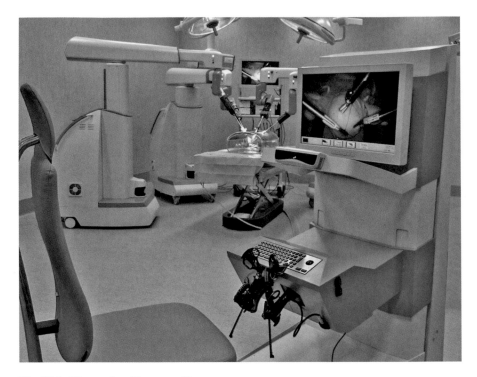

Fig. 13.8 3D console with eye-tracking system

combined with haptic sensation. This, with the advantages of no abdominal scars with all their disadvantages, is another step toward future optimal surgery.

The integration of this concept and system, which besides the technical development comes with state-of-the-art evidence-based optimized surgical methods created by surgical opinion leaders, will secure the accuracy, safety, and acceptance of this surgical system in the twenty-first century. It seems that with the same surgical system, other nonabdominal procedures, such as transoral operations, will become possible when the development of novel approaches and methodologies become prevalent in this century [91–93].

References

1. Arab SM. Medicine in ancient Egypt. http://www.arabworldbooks.com/articles8c.htm.
2. Keagy RD. Chopart amputations. Orthopedics. 1997;20(5):388.
3. Sanders LJ. Transmetatarsal and midfoot amputations. Clin Podiatr Med Surg. 1997;14(4): 741–62.
4. Othersen Jr HB. Ephraim McDowell: the qualities of a good surgeon. Ann Surg. 2004;239(5): 648–50.

5. Cottineau C, Cocaud J, Jacob JP. The beginning of anaesthesia. Allerg Immunol (Paris). 1998;30(5):135–7.
6. Busman DC. Theodor Billroth 1829–1894. Acta Chir Belg. 2006;106(6):743–52.
7. Köhler G. 100 years of the Wertheim operation: Ernst Wertheim between myth and reality. Zentralbl Gynakol. 1999;121(3):121–5.
8. Pfannenstiel J. On the advantages of a transverse cut of the fascia above the symphysis for gynecological laparotomies and advice on surgical methods and indications. Samml Klin Votr Gynäkol. 1987;68:1–22.
9. Mowat J, Bonnar J. Abdominal wound dehiscence after caesarean section. BMJ. 1971;2(5756): 256–7.
10. Lauter DM. Midline laparotomy and right retroperitoneal dissection is an alternative exposure for routine aortic surgery. Am J Surg. 2003;186(1):20–2.
11. Joel-Cohen S. Abdominal and vaginal hysterectomy. London: William Heinemann Medical Books; 1972.
12. Hatzinger M, Badawi JK, Häcker A, Langbein S, Honeck P, Alken P. Georg Kelling (1866–1945): the man who introduced modern laparoscopy into medicine. Urologe A. 2006;45(7):868–71.
13. Baggot MG. The endotracheal tube in situ as a foreign body: the master key to general anesthesia, its mechanism and inherent (though not peculiar) complications and to effective 'life support'. Med Hypotheses. 2002;59(6):742–50.
14. Dukanović S, Canić T. The value of hysteroscopy in perimenopausal women. Acta Med Croatica. 2007;61(2):185–90.
15. Anteby SO, Schenker JG, Polishuk WZ. The value of laparoscopy in acute pelvic pain. Ann Surg. 1975;181(4):484–6.
16. Wheeless Jr CR. Outpatient laparoscope sterilization under local anesthesia. Obstet Gynecol. 1972;39(5):767–70.
17. Moore DT. Laparoscopy: the "eyes" of gynecology. J Natl Med Assoc. 1975;67(2):145–8.
18. Nezhat C. Operative endoscopy will replace almost all open procedures. JSLS. 2004;8(2): 101–2.
19. Reynolds Jr W. The first laparoscopic cholecystectomy. JSLS. 2001;5(1):89–94.
20. Mettler L, Ahmed-Ebbiary N, Schollmeyer T. Laparoscopic hysterectomy: challenges and limitations. Minim Invasive Ther Allied Technol. 2005;14(3):145–59.
21. Parkar RB, Kamau WJ, Otieno D, Baraza R. Total laparoscopic hysterectomy at the Aga Khan University Hospital, Nairobi. East Afr Med J. 2007;84(11):508–15.
22. Ng SS, Li JC, Lee JF, Yiu RY, Leung KL. Laparoscopic total colectomy for colorectal cancers: a comparative study. Surg Endosc. 2006;20(8):1193–6.
23. Rashid P, Goad J, Aron M, Gianduzzo T, Gill IS. Laparoscopic partial nephrectomy: integration of an advanced laparoscopic technique. ANZ J Surg. 2008;78(6):471–5.
24. Yong JL, Law WL, Lo CY, Lam CM. A comparative study of routine laparoscopic versus open appendectomy. JSLS. 2006;10(2):188–92.
25. Pattenden CJ, Mann CD, Metcalfe MS, Dyer M, Lloyd DM. Laparoscopic splenectomy: a personal series of 140 consecutive cases. Ann R Coll Surg Engl. 2010;92(5):398–402.
26. Ford J, Grewal J, Mikolajczyk R, Meikle S, Zhang J. Primary cesarean delivery among parous women in the United States, 1990–2003. Obstet Gynecol. 2008;112(6):1235–41.
27. Stark M, Chavkin Y, Kupfersztain C, Guedj P, Finkel AR. Evaluation of combinations of procedures in cesarean section. Int J Gynaecol Obstet. 1995;48(3):273–6.
28. Holmgren G, Sjöholm L, Stark M. The Misgav Ladach method for cesarean section: method description. Acta Obstet Gynecol Scand. 1999;78(7):615–21.
29. Kresch AJ, Lyons TL, Westland AB, Wiener WK, Savage GM. Laparoscopic supracervical hysterectomy with a new disposable morcellator. J Am Assoc Gynecol Laparosc. 1998;5(2): 203–6.
30. Casanova N, Wolf JS. The alternative to laparoendoscopic single-site surgery: small strategic laparoscopic incision placement (SLIP) nephrectomy improves cosmesis without technical restrictions. J Endourol. 2011;25(2):265–70.

31. Goo TT, Goel R, Lawenko M, Lomanto D. Laparoscopic transabdominal preperitoneal (TAPP) hernia repair via a single port. Surg Laparosc Endosc Percutan Tech. 2010;20(6):389–90.
32. Ham WS, Im YJ, Jung HJ, Hong CH, Han WK, Han SW. Initial experience with laparoendoscopic single-site nephrectomy and nephroureterectomy in children. Urology. 2011;77(5): 1204–8.
33. Yuge K, Miyajima A, Hasegawa M, Miyazaki Y, Maeda T, Takeda T, et al. Initial experience of transumbilical laparoendoscopic single-site surgery of partial adrenalectomy in patient with aldosterone-producing adenoma. BMC Urol. 2010;10:19.
34. Hart S, Yeung P, Sobolewski CJ. Laparo-endoscopic single site hysterectomy in gynecologic surgery. Surg Technol Int. 2010;20:195–206.
35. Lin T, Huang J, Han J, Xu K, Huang H, Jiang C, et al. Hybrid laparoscopic endoscopic single-site surgery for radical cystoprostatectomy and orthotopic ileal neobladder: an initial experience of 12 cases. J Endourol. 2011;25(1):57–63.
36. De Sousa EM, Vermeulen L, Richel D, Medema JP. Targeting Wnt signaling in colon cancer stem cells. Clin Cancer Res. 2011;17(4):647–53.
37. Taran FA, Tempany CM, Regan L, Inbar Y, Revel A, Stewart EA, et al. Magnetic resonance-guided focused ultrasound (MRgFUS) compared with abdominal hysterectomy for treatment of uterine leiomyomas. Ultrasound Obstet Gynecol. 2009;34(5):572–8.
38. Legent F. Evolution of tonsillectomy. Bull Acad Natl Med. 2009;193(8):1885–94.
39. Maurer JT. Surgical treatment of obstructive sleep apnea: standard and emerging techniques. Curr Opin Pulm Med. 2010;16(6):552–8.
40. Stark M, Gerli S, Di Renzo GC. The importance of analyzing and standardizing surgical methods. J Minim Invasive Gynecol. 2009;16(2):122–5.
41. Kovac SR. Hysterectomy outcomes in patients with similar indications. Obstet Gynecol. 2000;95(6 Pt 1):787–93.
42. Burghardt J, Buess G. Transanal endoscopic microsurgery (TEM): a new technique and development during a time period of 20 years. Surg Technol Int. 2005;14:131–7.
43. Tilney HS, Heriot AG, Simson JN. Transanal endoscopic microsurgery: a necessary requirement? Colorectal Dis. 2006;8:710–4.
44. Guiot J, Rougerie J, Fourestier M, Fournier A, Comoy C, Vulmiere J, et al. Intracranial endoscopic explorations. Presse Med. 1963;71:1225–8.
45. Kalloo AN, Singh VK, Jagannath SB, Niiyama H, Hill SL, Vaughn CA, et al. Flexible transgastric peritoneoscopy: a novel approach to diagnostic and therapeutic interventions in the peritoneal cavity. Gastrointest Endosc. 2004;60(1):114–7.
46. Stark M, Benhidjeb T. Transcolonic endoscopic cholecystectomy: a NOTES survival study in a porcine model. Gastrointest Endosc. 2007;66(1):208–9.
47. Kantsevoy SV, Jagannath SB, Niiyama H, Isakovich NV, Chung SS, Cotton PB, et al. A novel safe approach to the peritoneal cavity for per-oral transgastric endoscopic procedures. Gastrointest Endosc. 2007;65(3):497–500.
48. Richards WO, Tattner DW. Endoluminal and transluminal surgery: no longer if but when. Surg Endosc. 2005;19:461–3.
49. Rattner D, Kalloo A. ASGE/SAGES working group on natural orifice transluminal endoscopic surgery. Surg Endosc. 2006;20:329–33.
50. Lee G, Sutton E, Clanton T, et al. Higher physical workload risks with NOTES versus laparoscopy: a quantitative ergonomic assessment. Surg Endosc. 2011;25(5):1585–93.
51. Ternamian AM, Vilos GA, Vilos AG, Abu-Rafea B, Tyrwhitt J, MacLeod NT. Laparoscopic peritoneal entry with the reusable threaded visual cannula. J Minim Invasive Gynecol. 2010;17(4):461–7.
52. Hauser J, Lehnhardt M, Steinau HU, Homann HH. Trocar injury of the retroperitoneal vessels followed by life-threatening postischemic compartment syndrome of both lower extremities. Surg Laparosc Endosc Percutan Tech. 2008;18(2):222–4.
53. Lima E, Rolanda C, Autorino R, et al. Experimental foundation for natural orifice transluminal endoscopic surgery and hybrid natural orifice transluminal endoscopic surgery. BJU Int. 2010;106(6 Pt B):913–8.

54. Hookey LC, Khokhotva V, Bielawska B, Samis A, Jalink D, Hurlbut D, et al. The Queen's closure: a novel technique for closure of endoscopic gastrotomy for natural-orifice transluminal endoscopic surgery. Endoscopy. 2009;41(2):149–53.
55. Kratt T, Küper M, Traub F, Ho CN, Schurr MO, Königsrainer A, et al. Feasibility study for secure closure of natural orifice transluminal endoscopic surgery gastrotomies by using over-the-scope clips. Gastrointest Endosc. 2008;68(5):993–6.
56. Watrelot A, Nassif J, Law WS, Marescaux J, Wattiez A. Safe and simplified endoscopic technique in transvaginal NOTES. Surg Laparosc Endosc Percutan Tech. 2010;20(3):e92–4.
57. Tsin DA. Culdolaparoscopy: a preliminary report. JSLS. 2001;5(1):69–71.
58. Tsin DA, Sequeria RJ, Giannikas G. Culdolaparoscopic cholecystectomy during vaginal hysterectomy. JSLS. 2003;7(2):171–2.
59. Zorrón R, Filgueiras M, Maggioni LC, Pombo L, Lopes Carvalho G, Lacerda Oliveira A. NOTES. Transvaginal cholecystectomy: report of the first case. Surg Innov. 2007; 14(4):279–83.
60. Bessler M, Stevens PD, Milone L, Parikh M, Fowler D. Transvaginal laparoscopically assisted endoscopic cholecystectomy: a hybrid approach to natural orifice surgery. Gastrointest Endosc. 2007;66(6):1243–5.
61. Marescaux J, Dallemagne B, Perretta S, Wattiez A, Mutter D, Coumaros D. Surgery without scars: report of transluminal cholecystectomy in a human being. Arch Surg. 2007;142(9): 823–6.
62. Harlaar JJ, Kleinrensink GJ, Hop WC, Stark M, Schneider AJ. The anatomical limits of the posterior vaginal vault toward its use as route for intra-abdominal procedures. Surg Endosc. 2008;22(8):1910–2.
63. Hackethal A, Sucke J, Oehmke F, Münstedt K, Padberg W, Tinneberg HR. Establishing transvaginal NOTES for gynecological and surgical indications: benefits, limits, and patient experience. Endoscopy. 2010;42(10):875–8.
64. Burghardt J, Federlein M, Müller V, Benhidjeb T, Elling D, Gellert K. Minimal invasive transvaginal right hemicolectomy: report of the first complex NOS (natural orifice surgery) bowels operation using a hybrid approach. Zentralbl Chir. 2008;133(6):574–6.
65. Aminsharifi A, Taddayun A, Shakeri S, Hashemi M, Abdi M. Hybrid natural orifice transluminal endoscopic surgery for nephrectomy with standard laparoscopic instruments: experience in a canine model. J Endourol. 2009;23(12):1985–9.
66. Porpiglia F, Fiori C, Morra I, Scarpa RM. Transvaginal natural orifice transluminal endoscopic surgery-assisted minilaparoscopic nephrectomy: a step towards scarless surgery. Eur Urol. 2010; [Epub ahead of print].
67. Chouillard EK, Al Khoury M, Bader G, Heitz D, et al. Laparoscopic Surgery (i-NOELS), Poissy, France. Combined vaginal and abdominal approach to sleeve gastrectomy for morbid obesity in women: a preliminary experience. Surg Obes Relat Dis. 2010; [Epub ahead of print].
68. Stark M, Benhidjeb T. Natural orifice surgery: transdouglas surgery—a new concept. JSLS. 2008;12(3):295–8.
69. Tinelli A, Malvasi A, Istre O, Keckstein J, Stark M, Mettler L. Abdominal access in gynaecological laparoscopy: a comparison between direct optical and blind closed access by Veress needle. Eur J Obstet Gynecol Reprod Biol. 2010;148(2):191–4.
70. Tinelli A, Malvasi A, Guido M, Istre O, Keckstein J, Mettler L. Initial laparoscopic access in postmenopausal women: a preliminary prospective study. Menopause. 2009;16(5):966–70.
71. Delvaux G, Devroey P, De Waele B, Willems G. Transvaginal removal of gallbladders with large stones after laparoscopic cholecystectomy. Surg Laparosc Endosc. 1993;3(4):307–9.
72. McGowan L. Incidental appendectomy during vaginal surgery. Am J Obstet Gynecol. 1966;95:588.
73. Pelosi 3rd MA, Pelosi MA. Vaginal appendectomy at laparoscopic-assisted vaginal hysterectomy: a surgical option. J Laparoendosc Surg. 1996;6:399–403.
74. Magos AL, Bournas N, Sinha R, Richardson RE, O'Connor H. Vaginal myomectomy. Br J Obstet Gynaecol. 1994;101:1092–4.

75. Wei FH, Zhao XD, Zhang Y. Feasibility and safety of vaginal myomectomy: analysis of 90 cases. Chin Med J (Engl). 2006;119:1790–3.
76. Federlein M, Borchert D, Müller V, Atas Y, Fritze F, Burghardt J, et al. Transvaginal video-assisted cholecystectomy in clinical practice. Surg Endosc. 2010;24(10):2444–52.
77. Miccoli P, Berti P, Coute M, Bendinelli C, Marcocci C. Minimally invasive surgery for thyroid small nodules: preliminary report. J Endocrinol Invest. 1999;22:849–51.
78. Benhidjeb T, Anders S, Bärlehner E. Total video-endoscopic thyroidectomy via Axillo-Bilateral-Breast-Approach (ABBA). Langenbeck's Arch Surg. 2006;391:48–9.
79. Bärlehner E, Benhidjeb T. Cervical scarless endoscopic thyroidectomy: axillo-bilateral-breast approach (ABBA). Surg Endosc. 2008;22:154–7.
80. Shimazu K, Shiba E, Tamaki Y, Takiguchi S, Taniguchi E, Ohashi S, et al. Endoscopic thyroid surgery through the axillo-bilateral-breast approach. Surg Laparosc Endosc Percutan Tech. 2003;13:196–201.
81. Choe JH, Kim SW, Chung KW, Park KS, Han W, Noh DY, et al. Endoscopic thyroidectomy using a new bilateral axillo-breast approach. World J Surg. 2007;31:601–6.
82. Kang SW, Lee SC, Lee SH, Lee KY, Jeong JJ, Lee YS, et al. Robotic thyroid surgery using a gasless, transaxillary approach and the da Vinci S system: the operative outcomes of 338 consecutive patients. Surgery. 2009;146(6):1048–55.
83. Wilhelm T, Harlaar J, Kerver A, Kleinrensink GJ, Benhidjeb T. Transoral endoscopic thyroidectomy. Part 1: rationale and anatomical studies. Chirurg. 2010;81(1):50–5.
84. Witzel K, von Rahden BHA, Kaminski C, Stein HJ. Transoral access for endoscopic thyroid resection. Surg Endosc. 2008;22(8):1871–5.
85. Benhidjeb T, Wilhelm T, Harlaar J, Kleinrensink GJ, Schneider TA, Stark M. Natural orifice surgery on thyroid gland: totally transoral video-assisted thyroidectomy (TOVAT): report of first experimental results of a new surgical method. Surg Endosc. 2009;23:1119–20.
86. Benhidjeb T, Witzel K, Burghardt J, Bärlehner E, Stark M, Mann O. Endoscopic minimally invasive thyroidectomy: ethical and patients safety considerations on the first clinical experience of an innovative approach. Surg Endosc. 2010; [Epub ahead of print].
87. Früh S, Knirsch W, Dodge-Khatami A, Dave H, Prêtre R, Kretschmar O. Comparison of surgical and interventional therapy of native and recurrent aortic coarctation regarding different age groups during childhood. Eur J Cardiothorac Surg. 2011;39(6):898–904.
88. Deroee AF, Younes AA, Friedman O. External nasal valve collapse repair: the limited alar-facial stab approach. Laryngoscope. 2011;121(3):474–9.
89. Shimachi S, Hirunyanitiwatna S, Fujiwara Y, Hashimoto A, Hakozaki Y. Adapter for contact force sensing of the da Vinci robot. Int J Med Robot. 2008;4(2):121–30.
90. Stark M, Di Renzo GC, Benhidjeb T. Natural orifice surgery (NOS)—toward a single-port transdouglas approach for intra-abdominal procedures. Eur J Obstet Gynecol Reprod Biol. 2010;148(2):114–7.
91. Tinelli A, Malvasi A, Buscarini M, Ruiz Morales E, Stark M. Laparoscopy and robotics in cervical cancer treatment: current insights, novel approaches and future perspectives in the new era of gynecological surgery. In: Salvatti EK, editor. Brain cancer, tumor targeting and cervical cancer. New York: Nova; 2011.
92. Richmon JD, Pattani KM, Benhidjeb T, Tufano RP. Transoral robotic-assisted thyroidectomy: a preclinical feasibility study in 2 cadavers. Head Neck. 2011;33(3):330–3.
93. Wilhelm T, Harlaar JJ, Kerver A, Kleinrensink GJ, Benhidjeb T. Surgical anatomy of the floor of the oral cavity and the cervical spaces as a rationale for trans-oral, minimal-invasive endoscopic surgical procedures: results of anatomical studies. Eur Arch Otorhinolaryngol. 2010;267(8):1285–90.

Chapter 14
Access in Natural Orifice Transvaginal Endoscopic Surgery

Daniel A. Tsin

Introduction of Anatomical Considerations

The knowledge of the topographic anatomy of the rectouterine pouch is a pivotal point for the understanding of the inclusion and exclusion criteria in this surgical approach [1].

The vagina extends from the vulva to the uterine cervix. Anteriorly it is in contact with the urethra and bladder and posteriorly with the rectum and peritoneum. The average length is 8.5 cm from the vulva to the posterior fornix. The elasticity of the vaginal tissues allows for stretching, as is noticed during the introduction of a vaginal port (Fig. 14.1) [2].

The vaginal elasticity decreases with age in reproductive women; this becomes more evident after menopause. The vaginal superior segment is located above the elevators muscles. This segment is in contact with the peritoneum of the pouch of Douglas. Below this segment the vagina remains in contact with the rectum, separated by the Denonvilliers fascia.

The posterior vaginal fornix makes contact with the cul-de-sac in a surface area of approximately 1.5–2 cm in length. This area increases several centimeters when the uterus is pushed anterior and cephalic. This is important in the placement of a vaginal port [3].

The description of the recto-uterine pouch is credited to the work of Dr. James Douglas "A description of the peritoneum and that part of the membrane cellularis which lies outside" (London, 1730).

This lower point in the female peritoneum is a virtual cavity limited in the front by the uterus and vagina, in the back by the rectum, and cephalic by the uterosacral ligaments.

D.A. Tsin
Division of Minimal Invasive Endoscopy, Department of Gynecology,
The Mount Sinai Hospital of Queens, New York, USA

A. Tinelli (ed.), *Laparoscopic Entry*,
DOI 10.1007/978-0-85729-980-2_14, © Springer-Verlag London Limited 2012

Fig. 14.1 Excavatio
recto-uterina is a peritoneal
cul-de-sac also known as the
Pouch of Douglas

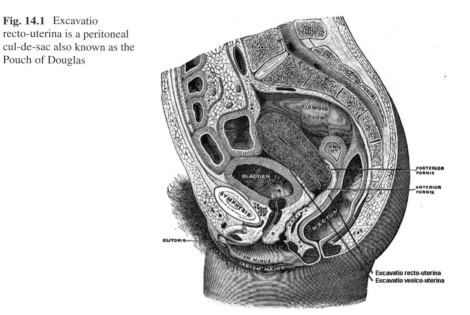

The uterosacral ligaments are easily identified when the uterus is pushed upward
and cephalic, exposing the pouch of Douglas. The ligaments start at the isthmus of
the uterus and extend to the both sides of the rectum. The ligament that began in the
posterior aspect of the uterus, travels lateral to the rectum, and then reaches the
parietal peritoneum in front of the sacrum. The ligament consists of muscle fibers,
rich in nerves and with few vessels. The posterior aspect of the uterus is covered by
the peritoneum, which extends in the cul-de-sac till its bottom is in contact with a
posterior vaginal fornix.

Patient Selection

The selection begins with a complete history and physical examination, including
routine blood tests, and when needed an electrocardiogram and imaging studies.
When necessary, medical consultations are obtained for a preoperative assessment. Attention is given to all medications, including prescription and nonpre-
scription, vitamins, and herbal medicine, some of which must be suspended days
or even weeks before surgery. All patients undergo bimanual pelvic examinations.
Papanicolaou tests are done in all patients with a uterus, and must be reported negative.
The exclusion criteria include the obliteration of the pouch of Douglas and/or vaginal narrowing. Adequate vaginal access confirms the width of the posterior fornix,
which must allow the introduction of two fingers; the middle finger and index must
be able to move freely during the vaginal examination. The uterus must be mobile.

Patients with one of either of the above findings are not considered candidates for the transvaginal approach. Patients have to pass the same criteria requirements used for laparoscopic procedures. All women must be ordered to receive intravenous antibiotic prophylaxis with metronidazole 500 mg and cephalosporin 1 g to be given within 1 h before the time of incision. In elective patients, bowel preparation is performed.

Informed Consent

This is a new approach in general surgery. Informed consent must be provided in accordance with the protocol for Minilaparoscopy Assisted Natural Orifice Surgery [4], MANOS, and Natural Orifice Transluminal Endoscopic Surgery [5] NOTES, approved by each institution. This must include an explanation to the patient of the different options and the patient must understand the risks, possible laparotomy conversion, benefits, and alternatives. Gynecologists who have the privilege of operative culdoscopy and advanced gynecological laparoscopy [6], and who intend to use MANOS or NOTES in gynecological pathologies must obtain approval by the head of the department.

The Team

MANOS and NOTES are evolving approaches that require expertise taught in different disciplines, such as gastroenterology, general surgery, and gynecology. A multi-specialist team would be advised till task groups of natural orifice surgery come up with a practical education solution. The team includes surgeons, assistants, operating room nurse, and technical personnel. The team must develop expertise in advanced laparoscopy and transvaginal surgery. This expertise is achieved by practicing in the laboratory as well to understand the conceptual design of the surgery based on previous experience adapted for the new approach.

MANOS requires additional team training and orientation in gynecological procedures, and appendectomies. The assistant handles the laparoscope and mini-instruments from the abdominal ports.

Meanwhile the surgeons view operating between the patient's legs is in a two-dimensional mirror image. The team coordination should be tried first in the laboratory and the commands should not be directed to right or left, but must be target specific. I advise that surgeons and assistant move one instrument at a time. The orientation and operation of flexible instruments of NOTES require additional skills and a longer learning curve than with rigid instruments. Today the use of magnets in natural orifice surgery in humans is in its infancy and radio-controlled robots are at experimental levels. This is an exciting time for minimally invasive new frontiers that require a trained team to safely implement this technology.

Operating Room Assembly

The operating room is assembled following the standards for gynecological laparoscopic surgery; the differences are the position of the monitors: one of them is placed in cephalic position, by the patient's right shoulder and the other by the patient's left foot. This disposition of the monitors is essential to allow proper visualization throughout the surgery, especially when the surgeon is operating from the vaginal port. Both monitors are movable, facilitating the view when the surgeon changes positions. The operating table must have a large perineal cutout to facilitate operating from the vaginal port.

I advise the use of Allen-type telescopic stirrups. This provides an easy way for the adjustment from lythotomy to semi-dorsoliththomy position, by changing stirrups from 90–15° angles from the horizontal. A careful positioning of legs and the separation of legs must provide enough room to operate between the patient's legs and avoids hyperextension, and one must observe safety in regard to the prevention of nerve injury of the sciatic, perineal, or femoral nerve.

Thromboembolic prophylaxis has to be considered. In low-risk patients, it is handled by pneumatic boots. High-risk patients should follow the standard thromboembolic prevention protocol with unfractionated or low-molecular-weight heparin. All procedures were performed under general anesthesia with endotracheal intubation. Patients were placed in a semi-dorsolithotomic position (Fig. 14.2).

A pelvic examination is carried out under anesthesia, to confirm that there is no obstruction of the posterior cul-de-sac. The bimanual examination under anesthesia is necessary to confirm previous findings of awake bimanual examinations or obtain a more detailed palpation in a paralyzed situation. Once again the width of the vaginal port, the empty cul-de-sac, the elasticity of the vagina, and the mobility of the uterus is assessed. A combined abdominal, perineal, and vaginal cleansing is done with 10% povidone iodine.

The patient is kept in the lithotomic position to place the uterine manipulator. A weighted speculum is placed to retract the posterior wall—we use Sims or Deaver retractors to further expose the uterine cervix—a Pozzi's tenaculum is placed in the anterior lip of the cervix. With the cervix exposed, the cavity is measured with a probe. A dilation of the cervix of the uterus is done progressively till 6 mm. In rare cases large dilators are needed. We used 4.5- and 5-mm diameter manipulators, such as the ZUMI 4.5 or Kroner Manipulator (Cooper Surgical, Trumbull, CT) (Fig. 14.3).

We adjust the length of the intrauterine portion of the manipulator to approximately 1 cm less than the measurements obtained by the uterine probe. Both uterine manipulators have inflatable catheters that are filled with air. Check that the manipulator is fixed in position. A Foley catheter is placed in all cases (Fig. 14.4).

Proper placement is necessary to mobilize the uterus and expose the pouch of Douglas. Poor placement or displacement is frustrating because this maneuver must be redone again at an unforeseeable time during the operation. Vaginal retractors should be temporarily removed and kept available for later uses during the procedure.

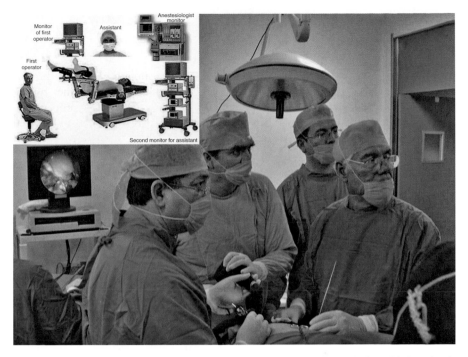

Fig. 14.2 The position of the monitors are the following: one is placed cephalic in line with the patient's right shoulder and the other is placed caudal in line with the patient's left foot [20]

Fig. 14.3 ZUMI (*white*) and Kroner (*green*) uterine manipulators

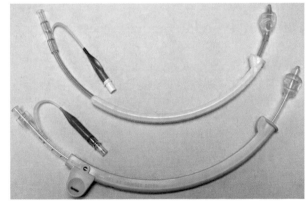

Fig. 14.4 The surgeon adjusts the length of the intrauterine portion of the manipulator to approximately 1 cm less than the measurements obtained by the uterine probe and inflate manipulator's catheters filling with air to fix it in uterus. Then a Foley catheter is placed in all cases after manipulator insertion

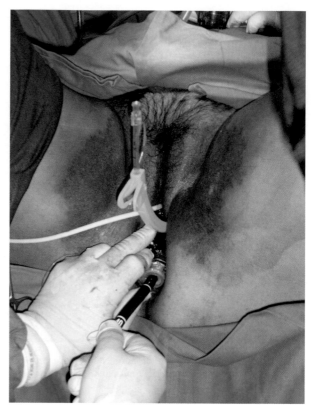

Different Types of Vaginal Access

The following are three types of vaginal access:
1. The minilaparoscopy assisted natural orifice surgery (MANOS).
2. Colpotomy could be used in MANOS [4] or in natural orifice transluminal endoscopic surgery (NOTES) [7].
3. Simultaneous procedures during vaginal hysterectomies could also be used in MANOS and NOTES [5–8].

Minilaparoscopy Assisted Natural Orifice Surgery (MANOS)

This transvaginal approach is also known as culdolaparoscopy [9]. This surgical concept uses minilaparoscopy as a safer entry for natural orifice peritoneoscopy. The pneumoperitoneum is developed with a Veress needle inserted in the umbilical area.

The minilaparoscope is introduced in most cases through a 3-mm umbilical port with two additional 3-mm ports. The posterior cul-de-sac is visualized with the minilaparoscope. A plastic rod that is 10 mm in diameter and 46 cm in length

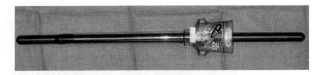

Fig. 14.5 A plastic rod 10 mm in diameter and 46 cm in length is mounted inside an insufflating cannula 12 mm in diameter and 15 cm in length (PortSaver, ConMed, Utica, NY)

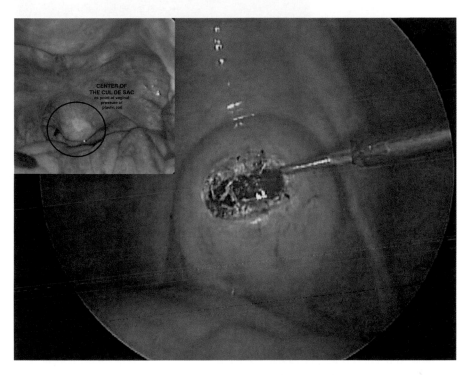

Fig. 14.6 The point of pressure made by plastic rod is in the center of the cul-de-sac and clearly identifiable with the umbilical minilaparoscope

(PortSaver, ConMed, Utica, NY) is mounted inside an insufflating cannula of 12 mm in diameter and 15 cm in length (Fig. 14.5). The plastic rod and the cannula are placed against the posterior fornix. The weighted speculum is removed and the uterine manipulator, together with the rod, is pushed upward and anterior. It is important that the point of pressure made by the rod is in the center of the cul-de-sac and clearly identifiable with umbilical minilaparoscope (Fig. 14.6).

When necessary, the bowel is pushed aside with a probe. A small incision is done via minilaparoscopy at the tip of the pressure point to aid the penetration of the rod and the cannula. Under minilaparoscopic surveillance, the trocar is inserted into the cul-de-sac with gentle, steady pressure. At this time, the insufflation line is attached to the vaginal port. The patient's thighs are brought to about 15° above the horizon-

Fig. 14.7 An Endobag is
introduced into the pouch of
Douglas, by the plastic
vaginal rod, to safely remove
the ovarian cyst

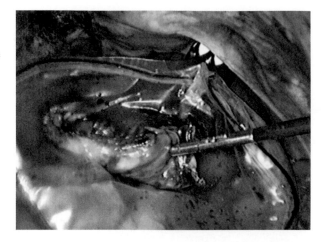

tal position while keeping the knees flexed. Culdolaparoscopy is then performed
with 3-mm abdominal instruments and a large vaginal port. The function of the
ports change, depending on the nature or stage of the procedure. The vaginal port is
used for placement of instruments larger than 3 mm, such as endoscopic gastric
anastomosis clamp, clip applier, grasper, and morcellator. The vaginal port is used
as a visual and an operative port for placing laparoscopes and gastroscopes [10].

The vaginal port is reintroduced and irrigation and suction are carried out through
it. For suction-irrigation we use probes from 5 to 10 mm. For the extraction we use
a 10-mm endoscopic bag (Fig. 14.7), graspers, or gastroscopes [3].

The incision in the posterior fornix is closed with a 2-0 chromic suture placed
inside the vagina. The abdominal ports are used to introduce the minilaparoscope,
scissors, graspers and dissectors.

The vaginal port could be also placed with a sharp trocar, although this is not as
safe as the blunt trocar entry described in the preceding. A meticulous technique is
essential. Whenever this approach is used a major concern is bowel perforation. The
protruding point must be clearly identified in position in the middle of the pouch of
Douglas. The insertion needs to be precise. Attention should be kept to avoid lateral
movements because the trocar has a tendency to slide laterally under pressure.
I advise not to attempt to use this armed sharp trocar entry until enough experience
is gathered with a blunt trocar entrance [2]. Patients with previous hysterectomy
could benefit from this approach with a modification. In such cases the vaginal port
is introduced by placing the trocar against the vaginal dome and guided inside the
abdomen with minilaparoscopic surveillance.

Colpotomy

The technique that the author uses is different than the approach used for the drain-
age of pelvic abscess. It is similar to exploratory colpotomy yet smaller since the
need is limited to make an endoscopic operating entrance into the posterior vaginal
fornix and in the pouch of Douglas.

Fig. 14.8 The posterior
vaginal fornix is tented for a
colpotomy

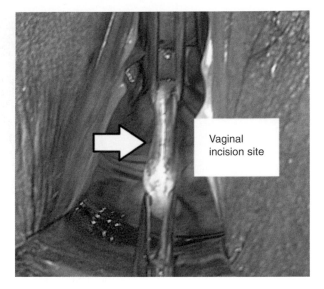

Vaginal
incision site

   A weighted speculum is placed in the posterior vaginal wall. Additional Sims or
Deaver retractors are used for exposure. The cervix is grasped with a tenaculum at
the posterior lip. The cervix is elevated anteriorly. We identified the area in the posterior fornix where the posterior vaginal wall meets the cervix. Approximately
1–2 cm posterior to this junction is the area for the colpotomy. We use two Allis
clamps to elevate the area and allow for making a transversal cut of 2 cm in length
with curved Mayo scissors. The point of the curved scissor is oriented anteriorly.
Most cases require only one cut to reach the cul-de-sac. In the event that the entrance
in the peritoneum is not achieved in one step, a careful relocation of the clamps in a
deeper layer, in most cases the peritoneum, is done and the cut is done with scissors
or scalpel. Hemostasis is achieved in the operative area before moving on to the next
step. The tenaculum is reapplied in the anterior cervical lip, then the surgeon places
the uterine manipulator as previously described. Colpotomy is the way to access for
a pure natural orifice surgery.
   We prefer the minilaparoscopy-guided introduction of the port in MANOS; it is
faster, less bloody, and is a better-coordinated step. The closure of the colpotomy is
done as previously described using a 2-0 chromic suture (Fig. 14.8).

During Vaginal Hysterectomy

Historically vaginal hysterectomy is preferred over abdominal because of less morbidity. This belief was recently validated by a Cochrane review [11].
   The selection and indication for a vaginal hysterectomy is beyond the intention
of this chapter. Nonetheless the previous validation criteria serve to prove the advantages as well as safety of transvaginal peritoneoscopy. These studies prove that the

Fig. 14.9 Extraction of a gallbladder via the vaginal port

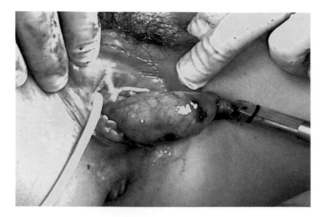

vaginal hysterectomy has less peritoneal irritation, ileus, and hernias when compared with abdominal and fewer ureter complications and a shorter operating time when compared with laparoscopic access. There is no increase in morbidity when simultaneous appendectomy or cholecystectomy is done during hysterectomy.

During vaginal hysterectomy a circular colpotomy is done to remove the uterus.

After the uterus is extracted, there is limited vision of the pelvis, but enough to perform oophorectomies and in some cases incidental appendectomies. Dr. Ott reported the endoscopic vision during vaginal hysterectomy under the name of ventroscopy in 1901 [12].

We have used this approach to perform simultaneous cholecystectomies [8] and difficult oophorectomies [5]. The sleeve of a trocar is secured with a pursestring suture. The vagina is packed with soaked gauze. The insufflation is done via the vaginal port until pneumoperitoneum is achieved. Then a 10-mm diameter 30° angle laparoscope is placed in the vaginal port for visualization. The abdominal ports are then placed under culdoscopic surveillance. Oophorectomy is performed by applying bipolar coagulation and by cutting the mesovarium with 5-mm laparoscopic scissors, introduced through the vaginal port. When necessary, 3-mm forceps and scissors are inserted through the abdominal trocars. The ovaries are extracted through the vaginal port using a 5-mm grasper and hemostasis is secured. The abdominal ports are removed under culdoscopic surveillance, and finally the vaginal cannula is extracted. The closure of the vaginal port is done through the vagina.

Technical Results

From 1998 to 2008 I participated in 130 cases, including minilaparoscopy assisted natural orifice surgeries, via colpotomy and during vaginal hysterectomy, including oophorectomies and salpingo-oophorectomies, ovarian cystectomies, myomectomies, appendectomies, and cholecystectomies (Fig. 14.9) [4–7].

We encountered only one complication; one patient with ovarian cystectomy developed a drug-related fever that improved after discontinuation of the antibiotics. No patients developed infection. Follow-up visits up to 2 months after surgery revealed no complications.

Discussion

Major concerns following the use of the vaginal route are the risk of pelvic infection, trauma to adjacent structures, dyspareunia, and cul-de-sac adhesion [9–13].

In our 10-year experience with culdolaparoscopy (1998–2008) we have not seen any of these complications. This is in agreement with previous reports demonstrating an extremely low incidence of complications with colpotomy [3] and culdoscopy [14].

It should be noted that with culdolaparoscopy the vaginal trocar is inserted under laparoscopic surveillance. This approach virtually eliminates the complications attributed to culdoscopy [15], in which instruments are blindly inserted. Nevertheless, in addition to insertion of the trocar under laparoscopic view, a meticulous endoscopic technique is essential. The trocar should not be introduced or forced into the cul-de-sac unless the protruding point is unquestionably under laparoscopic view.

The insertion should be done precisely in the midline of the posterior fornix [16].

The introduction of a new approach usually encounters resistance.

This surgery is questionable by the mainstream. Surgeons have to review the literature, attend courses, and learn in detail. A well-prepared team is essential for success. Be prepared to have few collaborators for a team willing to face long hours and sometimes tortuous training. Proactive anesthesiologist participation is important for patient position adjustments. The surgeon in charge must convince the head of the department, the medical director, and the hospital administrator that they should be buying new sets of expensive equipment. If no complications are found at the beginning of the project, the perception will improve. You may still feel some resistance, but with time I am quite sure that we will be able to prove the advantage of MANOS and NOTES.

Conclusion

Culdolaparoscopy is a feasible, simple, and safe technique for an experienced laparoscopist. MANOS avoids additional and larger abdominal ports, potentially decreasing the morbidity associated with conventional operative laparoscopy while overcoming the limitations of minilaparoscopy.

This approach enabled us to perform gynecological and nongynecological procedures using abdominal ports no larger than 3 or 5 mm. The progress in flexible technology magnetic platforms, secured independent tools [17], and robotics will facilitate the performance of major abdominal and pelvic procedures without any skin incision via a colpotomy. Until such technology becomes available and affordable and the learning of additional skill is achieved, MANOS should remain as an important step that should not be bypassed in the safe implementation of a pure natural orifice transvaginal operative peritoneoscopy [18–20].

References

1. Tsin DA. Culdolaparoscopy: a preliminary report. JSLS. 2001;5:69–71.
2. Tsin DA, Colombero LT, Mahmood D, Padouvas J, Manolas P. Operative culdolaparoscopy: a new approach combining operative culdoscopy and minilaparoscopy. J Am Assoc Gynecol Laparosc. 2001;8:438–41.
3. Ghezzi F, Raio L, Mueller MD, Gyr T, Buttarelli M, Franchi M. Vaginal extraction of pelvic masses following operative laparoscopy. Surg Endosc. 2002;16:1691–6.
4. Tsin DA, Colombero L, Lambeck J, Manolas P. Minilaparoscopy-assisted natural orifice surgery. JSLS. 2007;11:24–9.
5. Tsin DA, Bumaschny E, Helman M, Colombero L. Culdolaparoscopic oophorectomy with vaginal hysterectomy: an optional minimal-access surgical technique. J Laparoendosc Adv Surg Tech A. 2002;12:269–71.
6. Wagh M, Thompson C. Surgery insight; natural orifice transluminal endoscopic surgery. An analysis of work to date. Nat Clin Pract Gastroenterol Hepatol. 2007;4(7):386–92.
7. Zorrón R, Filgueiras M, Maggioni LC, Pombo L, Oliveira AL. NOTES. Transvaginal cholecystectomy: report of the first case. Surg Innov. 2007;14(4):279–83.
8. Tsin DA, Sequeira RJ, Giannikas G. Culdolaparoscopic cholecystectomy during vaginal hysterectomy. JSLS. 2003;7:171–2.
9. Tsin DA. Development of flexible culdoscopy (Letter to the editor). J Am Assoc Gynecol Laparosc. 2000;7:440.
10. Gómez N, Tsin D, Cabezas G, et al. Transvaginal cholecystectomy assisted by minilaparoscopy. Poster presentation at the 2008, AHPBA meeting Mar 26–30, Fort Lauderdale.
11. Johnson N, Barlow D, Lethaby A, Tavender E, Curr F, Garry R. Surgical approach for hysterectomy for benign gynecological disease. Cochrane Database Syst Rev. 2006; (2): CD003677.
12. Ott V. Ventroscopia. Zhurnal Akusherstva I Zhenskikh Boleznel. 1901;15:1045–9.
13. Miller CE. Methods of tissue extraction in advanced laparoscopy. Curr Opin Obstet Gynecol. 2001;13:399–405.
14. Copenhaver EH. A critical assessment of culdoscopy. Surg Clin North Am. 1970;50:713–8.
15. Decker A, Cherry T. Culdoscopy, a new method in diagnosis of pelvic disease. Am J Surg. 1944;64:40–4.
16. Neely MR, McWilliams R, Makhlouf HA. Laparoscopy: routine pneumoperitoneum via the posterior fornix. Obstet Gynecol. 1975;45:459–60.
17. Tsin DA, Davila F, Dominguez G, Manolas P. Secured independent tools in peritoneoscopy. JSLS. 2010;14:256–8.
18. Christian J, Barrier BF, Miedema BW, Thaler K. Culdoscopy: a foundation for natural orifice surgery past, present and future. J Am Coll Surg. 2008;207:417–22.
19. Tsin DA. Culdoscopy via MANOS as a prelude for NOTES. Contemp Surg. 2008;64:390–1.
20. Davila F, Tsin DA, Dominguez G, Jesus R, Arteche AG. Transvaginal cholecystectomy without abdominal ports. JSLS. 2009;13:213–6.

Index